S0-BQI-264

Transfer of Cell Constituents into Eukaryotic Cells

NATO ADVANCED STUDY INSTITUTES SERIES

A series of edited volumes comprising multifaceted studies of contemporary scientific issues by some of the best scientific minds in the world, assembled in cooperation with NATO Scientific Affairs Division.

Series A: Life Sciences

Recent Volumes in this Series

Volume 22 – Plant Regulation and World Agriculture
edited by Tom K. Scott

Volume 23 – The Molecular Biology of Picornaviruses
edited by R. Pérez-Bercoff

Volume 24 – Humoral Immunity in Neurological Diseases
edited by D. Karcher, A. Lowenthal, and A. D. Strosberg

Volume 25 – Synchrotron Radiation Applied to Biophysical and Biochemical Research
edited by A. Castellani and I. F. Quercia

Volume 26 – Nucleoside Analogues: Chemistry, Biology, and Medical Applications
edited by Richard T. Walker, Erik De Clercq, and Fritz Eckstein

Volume 27 – Developmental Neurobiology of Vision
edited by Ralph D. Freeman

Volume 28 – Animal Sonar Systems
edited by René-Guy Busnel and James F. Fish

Volume 29 – Genome Organization and Expression in Plants
edited by C. J. Leaver

Volume 30 – Human Physical Growth and Maturation: Methodologies and Factors
edited by Francis E. Johnston, Alex F. Roche, and Charles Susanne

Volume 31 – Transfer of Cell Constituents into Eukaryotic Cells
edited by J. E. Celis, A. Graessmann, and A. Loyter

Volume 32 – The Blood–Retinal Barriers
edited by Jose G. Cunha-Vaz

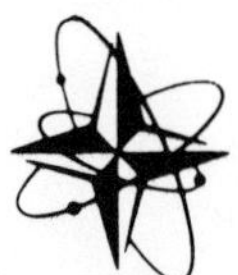

The series is published by an international board of publishers in conjunction with NATO Scientific Affairs Division

A Life Sciences B Physics	Plenum Publishing Corporation New York and London
C Mathematical and Physical Sciences	D. Reidel Publishing Company Dordrecht and Boston
D Behavioral and Social Sciences	Sijthoff International Publishing Company Leiden
E Applied Sciences	Noordhoff International Publishing Leiden

Transfer of Cell Constituents into Eukaryotic Cells

Edited by

J. E. Celis
Aarhus University
Aarhus, Denmark

A. Graessmann
Free University of Berlin
Berlin, German Federal Republic

and

A. Loyter
The Hebrew University of Jerusalem
Jerusalem, Israel

PLENUM PRESS • NEW YORK AND LONDON
Published in cooperation with NATO Scientific Affairs Division

Lectures presented at a NATO Advanced Study Institute
on Transfer of Cell Constituents into Eukaryotic Cells, held in
Sintra-Estoril, Portugal, September 2-14, 1979 and sponsored by
NATO and The Gulbenkian Foundation

A Division of Plenum Publishing Corporation
227 West 17th Street, New York, N.Y. 10011

Printed in the United States of America

PREFACE

This book is a record of the proceedings of a NATO Advanced Study Institute on "Transfer of Cell Constituents into Eukaryotic Cells" held September 2-14, 1979, at Sintra-Estoril, Portugal.

Transfer of cell constituents into living cells can be brought about by a variety of ways, namely by microinjection with micropipettes (small somatic cells, oocytes and plant cells), by microinjection using fusion methods (red cell mediated microinjection, liposome mediated transfer, transfer of membrane components, cell hybridization and fusion of cell fragments) and by means of uptake (DNA and chromosome gene transfer).

Prompted by the developments in this exciting and expanding field of cell biology it seemed timely to meet to review the existing knowledge and to speculate on future research applications. The lectures published here reflect the diversity of research currently underway using these techniques. The final outcome of the meeting was positive as it promoted collaboration between laboratories and, most important, created strong scientific and social links between individuals.

We wish to express our appreciation to Dr. Maria C. Lechner and Mrs. Helena Gata for providing valuable advice and help through the initial planning stages of this meeting. Finally, we are indebted to Ms. Lisbeth Heilesen for her outstanding organization and administration of the meeting and for typing all the manuscripts of this book. The meeting was held under the sponsorship of NATO with partial support from the Gulbenkian Foundation.

J.E. Celis

A. Graessmann

November 1979 A. Loyter

CONTENTS

MICROINJECTION OF SOMATIC CELLS WITH MICROPIPETTES

GHOST MEDIATED MICROINJECTION AND TRANSFER OF MEMBRANE COMPONENTS

MICROINJECTION OF SOMATIC CELLS WITH MICROPIPETTES AND PEG-ERYTHROCYTE GHOST MEDIATED MICROINJECTION

J.E. Celis, K. Kaltoft and R. Bravo

Division of Biostructural Chemistry
Department of Chemistry
Aarhus University
8000 Aarhus C, Denmark

1. INTRODUCTION

The development of techniques to introduce macromolecules into living somatic cells such as the direct microinjection with micropipettes (1, 2), the red cell mediated microinjection (3-7) and the liposome mediated injection (8-10) has opened the possibility of using the cell as a test tube to study complex biological phenomena that are not amenable to experimentation using conventional *in vitro* systems (11-25).

It is the purpose of this article to describe and compare the techniques of direct microinjection with micropipettes and the PEG-erythrocyte ghost mediated microinjection. The first part of this article describes the microinjection set-up we have used to inject somatic cells with glass micropipettes (13, 22) as well as recent data concerning the detection of [^{35}S]-methionine labelled globin synthesized in 100 mouse 3T3 cells microinjected with total rabbit globin mRNA (26-28, see also article by Huez *et al.* in this volume).

The second part describes the PEG-erythrocyte ghost mediated microinjection as it was developed to transfer HGPRT into HGPRT deficient cells (7, 28), and the third presents a brief comparison between the two microinjection techniques.

2. MICROINJECTION OF SOMATIC CELL WITH MICROPIPETTES

The technique of microinjection of somatic cells with micropipettes was developed independently by Graessmann (1) and by Diacumakos *et al.* (2). This technique has been used successfully to microinject DNAs (11, 29, 30), chromosomes (31), mRNAs (16, 25, 26, 28, 30, 32), tRNAs (13, 22), proteins (17-19, 23, 24) and small molecules (33, 34). The small number of cells that can be injected with this technique limits the assays that can be used to assess the success of the microinjection and to date only immunofluorescent, autoradiographic and virus plaques assays have been used.

In this section we will present evidence indicating that at least some biochemical assays can be used to assess the effect of the microinjected material. Specifically we will show that microinjection of total rabbit globin mRNA into as few as 100 mouse 3T3 cells followed by [^{35}S]-methionine labelling results in the synthesis of a globin like protein (27, 28) that can be easily detected by two dimensional gel electrophoresis (NEPHGE) (35).

The results of these experiments as well as a detailed description of the apparatus and manipulations neeeded to microinject somatic cells grown attached to a surface are given below.

(i) Microinjection set-up and preparation of micropipettes

The equipment we have used to microinject somatic cells (13, 22) grown attached to a surface is similar to that described by Graess-

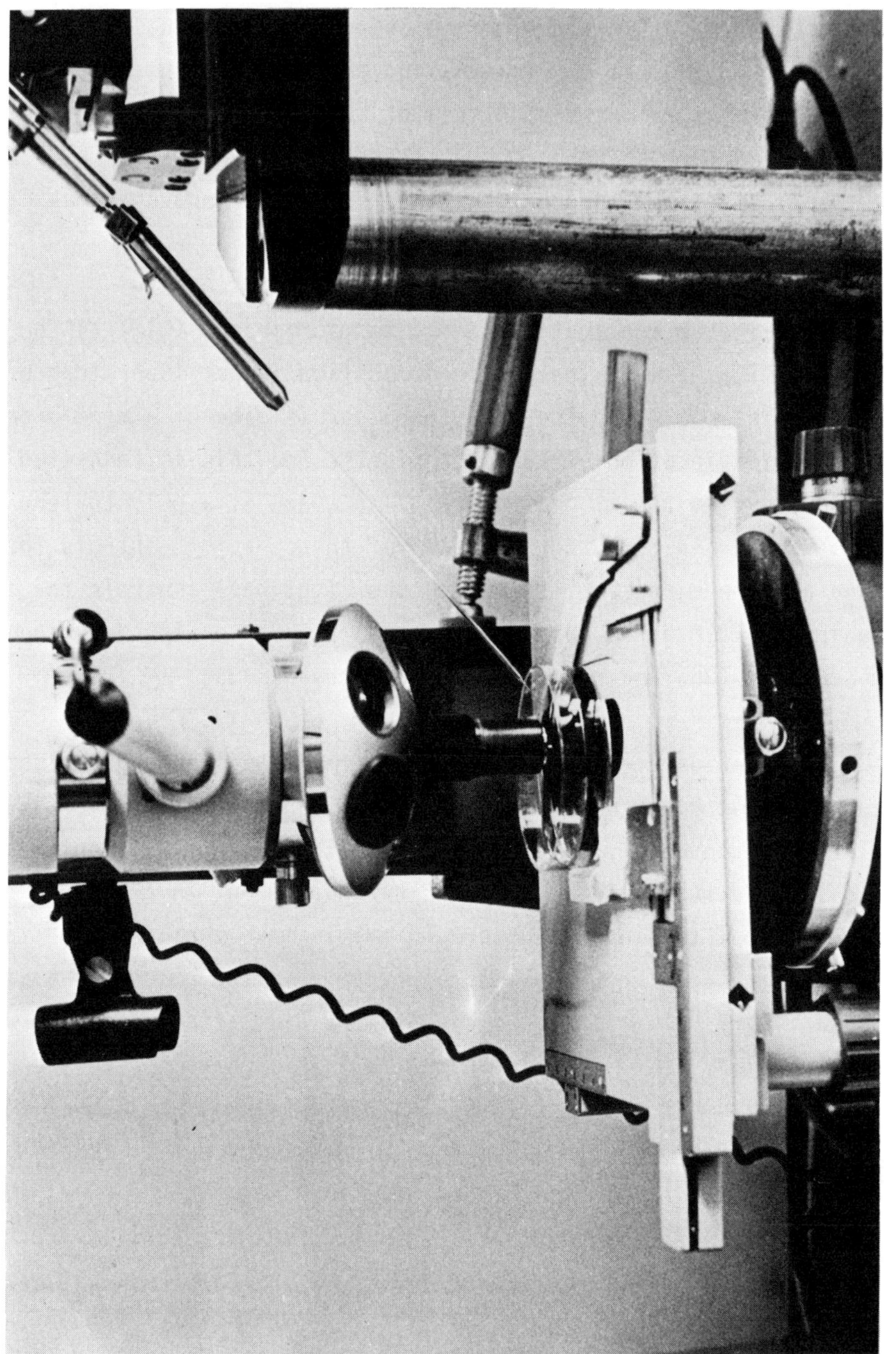

Fig. 1. *Microinjection set-up*. From Celis *et al.* (28).

mann and Graessmann (32). The equipment consists of a Carl Zeiss Jena Microsurgery equipment of which only the right hand micromanipulator is used (13, 22). A television camera, a Philips video cassette recorder and a television monitor have been attached to the microscope in order to keep record of the experiments (22, 28). Some video tape cassette recorders can take time lapse sequences making it possible to follow the cells after injection.

To obtain the inclination needed to microinject (Fig. 1) the right hand micromanipulator has been modified in our laboratory by Mr. B. Thomsen (13, 28). The pipette holder is made of a 6 cm bronze piece to avoid vibration of the micropipette and this is connected to a pressure system (50 ml glass syringe) by means of a polyethylene tubing. To microinject, the left hand of the operator controls the syringe and the microscope stage and the right hand controls the micromanipulator. Other microinjection apparatus have been described by Diacumakos (36) and by Yamamoto and Furusawa (33).

Micropipettes are made from 1.3-1.5 mm borosilicate glass capillaries (2G-100, Bie & Berntsen, Denmark) cleaned with chromic mixture, rinsed thoroughly with double distilled H_2O and siliconized with silicote. The capillaries are first pulled out in a microburner to give a local thining of about 0.16 mm. To make the micropipette the preformed capillary is placed vertically in the holder of a Carl Zeiss capillary puller and a weight of 4.75 g is attached to one end of the capillary (28). The platinum wire is brought close to the capillary and it is heated until the capillary breaks. The tip of the micropipette is broken off under the puller microscope by touching it with another micropipette. This operation is monitored by dipping the tip of the pipette in H_2O. Micropipettes made under these conditions have a tip diameter of approximately 1μ and are suitable to inject a wide range of somatic cells. Before use, the micropipettes are washed in double distilled H_2O, ethanol, dried at 145°C for 60 min and stored in a close container away from dust (11). To load the micropipettes with solution the tip of the pipette is introduced into a drop of the solution placed on a cold object glass and the liquid is aspirated with the aid of a syringe (11). To avoid clogging of the micropipette the solution to be injected is centrifuged in small capillaries at 20,000 rpm for 20 min in the SS-34 rotor of the Sorval centrifuge. An alternative way to load micropipettes has been described by Stacey and Alfrey (26)

(ii) Growth of somatic cells for microinjection and [^{35}S]-methionine labelling

Two types of coverslips have been used to grow cells depending on the assay to be used after microinjection. If microinjected cells are to be assayed by immunofluorescence or autoradiography the cells are grown in 144 mm^2 coverslips placed in 5 cm Petri dishes containing 8 ml of complete Dulbecco's modified Eagle's medium (DMEM). To help finding the cells after injection the coverslips are gridded in 1 mm^2 squares with a diamond pen (11) or are marked with a small circle in the center of the slide. If the microinjected cells are to be labelled with [^{35}S]-methionine they are plated in 9 mm^2 sterile coverslips (Microcover glass, Bellco Glass, Inc) placed in NUNC Microtest plates (NUNC, catalog no. 1480, Denmark) containing 0.2 ml of complete DMEM. The density of cells is adjusted as to obtain 100-150 cells per coverslip (28). To label the cells the coverslips are placed in 0.25 ml round bottomed NUNC Microtest plates (NUNC, catalog no. 163320, Denmark) containing 0.1 ml of home-made DMEM-methionine (1 g/l, $NaHCO_3$), supplemented with 10% dialyzed fetal calf serum and containing 100 μCi of [^{35}S]-methionine (Amersham, England). The labelling period is for 12 to 16 hrs at 37°C. Under these conditions about 1000 TCA precipitable cpm incorporate per cell

(28). At the end of the labelling period the cells are counted under the microscope, washed four times by dipping in Hank's buffered solution and resuspended in 20 μl of lysis buffer (37).

(iii) Microinjection

All operations are carried out in a sterile room or inside a laminar flow hood. The glass coverslip (144 or 9 mm^2) containing the attached cells is placed in a 5 cm Petri dish containing 8 ml of warm media without serum or Hanks's buffered solution (Fig. 1). The cells are viewed under phase contrast (x 300). First the cells are focused and then the tip of the micropipette is lowered until it is in the same focal plane as the cells. To microinject the tip of the micropipette is positioned so that it lies just outside the cell. It is enough just to touch the cell in order to penetrate. The pipette is connected to a 50 ml glass syringe to assist the injection of liquid (11). Injection is assessed visually. Once a cell has been injected, the micropipette is raised and moved closer to the next cell to be injected. The procedure is simple and about 100 cells can be injected in 15 min.

The microinjection as seen in the television monitor is shown in Fig. 2. In this case the tip of the micropipette has been introduced into the cytoplasm of a 3T3 cell. The volume injected per cell has been calculated to be about 5×10^{-11} ml (13, 22, 26), but this value depends on the size of the cell to be injected. In our experience volumes of up to 10% of the cell can be injected without any significant effect on the cell viability or macromolecular synthesis (22).

(iv) Microinjection of total rabbit globin mRNA into 100 mouse 3T3 cells

3T3 cells grown attached to 9 mm^2 coverslips were microinjected

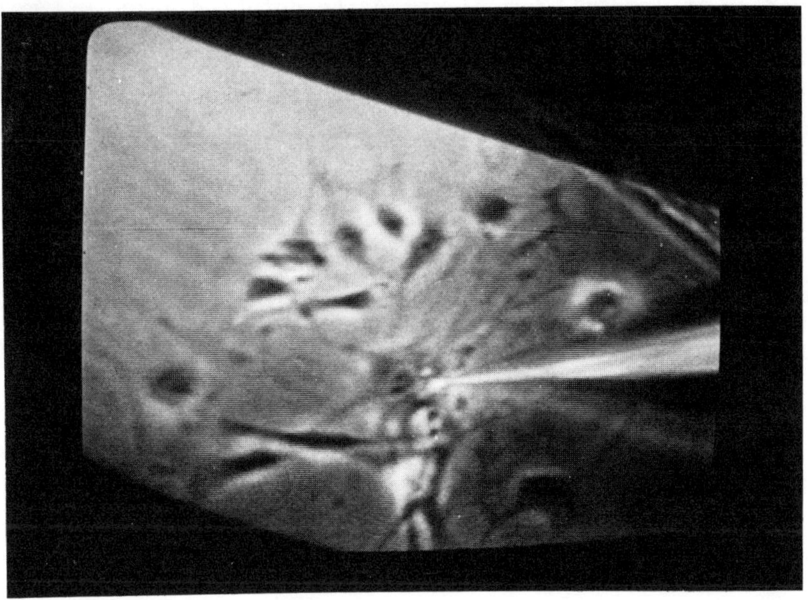

Fig. 2. *Microinjection of 3T3 cells.* Photograph taken from the television monitor.

in the cytoplasm with total rabbit globin mRNA and the polypeptides synthesized after injection were labelled with [^{35}S]-methionine under conditions in which the product of as few as 100 cells (27, 28, 38) could be analyzed by high resolution two dimensional gel electrophoresis (35, 37) followed by 10 days fluorography (39).

Fig. 3 shows fluorograms of two dimensional gels of basic polypeptides (NEPHGE, (27, 28, 35)) from approximately 100 mouse 3T3 cells injected with Hank's buffered solution (Fig. 3a) and with total rabbit globin mRNA (Fig. 3c; 0.5 mg/ml; about 7000 mRNA molecules injected per cell). About 125 basic polypeptides can be visually detected in the fluorograms. The only consistent difference between the control and the mRNA injected cells is one basic polypeptide of MW 15K (indicated with an arrow in Fig. 3c) that is present only in the mRNA injected cells. The intensity of this spot increases with increasing concentration of injected rabbit globin mRNA (we have analyzed up to 1 mg/ml) but it cannot be detected below 0.1 mg/ml (results not shown). That the 15K basic polypeptide may correspond to globin is suggested by the fact that it comigrates with [^{3}H]-leucine labelled rabbit globin synthesized *in vitro* (Fig. 3 b and c).

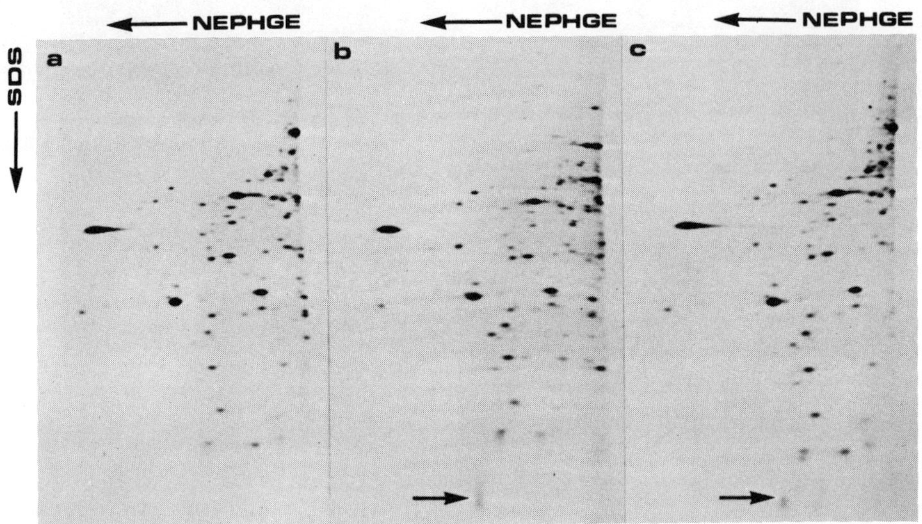

Fig. 3. *Synthesis of rabbit globin in 3T3 cells microinjected with total rabbit globin mRNA.* Two dimensional gel electrophoresis (NEPHGE) (35). a) control cells; b) control cells plus [^{3}H]-labelled globin synthesized *in vitro*; and c) cells injected with total globin mRNA (0.5 mg/ml). The arrows indicate the position of globin. From Celis *et al.* (28).

Due to the low amount of radioactivity contained in the 15K spot we have been unable to carry out immunoprecipitation or tryptic peptide analysis. Recently Huez *et al.* (40, this volume) have obtained similar results in HeLa cells microinjected with rabbit globin mRNA. In their case they fused many HeLa cells (40, 41) previous to microinjection of rabbit globin mRNA. Due to the large number of cells fused to form the homokaryons these workers could obtain enough counts to demonstrate by means of immunoprecipitation that the radioactive product synthesized *in vivo* corresponded to a

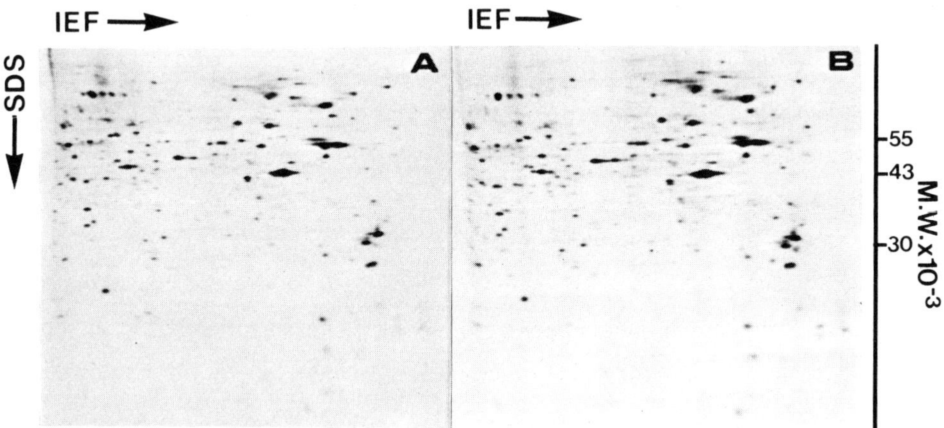

Fig. 4. *Two dimensional gel electrophoresis (IEF, 37) of [^{35}S]-methionine labelled polypeptides from control (A) and globin mRNA injected (0.5 mg/ml) mouse 3T3 cells (B).* Note that there is no apparent differences between the two patterns.

globin like protein. Also Ostro *et al.* (42) and Dimitriadis (43) have shown that rabbit globin mRNA inserted by liposomes into somatic cells can be translated, giving rise to a polypeptide closely related to rabbit globin as determined by immunoprecipitation.

Careful analysis of the fluorograms from acidic (IEF) (Fig. 4a and b) (NEPHGE) gels (FIG. 3a-c) of control as well as of mRNA injected 3T3 cells indicated that the microinjection of globin mRNA (0.5 mg/ml) does not alter significantly the relative intensity of the major [^{35}S]-methionine labelled polypeptide spots detected in the gels. These data are in line with the fact that we are microinjecting between 0.5-1% of the estimated relative mRNA population of the cell (44).

(v) Conclusions

It must be stressed that the experiments we have presented

were carried out under conditions in which more than 85% of the injected cells remained viable after injection. The fact that we can detect the translation product of 7000 molecules of globin mRNA microinjected per cell (about 0.5-1% of the total native population of cell mRNA (44)) in as few as 100 mouse cells opens new possibilities to study the effect of injected macromolecules on gene expression at the level of polypeptide synthesis.

Recently, we have been able to detect the major [^{35}S] methionine labelled cytoarchitecture polypeptides synthesized by 10 HeLa cells using high resolution two dimensional gel electrophoresis. As seen in Fig. 5 B at least five major cytocarchitectural proteins including total actin, β-tubulin and the subunit of the intermediate filaments are detected under normal running and exposure conditions. This result clearly illustrates the potentiality of using a combination of [^{35}S]-methionine labelling techniques and high resolution two dimensional gel electrophoresis to assay the effect of microinjected macromolecule on gene expression.

Even though it is possible to microinject with micropipettes up to 1000 cells in a single experiment it is clear that if many more cells need to be injected it is necessary to use other microinjection techniques available. One such technique we have used in this laboratory is described in the next section.

3. PEG-ERYTHROCYTE GHOST MEDIATED MICROINJECTION

Furusawa *et al.* (3), Loyter *et al.* (4) and Schlegel and Rechsteiner (5) first described a technique to inject macromolecules into a large number of somatic cells containing receptors for *Sendai* virus. The method consists of two steps: first the macromolecules are incorporated into erythrocyte ghosts during hypotonic hemolysis and secondly, the resealed ghosts are fused with the recipient cells

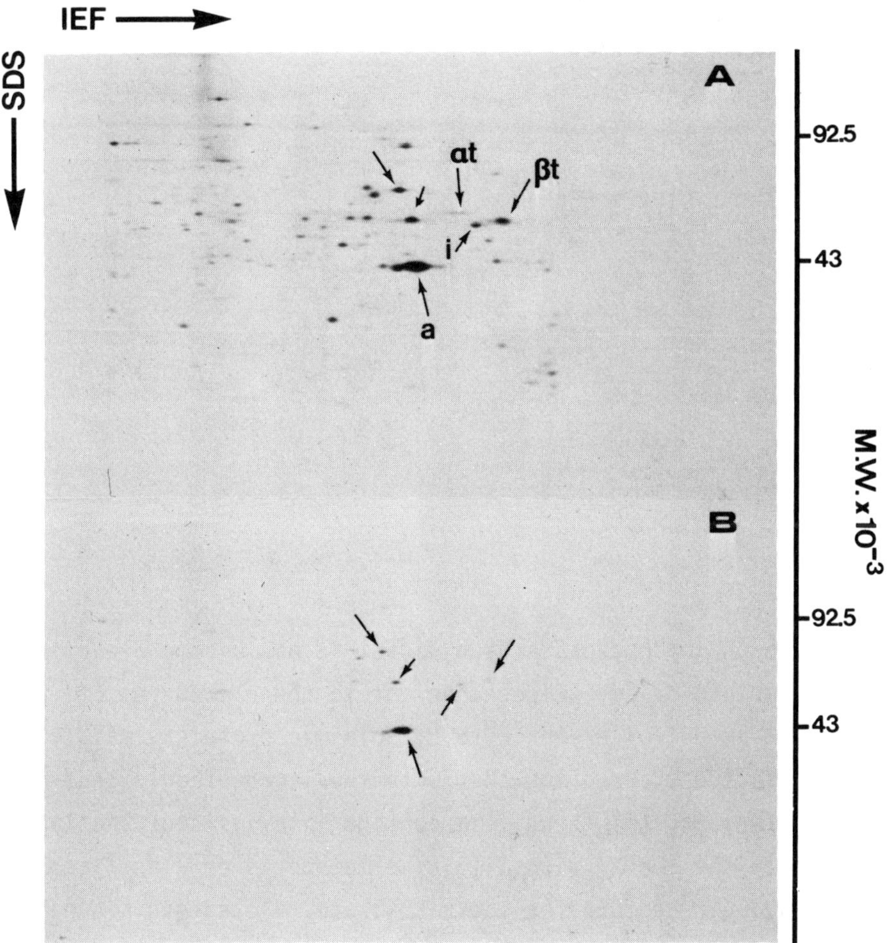

Fig. 5. *Two dimensional gel electrophoresis (IEF) of total* [^{35}*S*]-*methionine labelled polypeptides from HeLa cells.* A) Product of 50 cells; B) Product of 10 cells. Exposure time: 10 days at -80°C. αt = α-tubulin; βt = β-tubulin; i = intermediate filament (IFa55/1.16) and a = total actin.

using inactivated *Sendai* virus. A schematic representation of this method is shown in Fig. 6. Proteins such as albumin (5, 45, 46), antifragment A against Difteria toxin (47), ferritin (4), IgG (45, 47), nonhistone proteins (21, 48), thymidine kinase (5) and tRNA (12, 13, 22, 49) have been injected into mammalian cells using this me-

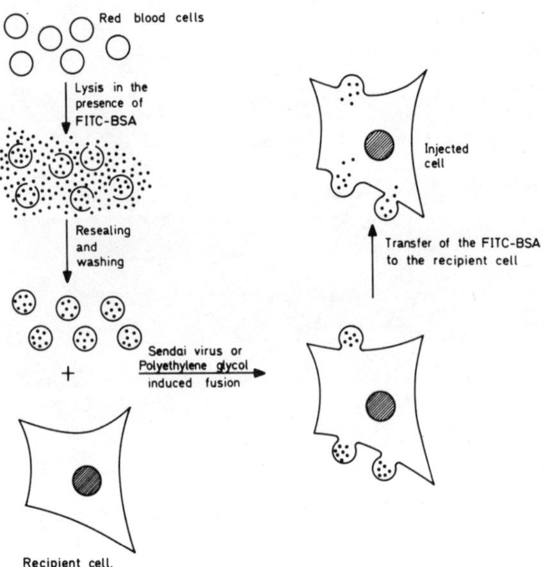

Fig. 6. *Erythrocyte ghost mediated microinjection.*

thod. Though the method has proven useful it has become clear that there are certain disadvantages inherent to the procedure: (1) a considerable amount of erythrocyte cytoplasmic proteins, mainly hemoglobin, are transferred together with the macromolecule that one wishes to transfer; (2) there is a considerable lysis of the loaded ghosts due to the *Sendai* virus; (3) the method is only applicable to cells having receptors for the virus, and (4) protein synthesis is severely reduced in the fused cells.

In view of the urgent need to have techniques to microinject large numbers of cells we have developed an alternative method in which hemoglobin free ghosts loaded with macromolecules are efficiently fused with recipient somatic cells (grown in monolayers) by means of polyethylene glycol (PEG) (7, 28). This procedure has at least four advantages over the *Sendai* virus induced fusion: (1) in theory it is applicable to all somatic cells; (2) it uses hemoglobin free ghosts; (3) the average number of ghosts fusing with recipient cells ranges between 5 and 10 (7) as compared to 1 or 2 found in

Sendai virus induced fusion (5, 12, 15); and (4) macromolecular synthesis is not significantly different in fused and non-fused cells. To develop this method we have chosen to microinject hypoxanthine guanine phosphorybosyl transferase (HGPRT) into ($HGPRT^-$) cells for the following reasons: (1) the enzyme and the mutant cells can be readily obtained; (2) the injection can be easily monitored and quantitated by autoradiography; and (3) a successful transfer demonstrates that the cells are actively engaged in nucleic acid synthesis suggesting that they have not been seriously affected by the fusion process. The procedure is described below (7, 28).

(i) Loading of erythrocyte ghosts with crude extracts containing HGPRT

Human erythrocytes collected in Ca^{2+}, Mg^{2+} free phosphate buffered saline (PBS) containing 2 mM EDTA are centrifuged at 500 g for 10 min and washed 3 times in the same buffer without EDTA. Hemoglobin-free ghosts are prepared by suspending the red cell pellet (1 vol) in 50 vol of 10 mM Na-phosphate buffer, 2 mM ATP pH 7.2 followed by centrifugation at 7.000 g for 10 min and three washes in the same buffer. The lysis can also be done in 20 vol of 2.0 mM ATP pH 7.2 followed by three washes in the same buffer. To load the ghosts with HGPRT the first supernatant after hemolysis is concentrated in an Amicon B15 to 1 vol and is added to half the volume of pelleted ghosts while vortex mixing. After 3 min at $0^{o}C$, 1/10 of the vol of 10 x PBS with reversed concentrations of KCl and NaCl is added to restore isotonicity and the ghosts are kept on ice for a further 5 min. At the end of this period the loaded ghosts are incubated at $37^{o}C$ for 30 min followed by three washes in PBS containing reversed concentration of KCl and NaCl. Ghosts loaded under these conditions contain 35% of the HGPRT activity found in normal human red blood cells (RBC). Mock loaded ghosts are prepared by adding buffer instead of the crude enzyme extracts. Loaded ghosts are usually fused with recipient cells within 1 hr of preparation, although longer storage (24 hrs at $4^{o}C$) does not affect the ghosts. In the case of precious samples we recommend to load 5 μl of pelleted ghosts with 5 μl of the sample. Under these conditions one obtains enough loaded ghosts to inject 3 x 10^{5} recipient cells at a ratio of 100 ghosts per cell.

(ii) PEG induced fusion of HGPRT loaded ghosts with CHO $HGPRT^{-}$ cells

CHO $HGPRT^{-}$ cells plated on a 144 mm^{2} coverslip and grown for 1 day to about 80% confluency to avoid too much self-to-self fusion are placed in a flat-bottomed centrifuge tube (20 mm in diameter) and covered with an excess of loaded ghosts in 100 μl of PBS. Three ml of complete DMEM are then added and the ghosts containing the HGPRT are pelleted onto the coverslip by centrifugation at 3,000 g for 5 min at room temperature in a bench centrifuge. The excess of medium is thoroughly removed and the coverslip is covered with 2 ml of 50% PEG 6000 (1 g of PEG 6000 (Koch-Light) + 1 ml of PBS) (50). After 1 min the coverslip is transferred to a Petri dish containing DMEM and the PEG is thoroughly removed by rocking the Petri dish for at least 1 min or by pipetting DMEM onto the coverglass. The coverglass in then transferred to another Petri dish with medium, and the washing is repeated. Thereafter, the coverslip is placed in a plastic Leighton tube or Petri dish containing complete DMEM plus 1 μCi/ml of [^{3}H]-hypoxanthine ([^{3}H]-hypoxanthine, 1.8 Ci/mmol, 0.5 μCi/μl, Amersham, England) and aminopterin (10^{-5}M) and the cells are incubated for further 24 hrs at $37^{o}C$. At the end of this period the coverslip is washed 3 times in PBS, fixed in 2.5% glutaraldehyde in PBS and washed twice in cold 2% perchloric acid. After washing with distilled water the coverslip is covered with Kodak NTB-3 emulsion and exposed for 18½ hrs before developing and staining with Giemsa. Alternatively, after washing with distilled water and drying the amount of [^{3}H]-hypoxanthine incorporated into nucleic acids can be estimated by scintilation counting. The coverslip can be recovered for autoradiography by washing it thoroughly in toluene.

To fuse cells grown in suspension (P3-X63 Ag8 - HGPRT$^-$) (51) the cell mixture (P3 cells plus loaded ghosts) is first spun down on top of a coverslip and then fused as described above. Under these conditions more than 50% of the myeloma cells adhere to the glass and remain attached for at least 18 hrs. This procedure enables one to do autoradiography on the attached cells. If the cells are to be kept in suspension the cell mixture is spun down in a round-bottomed centrifuge tube (NUNC N - 215-4). After thoroughly removing the medium, 2 ml of 50% PEG is added. After 1 min, 20 ml of complete DMEM is added and after carefully mixing, the cells are centrifuged and resuspended in complete DMEM.

(iii) <u>Microinjection of HGPRT into HGPRT$^-$ cells</u>

Fig. 7. shows an autoradiography of CHO-EMS 16.4 HGPRT$^-$ cells fused with mock loaded ghosts at a multiplicity of 100 ghosts/cell (7, 28). The grain density over CHO cells is not larger than that of the background indicating that little or no HGPRT remains in the ghosts after hemolysis (Fig. 7, control). The same results is obtained if the HGPRT containing extract is added together with the PEG solution during fusion or immediately after it, indicating that the enzyme does not enter the recipient cells directly from the PEG solution during the fusion. HGPRT activity is not affected by the high concentration of PEG. If, on the other hand, HGPRT loaded ghosts are fused at a ratio of 100 ghosts/CHO about 80% of the cells show grains above the background (Fig. 7, injected). A detailed analysis of the number of grains incorporated per cell under various conditions has been published elsewhere (7).

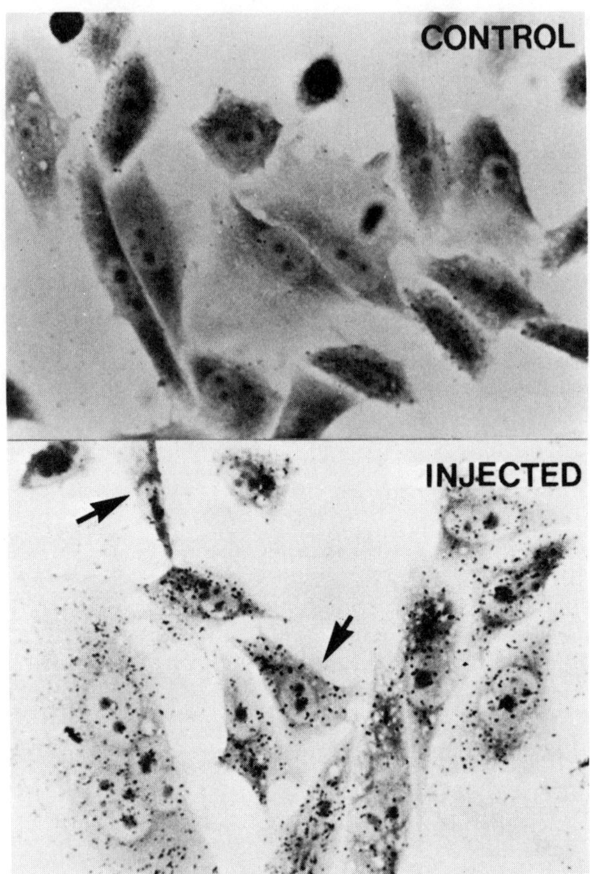

Fig. 7. *Autoradiography of CHO HGPRT⁻ cells fused with HGPRT loaded ghosts and labelled with* [^{3}H]*-hypoxanthine*. Control. HGPRT$^-$ cells fused with mock loaded ghosts at a ratio of 100 ghosts/CHO cell. Injected. HGPRT$^-$ CHO cells fused with HGPRT loaded ghosts at a ratio of 100 RBC/CHO cell.

(iv) Effect of PEG ghost mediated microinjection on cell viability, DNA, RNA and protein synthesis

When macromolecules are to be introduced into somatic cells the pertubation of the cell by the transfer procedure should be minimized as much as possible. For *Sendai* virus induced fusion there is a considerable cytotoxicity as protein synthesis is severely reduced in the recipient cells (45).

It was therefore of interest to test whether the PEG-induced fusion procedure suffers from the same limitations. The cytotoxicity of PEG has often been reported (52, 53). When the fusion procedure, however, is performed as described in this article we find no significant differences on cell parameters like cell viability (more than 90% viability as tested by tryphan blue staining), DNA, RNA and protein synthesis.

DNA synthesis has been estimated by measuring the incorporation of [^{3}H]-thymidine into DNA and by autoradiographic analysis of control cells and of cells fused with mock loaded ghosts. No difference was detected when labelling was performed at different times after PEG induced fusion (results not shown). This result is in agreement with data of Norwood *et al.* (54), which showed no significant decrease in cells entering S-phase after PEG induced fusion of human skin fibroblasts.

Total nucleic acid synthesis has been estimated by following the incorporation of [^{3}H]-hypoxanthine into macromolecules. Neither fusion of recipient cells with mock loaded ghosts nor among themselves results in apparent differences between PEG and non-PEG treated cells (7, 28).

Finally, protein synthesis has been monitored quantitatively by autoradiography (Fig. 8) and qualitatively by two dimensional gel electrophoresis (Fig. 9). As can be seen no significant changes are observed either in the number of grains (average number of grains per cm^2 = 15 in control cells and 15.5 in fused cells, Fig. 8) or the pattern of proteins synthesized (Fig. 9) following fusion. Other parameters of the tissue culture, like population doubling (starting from the same number of unfused cells) will, of course, differ in PEG treated and non-treated cells due most likely to the formation of multinucleated cells.

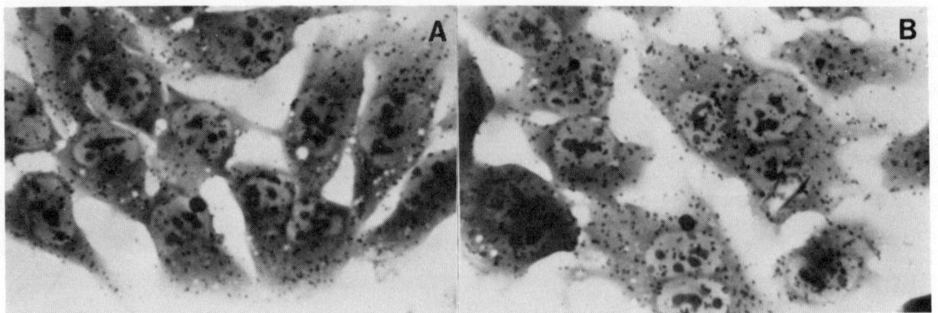

Fig. 8. *Autoradiography of CHO 16.4 cells fused with mocked loaded ghosts and labelled with [^{3}H]-methionine.* (A) Control cells labelled for 1 hr with 3 μCi/ml of [^{3}H]-methionine in complete DMEM containing 1 mg/l of cold methionine. (B) CHO 16.4 cells fused with mocked loaded ghosts at a ratio of 100:1 and labelled as described above.

(v) Macromolecules that have been injected using the PEG-erythrocyte ghost mediated microinjection

Several macromolecules have been injected into a variety of cell lines and these are summarized in Table 1. At present we do not know whether the published procedures (6, 7) can be used to microinject other cell lines although we suspect that it may be necessary to optimize the procedure for the cell line as well as for the macromolecules to be injected.

Preliminary experiments in our laboratory indicate that the amount of material transferred by the PEG mediated fusion procedure is about 5 times larger than the *Sendai* virus mediated fusion method.

(vi) Conclusions

The outstanding features of the PEG-erythrocyte ghost mediated microinjection are that a large number of cells can be injected and that it is possible to use biochemical assays to assess the effect of the microinjected material. The procedure is simple, does not re-

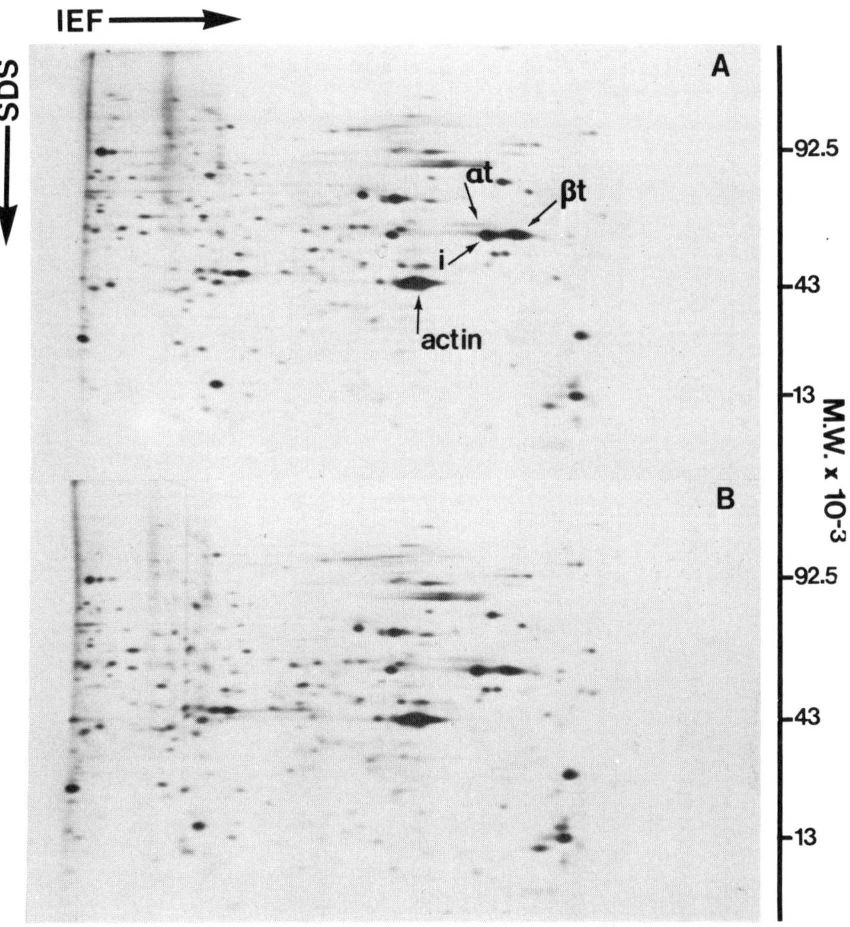

Fig. 9. *Two dimensional gel electrophoresis of total* [^{35}S]*-methionine labelled polypeptides from RJK39 cells.* (A) Control of cells. (B) Cells fused with mocked loaded ghost at a ratio of 100:1. αt = α-tubulin; βt = β-tubulin; i = intermediate filament (IFa 55/1.16).

quire any special equipment and with practice about 30 microinjection experiments can be performed per day. The main disadvantage of this technique is that nearly all the material to be injected (>95%) is waisted during the two step injection procedure. In the case of precious samples this disadvantage can be easily overcome by loading red cells in as few as 5 μl. Also large macromolecules like DNA can-

Table 1. *PEG-erythrocyte ghost mediated microinjection of macromolecules into different cell lines.*

Cell line	Macromolecules injected	Comments
CHO-16.4 (HGPRT$^-$); RJK39 (HGPRT$^-$); P3-X63-Azg8 (HGPRT$^-$)	Human HGPRT	Enzyme activity is greatly enhanced when aminopterin (10^{-5}M) is included in the media (Refs. 7, 28).
CHO-16.4 (HGPRT$^-$)	Mouse HGPRT	As above (Refs. 7, 28).
CHO-16.4 (HGRPT$^-$)	[^{125}I]-labelled non-histone proteins	The distribution of radioactivity between cytoplasm and nucleus is approximately equal 2 hrs after injection (Ref. 28).
CHO-16.4 (HGPRT$^-$); RJK39 (HGPRT$^-$); 3T3; CLID; primary and stablished amnion cells; HeLa and XP fibroblasts.	FITC-BSA	FITC-BSA is found exclusively in the cytoplasm shortly after fusion (Refs. 7, 28).
VICO, CV-IP	FITC-BSA	FITC-BSA is found in the nucleus (Ref. 6).
CV-IP	T-antigen	Injection of T-antigen causes complementation of the SV40 tsA mutant (Ref. 20).

not be loaded into erythrocyte ghosts using present procedures. Trapping of DNA into liposomes or direct microinjection with micropipettes are obvious alternatives in this case.

4. MICROINJECTION OF FITC-BSA INTO SOMATIC CELLS USING THE DIRECT MICROINJECTION WITH MICROPIPETTES AND THE PEG-ERYTHROCYTE GHOST MEDIATED MICROINJECTION

Even though both microinjection techniques have been widely used to inject a number of macromolecules there is yet little data concerning the comparative efficiencies of these techniques. Also it is of interest to determine whether macromolecules injected by both techniques reach the same compartment of the cell.

To answer these questions at least partially we have compared the microinjection of FITC-BSA into somatic cells using both techniques. As shown in Figs. 10 and 11, FITC-BSA microinjected by both techniques remains in the cytoplasm of somatic cells at least a few hrs after injection. This result differs from that of Kriegler and Livingston (6), who using a similar PEG fusion technique found that microinjected FITC-BSA is in the nucleus of the injected cells. At present we do not know the reason for this discrepancy. A complete report concerning the fate of fluorescent proteins microinjected with micropipettes has been published by Stacey and Alfrey (17).

Even though we have not yet determined the amount of FITC-BSA injected by both techniques visual comparison of the preparations by fluorescent microscopy indicates that at least 5-10 times more material is injected by the micropipette technique.

5. CONCLUDING REMARKS

We have described two techniques to microinject macromolecules into a wide range of somatic cells under conditions in which viabi-

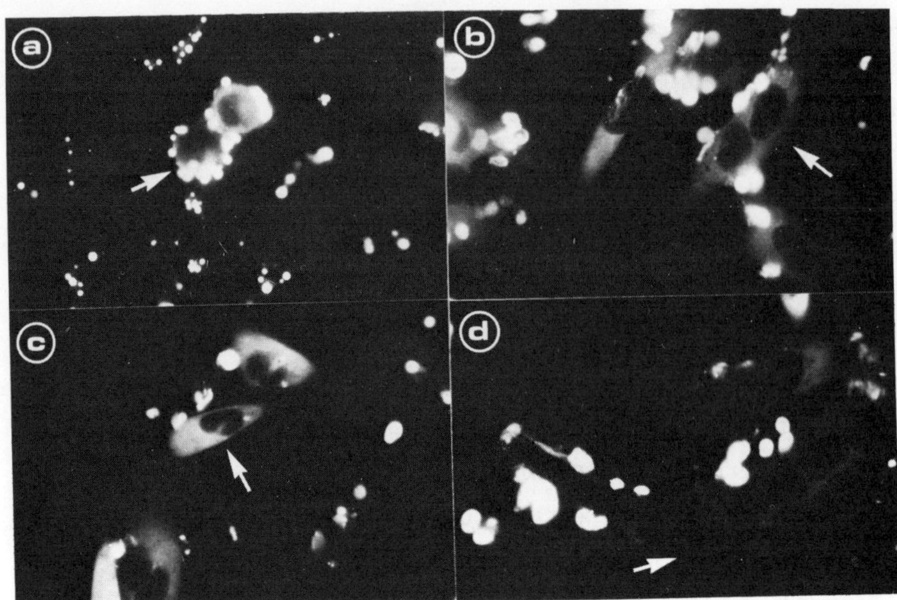

Fig. 10. *Fusion of CHO cells with human ghosts loaded with FITC-BSA (16OD$_{490}$/ml) as seen by immunofluorescence microscopy.* (a) 10 min after fusion; (b), (c) and (d) 2 hrs after fusion. Note that the fluorescence is excluded from the nucleus.

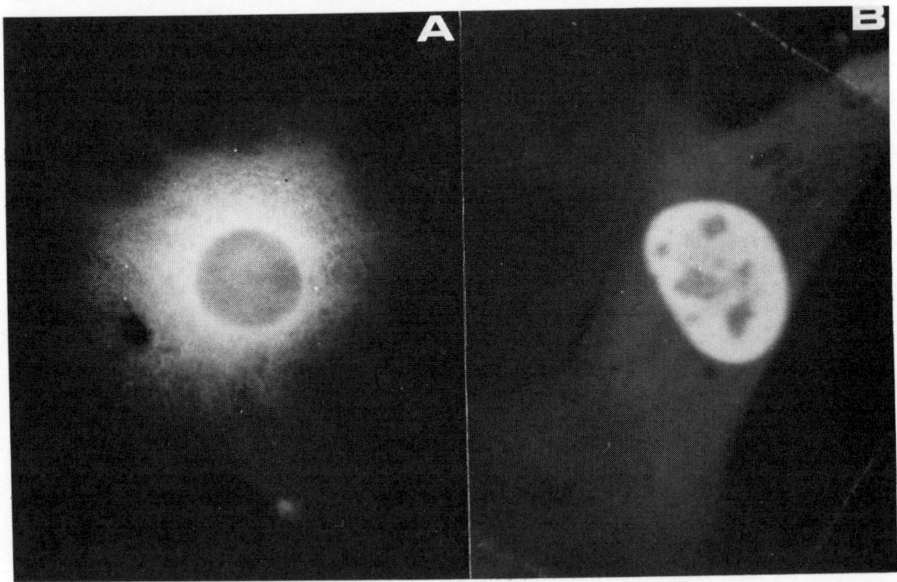

Fig. 11. *Microinjection with micropipettes of FITC-BSA (16OD$_{490}$/ml) into mouse 3T3 cells.* (A) Injection into the cytoplasm. (B) Injection into the nucleus.

lity and macromolecular synthesis do not seem to be impaired. Both techniques should complement each other and together they represent valuable tools to study biological phenomena *in vivo*. Currently, in this laboratory we are assessing the value of both techniques to study problems such as cell transformation and the isolation of nonsense mutations in somatic cells.

6. ACKNOWLEDGEMENTS

We would like to thank A. Celis, B. Thomsen and O. Jensen for expert assistance and to J. Bellatin and F. Baralle for samples of [^{3}H]-leucine labelled globin and total rabbit globin mRNA, respectivly. R. Bravo is a recipient of a long-term post-doctoral fellowship from EMBO. This work was supported in part by grants from the Danish Natural Science Research Council, Euratom and Novo.

7. REFERENCES

1) GRAESSMANN, A. (1968). Doctoral dissertation, Free University of Berlin.
2) DIACUMAKOS, E.G., HOLLAND, S. and PECORA, P. (1970). A microsurgical methodology for human cells *in vitro*: Evolution and applications. Proc. Natl. Acad. Sci., 65, 911.
3) FURUSAWA, M., NISHIMURA, T., YAMAIZUMI, M. and OKADA, Y. (1974). Injection of foreign substances into single cells by cell fusion. Nature, 249, 449.
4) LOYTER, A., ZAKAI, N. and KULKA, R.G. (1975). "Ultramicroinjection" of macromolecules or small particles into animal cells. J. Cell Biol., 66, 292.
5) SCHLEGEL, R.A. and RECHSTEINER, M.C. (1975). Microinjection of thymidine kinase and bovine serum albumin into mammalian cells by fusion with red blood cells. Cell, 5, 371.

6) KRIEGLER, M.P. and LIVINGSTON, D.M. (1977). Chemically facilitated microinjection of proteins into intact monolayers of tissue culture cells. Somat. Cell Genet., 3, 603.

7) KALTOFT, K. and CELIS, J.E. (1978). Ghost mediated transfer of human hypoxanthine-guanine phosphoribosyltransferase into deficient Chinese hamster ovary cells by means of polyethylene glycol-induced fusion. Exptl. Cell Res., 115, 423.

8) GREGORIADIS, G. (1976). Carrier potential of liposomes in biology and medicine. 1. Eng. J. Med., 295, 704.

9) TYRELL, D., HEATH, T., COLLEY, C. and RYMAN, B. (1976). New aspects of liposomes. Biochim., Biophys. Acta, 457, 259.

10) POSTE, G., PAPAHADJOPOULOS, D. and VEIL, W. (1976). In: Methods in Cell Biology. Lipid vesicles as carriers for introducing biologically active materials into cells (ed., D.M. Presscott), Academic Press, New York, 14, 33.

11) GRAESSMANN, M. and GRAESSMANN, A. (1976). "Early" simian-virus-40 specific RNA contains information for tumor antigen formation and chromatin replication. Proc. Natl. Acad. Sci., 73, 366.

12) KALTOFT, K., ZEUTHEN, J., ENGBÆK, F., PIPER, P.W. and CELIS, J.E. (1976). Transfer of tRNAs to somatic cells mediated by *Sendai* virus induced fusion. Proc. Natl. Acad. Sci., 73, 2793.

13) CELIS, J.E. (1977). Injection of tRNAs into somatic cells. Search for *in vivo* systems to assay potential nonsense mutations in somatic cells. Brookhaven Symp. Biol., 29, 178.

14) GRAESSMANN, A., GRAESSMANN, M. and MUELLER, C. (1977). Simian virus 40 gene expression in permissive, non-permissive and virus-resistant cells. Brookhaven Symp. Biol., 29, 197.

15) CAPECCHI, M.R., VONDER HAAR, R.A., CAPECCHI, N.E. and SVEDA, M.M. (1977). The isolation of a suppresible nonsense mutant in mammalian cells. Cell, 12,371.

16) STACEY, D.W., ALFREY, V.G. and HANAFUSA, H. (1977). Microinjection analysis of envelope-glycoprotein messenger activities of avian leukosis viral RNAs. Proc. Natl. Acad. Sci., 74, 1614.

17) STACEY, D.W. and ALFREY, V.G. (1977). Evidence for the autophagy of microinjected proteins in HeLa cells. J. Cell Biol., 75, 807.

18) McCLAIN, D.A., MANESS, P.F. and EDELMAN, G.M. (1978). Assay for early cytoplasmic effect of the *src* gene product of Rous sarcoma virus. Proc. Natl. Acad. Sci., 75, 2750.

19) TJIAN, R., FEY, G. and GRAESSMANN, A. (1978). Biological activity of purified simian virus 40 T antigen proteins. Proc. Natl. Acad. Sci., 75, 1279.

20) KRIEGLER, M.P., GRIFFIN, J.D. and LIVINGSTON, D.M. (1978). Phenotypic complementation of the SV40 ts A mutant defect in viral DNA synthesis following microinjection of SV40 T antigen. Cell, 14, 983.

21) RECHSTEINER, M. and KUEHL, L. (1979). Microinjection of the non-histone chromosomal protein HMG 1 into bovine fibroblasts and HeLa cells. Cell, 16, 901.

22) CELIS, J.E., KALTOFT, K., CELIS, A., FENWICK, R. and CASKEY, C.T. (1979). Microinjection of tRNAs into somatic cells. In: "Nonsense mutations and tRNA suppressors". (eds., J.E. Celis and J.D. Smith), Academic Press, London, p. 255.

23) FERAMISCO, J.R. (1979). Microinjection of fluorescently labelled α-actinin into living fibroblasts. Proc. Natl. Acad. Sci., 76, 3967.

24) KREIS, T.E., WINTERHALTER, K.H. and BIRCHMEIER, W. (1979). *In vivo* distribution and turnover of fluorescent labeled actin microinjected into human fibroblasts. Proc. Natl. Acad. Sci. USA, 76, 3814.

25) LIU, C.P., SLATE, D.L., GRAVEL, R. and RUDDLE, F.H. (1979). Biological detection of specific mRNA molecules by microinjection. Proc. Natl. Acad. Sci. USA, 76, 4503.

26) STACEY, D.W. and ALFREY, V.G. (1976). Microinjection studies of duck globin messenger RNA translation in human and avian cells. Cell, 9, 725.

27) BRAVO, R. and CELIS, J.E. (1979), Expt. Cell Res., in press.

28) CELIS, J.E., KALTOFT, K. and BRAVO, R. (1979). Microinjection of somatic cells. In: "Introduction of macromolecules into viable cells". (eds., G. Rovera, R. Baserga and C. Croce), Alan R. Liss. Inc., in press.

29) GRAESSMANN, A., GRAESSMANN, M. and MUELLER, C. (1977). Regulatory function of simian virus 40 DNA replication for late viral gene expression. Proc. Natl. Acad. Sci., 74, 4831.

30) GRAESSMANN, A., GRAESSMANN, M. and MUELLER, C. (1979). In:"Introduction of macromolecules into viable cells". (eds., G. Rovera and C. Croce), Alan K. Liss, Inc., in press.

31) DIACUMAKOS, E.G., HOLLAND, S. and PECORA, P. (1971). Chromosome displacement in and extraction from human cells at different mitotic stages. Nature, 232, 33.

32) GRAESSMANN, A. and GRAESSMANN, M. (1971). Über die Bildung von Melanin in Muskelzellen nach der direkten Übertragung von RNA aus Harding-Passey-Melanonomzellen. Hoppe-Seyler's Z. Physiol. Chem., 352, 527.

33) YAMAMOTO, F. and FURUWASA, M. (1978). A simple microinjection technique not employing a micromanipulator. Exptl. Cell Res., 117, 441.

34) WEHLAND, J., OSBORN, M. and WEBER, K. (1977). Phalloidin-induced actin polymerization in the cytoplasm of cultured cells interferes with cell locomotion and growth. Proc. Natl. Acad. Sci., 74, 5613.

35) O'FARRELL, P.Z., GOODMAN, H.M. and O'FARRELL, P.H. (1977). High resolution of two-dimensional electrophoresis of basic as well as acidic proteins. Cell, 12, 1133.

36) DIACUMAKOS, E.G. (1973). Methods for micromanipulation of human somatic cells in culture. Methods Cell Biol., 8, 287.

37) O'FARRELL, P.H. (1975). High resolution two-dimensional electrophoresis of proteins. J. Biol. Chem., 250, 4007.

38) BRAVO, R. and CELIS, J.E. (1979). A search for differential

polypeptide synthesis through the cell cycle of HeLa cells. J. Cell Biol., in press.

39) LASKEY, R.A. and MILLS, A.D. (1975). Quantitative film detection of ^{3}H and ^{14}C in polyacrylamide gels by fluorography. Eur. J. Biochem., 56, 335.

40) HUEZ, G.A., BRUCK, C., PORTETELLE, D. and CHEUTER, Y. (1979). Translation of rabbit globin mRNA upon injection into fused HeLa cells. FEBS Lett., in press.

41) GRAESSMANN, A., GRAESSMANN, M. and MUELLER, C. (1979). Fused cells are suited for microinjection. Biochem. Biophys. Res. Commun., 88, 428.

42) OSTRO, M.J., GIACOMON, D., LAVELLE, D., PAXTON, W. and DRAY, S. (1978). Evidence for translation of messenger-RNA after liposome-mediated insertion into a human cell line. Nature, 274, 923.

43) DIMITRIADIS, G.J. (1978). Evidence for translation of rabbit globin mRNA after liposome mediated insertion into a human cell line. Nature, 274, 921.

44) DARNELL, J.E. (1978). Ribonucelic acids from animal cells. Bacteriol. Rev., 32, 262.

45) WASSERMAN, M., ZAKAI, N., LOYTER, A. and KULKA, R.G. (1976). A quantitative study of ultramicroinjection of macromolecules into animal cells. Cell, 7, 551.

46) WILLE, W., and WILLECKE, K. (1976). Retention of purified proteins in resealed human erythrocyte ghosts and transfer by fusion into cultured murine recipient cells. FEBS Lett., 65, 59.

47) YAMAIZUMI, M., UCHIDA, T., OKADA, Y. and FURUSAWA, M. (1978). Neutralization of difteria toxin in living cells by microinjection of antifragment A contained within resealed erythrocyte ghosts. Cell, 13, 227.

48) YAMAIZUMI, M., UCHIDA, T., OKADA, Y., FURUSAWA, M. and MITSUI, H. (1978). Rapid transfer of non-histone chromosomal proteins to the nucleus of living cells. Nature, 273, 782.

49) SCHLEGEL, R.A., IVERSEN, P. and RECHSTEINER, M.C. (1978). The turnover of tRNAs microinjected into animal cells. Nucl. Acids Res., 5, 3715.

50) PONTECORVO, G., RIDDLE, P.N. and HALES, A. (1977). Time and mode of fusion of human fibroblasts treated with polyethylene glycol (PEG). Nature, 265, 257.

51) KÖHLER, G. and MILSTEIN, C. (1975). Continuous cultures of fused cells secreting antibody of predefined specificity. Nature, 256, 495.

52) MERCER, W.C. and SCHLEGEL, R.A. (1979). Phytohemagglutinin enhancement of cell fusion reduces polyethylene glycol cytotoxicity. Exp. Cell Res., 120, 417.

53) SCHNEIDERMAN, S., FARBER, J.L. and BASERGA, R. (1979). A simple method of decreasing the toxicity of polyethylene glycol in mammalian cell hybridization. Somat. Cell Genet., 5, 263.

54) NORWOOD, T.H., ZEIGLER, C.J. and MARTIN, G.M. (1976). Dimethyl sulfoxide enhances polyethylene glycol-mediated somatic cell fusion. Somat. Cell Genet., 2, 263.

MICROINJECTION OF CELLULAR AND VIRAL mRNAs

D.W. Stacey

Roche Institute of Molecular Biology
Nutley, New Jersey 07110, U.S.A.

1. INTRODUCTION

The technique of microinjection in cultured cells has been used to critically analyze the biological activities of purified mRNAs. Since microinjected RNA is translated within viable somatic cells, in competition with endogenous mRNAs and in the presence of cellular regulatory factors, its observed behavior is likely to represent the activity of the corresponding molecule *in vivo*. Furthermore, the biological activities of proteins translated from injected mRNAs can be studied in relation to the living cell. Activities such as induction of DNA synthesis and complementation of genetic mutants have proven particularly useful.

The results obtained following microinjection of three types of RNA will be discussed. First, duck globin mRNA was microinjected into HeLa cells. The avian messenger was translated well by the human cell line. Next, RNA copied from the "early" strand of SV40 and polyoma DNA was shown to be translated following microinjection into mammalian cells to produce viral T-antigen which then induced DNA synthesis within the injected cells. Finally, as an intracellular assay for avian retroviral envelope glycoprotein (*env*) messenger, RNAs were injected into chick embryo fibroblasts infected with the envelope-deficient Bryan strain of Rous sarcoma virus. The *env* messenger was identified along with its nuclear precursor within cells as well as virus particles. In the course of these studies unexpected observations were made relating to the infrequent participation of *env* mRNA in viral gene expression and recombination. These minor activities of the viral messenger, which have been obscured in traditional genetic analyses, suggest the possibility that retroviral infections might lead to the altered expression of endogenous genetic information.

2. GLOBIN mRNA

Polysomes were prepared from duck reticulocytes. These were either microinjected directly into HeLa cells or else (a) dissociated with high salt and puromycin to yield messenger ribonucleoprotein (RNP) particles, or (b) phenol extracted and passed over poly(U) Sepharose to obtain naked messenger RNA. All three preparations promoted the accumulation of large amounts of globin antigen following microinjection into HeLa cells (as detected by a specific fluorescent antibody stain). In each case the amount of globin antigen continued to increase within the injected cells for at least 24 hrs (1).

In order to roughly quantitate the amount of antigen which had accumulated following these injections, varying concentrations of purified duck hemoglobin were microinjected and the cells stained with the globin-specific antisera. Fluorescence negatives of mRNA and hemoglobin-injected cells were each scanned with a microdensitometer and the results compared in order to determine the amount of globin within mRNA-injected cells (Fig. 1). When 1.4×10^4 globin mRNA molecules were injected approximately 2.6×10^7 globin molecules had accumulated within each cell after 16 hrs, indicating that each injected messenger was translated at least 120 times each hr (1).

(i) Stability of globin mRNA

In order to determine the functional half-line of the injected globin mRNA the rate of turnover of globin antigen within the HeLa cell was studied. Various concentrations of duck hemoglobin were injected and at varying times thereafter the injected cells were fixed and stained for globin antigen. Very little injected antigen had disappeared from the cell within 20 hrs following injection indicating that turnover of globin could be neglected in determining mRNA stability (Fig. 2) (1, 2). The fact that antigen continued to accumulate for at least 25 hrs following mRNA injection, therefore, indicates that globin mRNA functions actively for at least 25 hrs and is likely to have a half-life of over 10 hrs within HeLa cells.

(ii) Translational control

When duck globin mRNA or polysomes were injected into either duck embryo cells or primary culture chick liver cells little or no globin antigen accumulated. Microinjected hemoglobin was stable within these cells which were also shown to survive the microinjection process well (1). Therefore, the failure of duck embryo and chick liver cells to accumulate globin following mRNA injections was not due either to rapid degradation of the globin antigen produced or to adverse effects of microinjection. Consequently, the injected mRNA was either less stable within the duck and chick cells than within the HeLa cells, or else the first two cell types were able to suppress the translation of the exogenous message. In either case it is interesting that a human line performed translation of duck globin mRNA more efficiently than a duck or chicken cell. Apparently the translational control mechanism which functioned within the first two cell types was absent from the HeLa cells.

The results with injected reticulocyte polysomal material with-

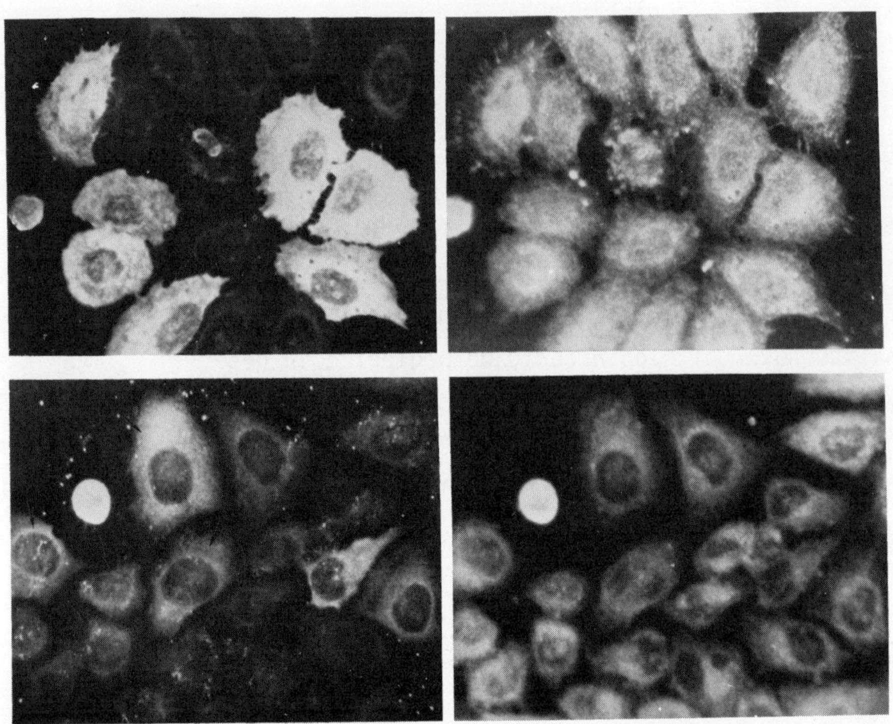

Fig. 1. *Correlation between hemoglobin content of HeLa cells and their uptake of specific fluorescent antibody.* Solutions containing 7.0 mg/ml (top) or 0.7 mg/ml (bottom) duck hemoglobin were microinjected into HeLa cells which were then fixed and stained with a specific, fluorescent antibody to duck globin. Fluorescene photographs (left) can be compared to duplicate dark-field photographs (right). From Ref. 19.

in HeLa cells emphasize the fact that injected mRNA in a variety of forms may be recognized by a recipient cell and subsequently translated with high efficiency. The results also demonstrate that the injected cells do survive. The approach used may be of great value for other studies. Since both the message and the product can be microinjected it is possible to relate the appearance of a translated product within the cell to its intracellular concentration. Then by determining turnover rate of the product, the intracellular translational efficiencies of injected mRNAs can be accurately determined. When these translation characteristics are then determined within

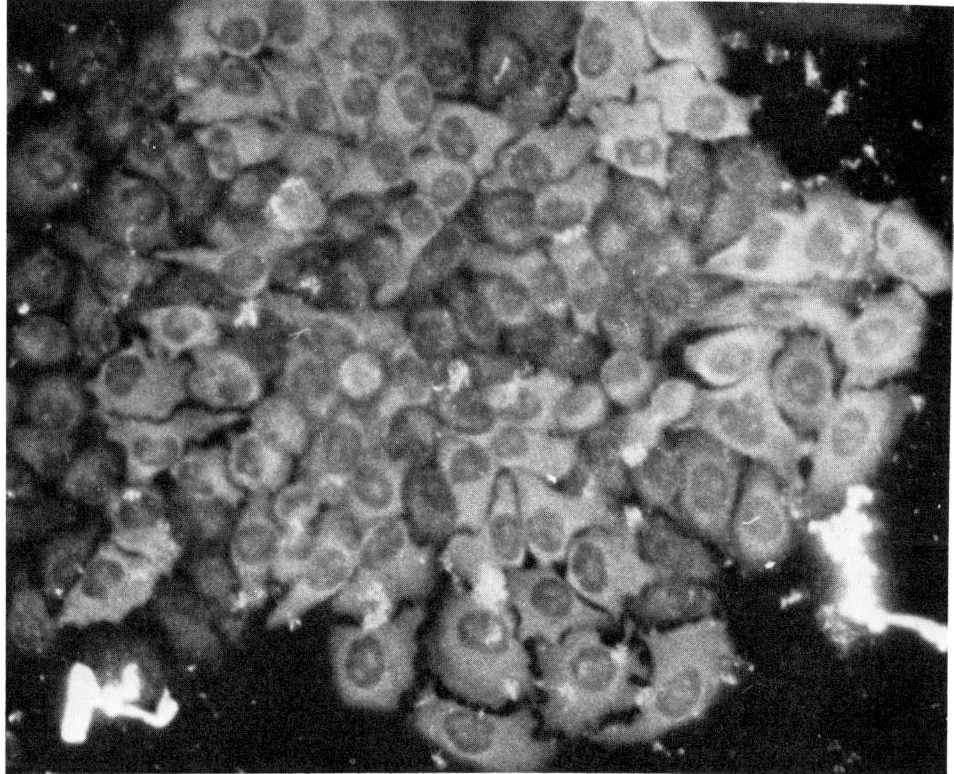

Fig. 2. *Stability of hemoglobin within HeLa cells.* A few cells within a small colony received an injection of duck hemoglobin (25 mg/ml) 3-$\frac{1}{2}$ days prior to fixation and staining with a globin-specific antibody. In this fluorescence photograph globin antigen is still apparent within the progeny of the originally injected cells. These progeny are arranged in wedge-shaped sectors of the colony which are separated by the progeny of uninjected cells. From Ref. 19.

different cell types under different conditions or in the presence of coinjected translation factors, definitive conclusions concerning the control of translation might become apparent.

3. T-ANTIGEN MESSAGE

The studies of Graessmann and coworkers have demonstrated that SV40 and polyoma large T-antigens are virus coded and are responsible for induction of DNA synthesis within virus-infected cells. Bacterial RNA polymerase is able to correctly copy the "early" DNA strand of both these viruses to yield cRNA analogous to viral early mRNA. When this cRNA preparation was microinjected into quiescent cells they accumulated T-antigen within their nuclei. Since the preparations had been rigorously tested to exclude the presence of any contaminating DNA, and since T-antigen accumulated in the presence of actinomycin D, this observation strongly supported the notion that T-antigen was virus coded and not a cellular function induced as the result of viral replication (3, 4).

Further analyses correlated the presence of T-antigen within a cell and induction of DNA synthesis. It was found that most cRNA-injected cells accumulated T-antigen and went on to incorporate thymidine. T-antigen was thus shown not only to be virus-coded, but also to be functional in the induction of cellular DNA synthesis (5).

These studies also provided an opportunity to analyze the effect of interferon upon viral RNA translation. Only 0.1% of interferon-treated cells accumulated T-antigen following injection of cRNA whereas 40% of the untreated cells did, indicating that interferon acted to block the translation of viral mRNA. In addition, when cRNA was coinjected with SV40 viral DNA the expression of viral capsid antigen (a late virus function) was observed in a much greater proportion of injected cells than when viral DNA was injected alone (6).

It is important to note, however, that cRNA is not the natural T-antigen messenger. It is not capped, spliced, associated with poly(A) or exclusively of the appropriate length. The fact that it functioned within the cell may indicate that the injected RNA was modified in some way by the cell. On the other hand, the characteristics required for mRNA function may be contained in the primary sequence of the RNA molecule such that modifications characteristic of messenger RNAs may not be required for translation in this system.

4. RETROVIRAL ENVELOPE GLYCOPROTEIN mRNA

The retroviral genome consists of two 30-40S "positive" strand RNA molecules each of which contains a 5' cap structure and 3' poly(A). Two such molecules associate together within the virus particle to form a 70S complex which is presumably the template for viral DNA synthesis. Within virus-infected cells an RNA species similar, if not identical, to the 35S virion molecule serves as messenger for the 5'-proximal *gag* (group-specific antigen) and *pol* (polymerase) genes (7, 8). In the Rous associated virus (RAV)-2-infected cell a second 21S viral-specific molecule is present. It contains the 3' third of the full-genomic molecule along with an identical 5' terminal sequence (9, 10). Since both the 35S and 21S cellular molecules contain the viral envelope glycoprotein (*env*) gene, experiments were performed to determine which molecule functioned as *env* messenger. For this determination cells infected by the envelope-deficient Bryan strain of Rous sarcoma virus [RSV(-) cells] were used.

Virus particles released by RSV(-) cells are not infectious due to their lack of envelope glycoprotein. When *env* mRNA was microinjected into these cells, however, the *env* deficiency was complemented and infectious virus were released (11). (These could be readily assayed by their ability to induce foci on chick fibroblasts.) It is important to point out that for complementation to occur the injected message had to be translated by a viable host cell and the envelope protein produced presumably had to be properly glycosylated and associated with the virus particle to be active. It is unlikely, under these circumstances, that an RNA molecule other than the natural *env* messenger would function well (as verified in part by the data to follow).

(i) Size of *env* mRNA

In order to determine the size of *env* mRNA, poly(A)-containing RNA from RAV-2-infected cells was fractionated on a sucrose gradient and size fractions were microinjected into RSV(-) cells. Only RNA in the 21S size region efficiently complemented the envelope deficiency of the injected cells and promoted the release of focus forming units (FFU), indicating that the 21S RNA species within infected cells functions as *env* mRNA. RNA in the 35S size fraction complemented RSV(-) cells very poorly indicating that the *env* gene near the 3' terminus of the full-genomic molecule was not translated (Fig. 4). In chf^+ cells (expressing endogenous *env* mRNA) which were infected by the polymerase deficient RSVα, however, 35S RNA from RAV-2-infected cells was found to complement the *pol* deficiency and, therefore, functioned as *pol* messenger. The 21S RNA did not complement RSVα cells (11).

These results stand as strong evidence against multiple initiation sites on eukaryotic mRNA. The *gag* and *pol* gene products are both translated from 35S RNA. Both of these appear as large proteins whose translation initiates near the 5' terminus of the 35S viral message (7, 8). There was no biological evidence that translation initiated internally within the molecule to yield envelope glycoprotein since the *env* gene product was only translated from a subgenomic messenger. This observation is made particularly significant since, as stated above, translation in these experiments took place under extremely rigorous conditions.

(ii) Stability and expression of *env* mRNA

The kinetics of infectious virus release following *env* mRNA injections indicated the stability of the message within the cell. There was a 3 hr lag in release of infectious virus immediately following injection (Fig. 3). This lag was not due to adverse effects of microinjection upon the cells (12). Apparently, 3 hrs was required for association of injected RNA with membrane-bound polysomes, synthesis and glycosylation of the envelope protein, migration of the glycoprotein to the membrane site of virus budding and association with the virus particle. After 3 hrs the rate of virus release increased sharply to a peak at 9 hrs, followed by a rapid decrease until at 24-36 hrs following injection a low rate of virus production existed. Virus production did not decrease to zero, however, and with time actually began to increase as will be discussed below (Fig. 3) (11). The decrease in the rate of virus production after 9 hrs indicates that the *env* mRNA must be relatively short lived. On two occasions, however, RNA preparations have been obtained which promoted the release of virus at a high rate for 24-36 hrs before a gradual decrease to near zero after 3 days (unpublished data; Fig. 4). This rare observation seemed not to be due to differences in the recipient cells and may indicate fundamental differences in the RNA molecules injected.

(iii) Fidelity of translation

Evidence that translation in this system took place with high fidelity came from the fact that the FFU released from injected RSV(-) cells expressed the same host range, interference and antibody neutralization characteristics as RAV-2 (which infected the cells from which the injected RNA was isolated) (11). In addition, the injected cell was shown to be highly selective in the type of RNA translated to produce viral envelope glycoprotein. 21S *env* mRNA appears to be the product of RNA splicing since it contains 5' and 3' termini identical to the 35S molecule (10). Fragments of the 35S molecule which contained the *env* gene but not the 5' spliced sequence were found to be totally inactive as *env* mRNA following injection into RSV(-) cells. This was the case whether the fragments were generated chemi-

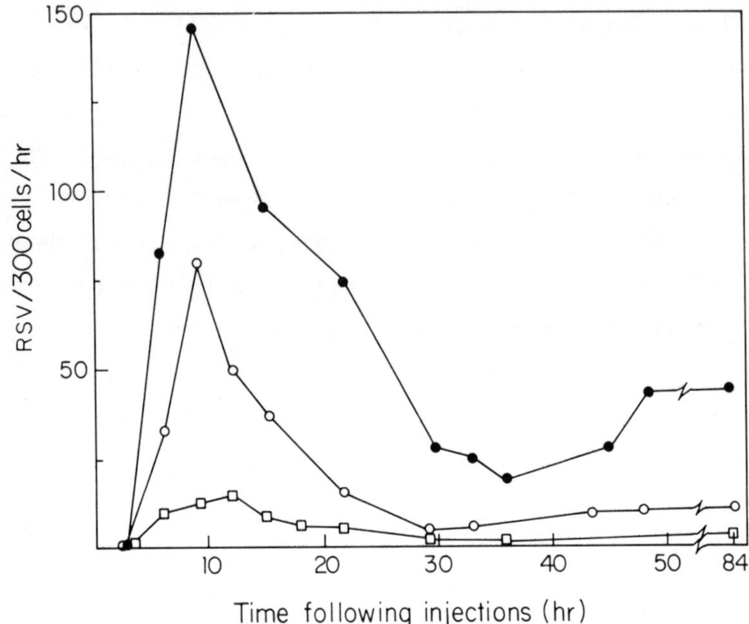

Fig. 3. *Time-course of virus release following injection of varying concentrations of env mRNA.* 21S poly(A)-containing RNA from RAV-2-infected cells in three concentrations (0.78, 0.30 and 0.08 mg/ml) were each injected into 300 RSV(-) cells. Transforming virus released a varying times thereafter were analyzed. Note the increase in virus released between 35 and 50 hrs. From Ref. 11.

cally or enzymatically. These same fragments were translated well, however, in a cell-free translation system to yield envelope protein (12, 13, 15).

(iv) Nuclear precursor to *env* mRNA

Since it is presumed that *env* mRNA is produced by nuclear RNA processing, nuclear injections were performed in order to identify the precursors. When 35S RNA from RAV-2 virus particles was injected cytoplasmically into RSV(-) cells no complementation occurred as

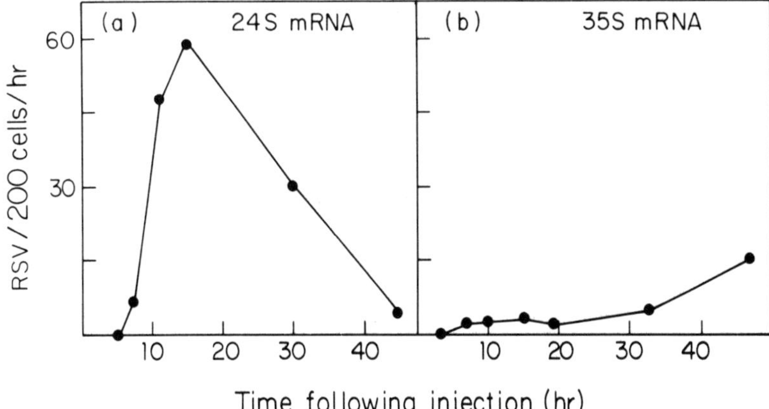

Fig. 4. *Unusual time-course of virus release.* (a) 21S mRNA from RAV-2-infected cells (0.7 mg/ml) was microinjected into RSV(-) cells. Transforming virus were actively released for over 30 hrs. This was an unusual result observed with individual mRNA preparations. (b) 35S RNA from RAV-2-virions (7.0 mg/ml) was microinjected into RSV(-) cells. Comparatively few virus were released within 30 hrs following injection.

expected on the basis of results obtained with the analogous 35S cellular species (Fig. 4). The *env* gene was not available for translation on the 35S molecule or any of its fragments generated by the cell. When 35S virion RNA was microinjected into the nuclei of RSV(-) cells, however, efficient complementation resulted in the release of numerous infectious virus. Apparently, the 35S virion molecule had served as nuclear precursor to *env* mRNA. As evidence that the nuclear conversion was efficient, the specific *env* mRNA activity of the 35S RNA preparation injected into the nucleus was greater than that of any cytoplasmically injected 21S mRNA preparation yet obtained from infected cells (13). (Cellular preparations would be expected to contain at most 10-15% viral-specific RNA).

From an analysis of the type of virus released following nuclear injection it appears that approximately one-half of the nuclear-injected virion RNA escaped from the nucleus without being processed to *env* mRNA. In addition, injected 35S virion RNA was efficiently encapsulated into virus particles so as to serve as virus genome upon subsequent infection (13).

(v) Virion RNA is sufficient for virus production

These results provide an interesting insight into the efficiency and simplicity of retroviral replication. The 35S viral RNA was shown to serve as messenger for viral polymerase and is known to be translated *in vitro* to form *gag* and *pol* proteins. This molecule is also encapsulated into virus particles to serve as genomic RNA. These facts are true of both virion and cellular 35S viral RNA suggesting that the two may be identical. In addition, it is clear from the above results that this same 35S virion molecule can also serve as the nuclear precursor to the messenger of the only other viral gene. Nuclear processing was only partial, however, making it possible that the nuclear precursor might have cytoplasmic functions of its own.

To determine if full-genomic viral RNA introduced into the nucleus was sufficient to promote virus release, 35S RNA from RAV-2 virus particles was microinjected into the nuclei of uninfected chick embryo cells (which were expressing no endogenous viral information). Within 9 hrs following injection (before any type of normal virus infection could have been responsible) fully infectious virus particles were released from injected cells. The release of virus from these uninfected cells was duplicated when both 35S virion RNA and 21S cellular *env* mRNA were coinjected into the cytoplasm of uninfected cells (13).

These experiments not only confirm the idea that 35S virion RNA within the nucleus is sufficient to enable a cell to release virus, they also serve to illustrate the value of microinjection in other viral systems. For example, when all the components required for release of any animal virus have been tentatively identified they can be combined and microinjected into the uninfected host cell. Subsequent release of virus particles (under circumstances precluding infection of injected cells) would confirm that no unidentified factors are required for virus production.

(vi) Characteristics of nuclear RNA processing

Basic information regarding the molecular biology of nuclear RNA processsing was also obtained from the nuclear injections described above. First, it is apparent that RNA processing does not exclusively involve nascent RNA molecules. In these experiments full-length, capped molecules with 3' poly(A) were substrates for RNA processing. Second, the kinetics of virus release revealed that nuclear processing must be rapid. When RAV-2 virion RNA was microinjected into the nuclei of RSV(-) cells, infectious virus were released with almost identical kinetics to that generally observed following cytoplasmic mRNA injections; with a 3 hr lag followed by a peak at 9 hrs and a subsequent decline. Since the time-course of virus release was indistinguishable whether *env* mRNA was injected into the cytoplams or its precursor was injected into the nucleus, the nuclear processing must have been very rapid in relation to the time required for expression of messenger formed (13). These experiments demonstrate, therefore, that nuclear processing occurs rapidly and can use preformed molecules as substrate. In addition, it is apparent that the technique of microinjection may be of great value in further studies of nuclear RNA processing.

(vii) Long-term *env* mRNA expression

The most unexpected observation made in the course of this work was the continued release of FFU even up to 12 days following injection of *env* mRNA into RSV(-) cells (11). The injected mRNA would not be expected to remain functional and promote virus release for more than 2 or 3 days at most. When injected cultures were treated to enhance growth of transformed cells (which were the recipients of injected RNA), the level of virus production actually increased after 6 days to a level four-fold greater than the peak in the rate of release observed at 9 hrs, and many-fold greater than the low level of virus production observed 2-3 days following injection (14). Careful observation revealed a distinct, although slight, increase in the level of virus production at 40-48 hrs (Fig. 3).

Extensive analysis proved that the release of virus several days after these injections could not be explained on the basis of any known genetics of the virus. These virus (which obviously contained envelope glycoprotein to render them infectious) did not express the *env* gene following infection of chick cells (except in an extreme case described below). If any virus containing the *env* gene had been present, the subsequently infected cells would have actively expressed the gene. The cells within the injected culture, therefore, expressed the *env* gene in the absence of its expression by any viral genome (manuscript in preparation). Perhaps the *env* genetic information had been converted within these cells to a stable form, presumably DNA, which could then be continuously transcribed and replicated.

(viii) Virus spread and long-term *env* expression

In an effort to understand the phenomenon of continued *env* mRNA expression several types of experiments were performed. First it was determined that virus spread within the injected culture was necessary for the long-term messenger expression. *Env* mRNA was injected into quail cells or chicken C/B cells transformed by *env* deficient Rous sarcoma virus. (Neither of these cell types were susceptible to infection by RAV-2 or FFU released by injected cells).

Following these injections the pattern of virus release was identical to the pattern described above except that after 50 hrs the injected quail or C/B cells stopped releasing FFU: they had failed to exhibit the long-term *env* expression. If the injected C/B cells were mixed with susceptible C/E cells following injection, on the other hand, long-term expression was again observed (manuscript in preparation). Apparently, the virus released by injected cells carried a factor which was responsible for long-term messenger expression within subsequently infected neighboring cells (15). Since the primary molecular process in a retroviral infection is the transcription of RNA into chromosomal DNA, it is not unreasonable to suppose that the factor responsible for long-term *env* expression was an RNA molecule which became transcribed into DNA and integrated into the host chromosome.

(ix) RNA promotes continued *env* expression

In order to demonstrate that the long-term virus production described above was not the result of viral-specific DNA injected as a contaminant of the *env* mRNA preparation, *env* mRNA was purified from DNA on a $CsSO_4$-DMSO gradient. Purified 21S *env* mRNA injected into RSV(-) cells promoted the release of FFU for up to 35 days. In one experiment the level of virus release was nearly 10^4-fold greater at 18-21 days than that observed 9 hrs following injection (manuscript in preparation). The release of FFU from these injected cultures ceased after transfer of the cells at 35 days post-injection, presumably due to the fact that chicken RSV(-) cells are short-lived in culture and that RAV-2 envelope glycoprotein has strong cytopathic effect upon RSV(-) cells.

(x) Tentative explanation for long-term *env* expression

On the basis of the above observations the following general model was proposed to explain long-term *env* expression following *env* mRNA injections into RSV(-) cells (15). (It is important to remember that the injected cells were producing non-infectious virus particles and contained all but the virus *env* gene prior to injection.) It is postulated that some of the *env* mRNA injected into the RSV(-) cells became encapsulated into infectious virus particles released by the injected cells. These *env* mRNA-containing virus then superinfected neighboring RSV(-) cells in such a way that the encapsualted *env* mRNA was transcribed into a DNA molecule independent of any other viral genes. This *env* DNA then behaved like a provirus by integrating into cellular DNA and serving constitutively as the template for mRNA synthesis. In this way the cell would express the *env* gene in a stable way. No full-genomic virion RNA within the cell would contain the *env* gene, however, so virus released by the cell would not express the envelope gene.

(xi) Virus encapsulation of *env* mRNA

Definitive proof for the above hypothesis has not been obtained. There are several observations, however, which support the hypothesis. First, it was proposed that the *env* mRNA had been encapsulated into the virus particle. It was, therefore, important to determine directly that *env* mRNA could be encapsulated into virus particles. When RAV-2 virion RNA is displayed on a sucrose gradient a major peak is observed at 35S followed by a gradual tailing resulting mainly from RNA degradation within the virion. When size fractions across such a gradient were injected into RSV(-) cells a sharp peak in *env* mRNA activity was observed at 21S (15). In addition, recent studies with agarose gels have revealed a poly(A)-containing RNA species in RAV-2 virion RNA with a sedimentation value close to 21S. This species may be the *env* mRNA responsible for the activity described. It comprises only a few percent of the total virion RNA (unpublished data). Evidence for *env* mRNA within the virus particle has also been obtained from hybridization experiments with specific cDNA probes (W.S. Hayward, personal communication).

In undenatured RAV-2 virion RNA 90% of the *env* mRNA activity sedimented with the virion 70S complex (15). The 70S complex is believed to be the template for RNA-dependent DNA synthesis. The mRNA contains 5' and 3' termini identical to the 35S genomic RNA molecule. These termini are directly involved in viral DNA synthesis (17). If *env* mRNA were intimately associated with the 70S complex, therefore, it might become involved in DNA synthesis leading to a DNA copy with termini identical to a normal provirus but containing only the *env* gene (as proposed in the above model).

In order to determine the type of association between the viral 70S complex and *env* mRNA, denaturation and careful sizing studies were performed. The dissociation temperature of *env* mRNA from the 70S complex was indistinguishable from the dissociation temperature of the complex itself, indicating that the association between the two was intimate and that the bond holding *env* mRNA within the 70S complex was similar to that which stabilized the complex itself. In addition, it was found that virion RNA complexes which contained *env* mRNA sedimented slightly more rapidly than the average suggesting that *env* mRNA might be added to an otherwise normal virion complex. The latter observation further indicates that the active messenger within the virus particle is actually *env* mRNA from the cell rather than a breakdown product of 35S virion RNA which, unlike *in vitro*-generated fragments, was active as *env* mRNA following injection (15).

(xii) Evidence for viral expression of *env* messenger

Since it appears from direct analysis that *env* mRNA is packaged into virus particles positioned appropriately for its involvement in

DNA synthesis, it was important next to obtain evidence that the packaged messenger could be genetically expressed upon virus infection. Such a demonstration could be performed if a virus stock were available which contained the *env* gene only in the form of the 21S messenger. Long-term expression of the *env* gene by cells infected with this virus stock would indicate that the messenger had been converted into chromosomal DNA as proposed.

The virus released after many days following *env* mRNA injection into RSV(-) cells appear to constitute the desired virus stock. They are released by cells which obviously contain *env* mRNA since the virus are infectious; and it is assumed that this messenger would be encapsulated into the virus released. There is no biological evidence that the *env* gene is contained within any genomic viral RNA, however, because the gene is not readily expressed following infection. Furthermore, evidence that the *env* gene within injected cultures is contained only on 21S molecules comes from the purity of injected material. 21S, poly(A)-containing RNA was purified up to 5 times by velocity sedimentation and two times by affinity chromatography on oligo(dT)-cellulose. The highly purified material was able to induce long-term *env* expression as well as any RNA preparation studied. It is unlikely, therefore, that the *env* gene associated with an RNA molecule much larger than 21S is responsible for the continued *env* expression described, or even present within the cultures.

Consequentely, the virus released long after *env* mRNA injection into RSV(-) cells was carefully analyzed for any evidence that the *env* mRNA could be genetically expressed by infected cells. When up to several hundred such FFU infected chick embryo cells the resulting transformed culture almost never released infectious virus even after multiple transfers. When 1000-4000 of these FFU infected chick cells, however, about 50% of the infected cultures went on to release

FFU. Virus were released for over 8 days and no *env*-containing (helper) virus were detected (manuscript in preparation). The *env* gene had therefore been genetically expressed by the virus stock which apparently contained only 21S *env* mRNA (within RSV(-) virions). The cells infected by numerous FFU were analogous to the injected cultures described above since the cells themselves expressed the *env* gene but the virus they released did not. This is the result predicted by the model proposed. In addition, this result constitutes added evidence that the factor responsible for long-term *env* expression is carried by a virus particle and is consistent with the quail and C/B experiments described previously.

(xiii) Participation of *env* mRNA in recombination

Added support for the contention that the *env* gene is present only as 21S messenger within RSV(-) cultures long after *env* mRNA injection comes from the structure of recombinants which arise within these cultures. It was pointed out previously that helper virus, which contain the *env* gene, were not responsible for any of the results described above. This type of virus did spontaneously arise in long-term cultures, however, at which time the analysis was of necessity terminated.

Preliminary evidence concerning the origin of these spontaneously arising viruses was obtained using RNase T-1 oligonucleotide mapping. Eight isolates were independently obtained. These each had oligonucleotide patterns which were identical to one another but different from either RAV-2 or RSV(-). The patterns were consistent with the suggestion that these spontaneous helper viruses were produced by recombination between *env* mRNA and RSV(-) genomic RNA. Furthermore, the recombination event appeared to occur in each case within a limited region near the 3' terminus of the RSV(-) *pol* gene (D.W. Stacey and L.-H. Wang, unpublished data). The result is strong evidence that *env* genetic sequences within the culture are present only as a 21S mRNA species consistent with the previously stated hypothesis. Otherwise, recombinants would have been expected which contained parts of the RAV-2 genome other than those contained in *env* mRNA. Furthermore, recombination involving molecules other than 21S *env* mRNA would not be expected to occur in such a limited region of the RSV genome.

(xiv) Conclusions

In summary, microinjection studies have shown that *env* messenger has a sedimentation rate of 21S and that its nuclear precursor may be identical to virion 35S RNA. This 35S molecule within the nucleus appears to be sufficient to promote virus release. When 21S *env* mRNA is injected into RSV(-) cultures the cultures express *env* mRNA for many days. The nature of virus released along with the fact that virus spread was required for the long-term phenomenon are the basis for the hypothesis that continued *env* expression by injected cultures occurs when *env* mRNA injected into RSV(-) cells is packaged into virus particles. Upon infection of neighboring cells the encapsulated messenger is then transcribed into DNA which is integrated into the host chromosome. This model is supported by the fact that *env* mRNA was found to be encapsulated into virus particles in close association with the viral 70S complex. Furthermore, in virus stocks which apparently contain the *env* gene only as the 21S message, the *env* gene was genetically expressed at a low frequency following infection. Finally, the *env* mRNA appears to be able to participate in viral recombination.

5. A MODEL FOR VIRAL EXPRESSION OF HOST GENES

While direct proof that *env* mRNA is copied into a proviral like DNA has not been obtained, the evidence presented in favor of this possibility is sufficient to warrant consideration of its implications. If *env* mRNA is gentically expressed by a retrovirus it is possible that a variety of RNAs other than viral genomic, 30-40S RNA could be similarly expressed (15). The critical question then is whether and how a host sequence might be expressed by an infecting retrovirus.

While *env* mRNA is not a typical genomic molecule it is nevertheless a viral molecule. Association with critical viral sequences may, therefore, be essential for the viral expression of any RNA molecule. There is no certainty, of course, that even if a host RNA sequence became associated with viral sequences it would be genetically expressed by the virus. This possibility is definitely raised by the data referred to above. Furthermore, the capacity of an RNA molecule to be expressed by a retrovirus appears not to be a function of the internal viral genes since mutants in each of the viral genes, and virus containing large insertions of foreign RNA yield molecules which are readily expressed by the virus. If the correct viral sequences became linked to a host RNA molecule, therefore, the hybrid molecule might behave just as *env* mRNA is postulated to behave by being encapsulated into the virus particle, copied into DNA, integrated into the host chromosome and then serve continuously as a template for transcription (15).

There are at least three mechanisms by which a host RNA molecule might be joined to a viral sequence. First, there may be genetic alterations, mutation or recombination within a virus-infected cell creating a hybrid host-viral gene which would be transcribed into a hybrid RNA molecule. Second, since some retroviral mRNAs are formed by nuclear RNA processing, it is possible that host and viral molecules on occasion might be joined together during an aberrant nuclear splicing event. Such a mistake in processing of RNAs would presumably be extremely rare and normally of little consequence to the cell. If the cell, by virtue of its infection with a retrovirus, were able to convert such a hybrid molecule into DNA the consequences of its formation would be much more important.

A third mechanism for joining host and viral sequences within an RNA molecule involve the redundant nature of proviral DNA. The 3' and 5' terminal sequences of retroviral RNA are both contained at each terminus of the integrated provirus. If a solid line represents viral structural genes the virion 35S RNA would have the structure 5'——3', and the integrated provirus the structure 3'5' ——3'5' (16). Transcription apparently initiates and terminates at the junction between the 3' and 5' terminal sequences of the provirus. It has been proposed that transcription not only initiates at the left-most 3'5' terminal junction to yield viral 35S RNA, but that transcription might also initiate at the right terminal junction yielding an RNA with the 5' viral sequences attached to the adjoining host sequences (18). If two proviruses were by chance integrated closely together within a chromosome an arrangement such as the following would result:

[- - - - 3'5' —— 3'5' - - - - 3'5' —— 3'5' - - - -]

where the dashed lines indicate cellular sequences. If transcription were to initiate at the second 3'5' junction and proceed through the cellular sequences to terminate at the third 3'5' junction an RNA molecule with the following structure would result 5' - - - - 3'. This molecule would have termini identical to viral RNAs. These termini would enclose a host genetic sequence. By virtue of its two viral termini, the resulting molecule might be encapsulated into and expressed by the virus particle resulting in the continuous expression of the enclosed host sequences just as is postulated for *env* mRNA.

The consequences of viral expression of host sequences would be profound even in an extremely rare event. If, for example, the host sequences abnormally expressed coded for a mitogenic factor the cell might become neoplastically transformed. Such an occurrence would be extremely rare and would probably be observed only following a massive number of virus infections. It is interesting to note that induction of leukemia by retroviruses (which lack an oncogene) is an event which requires long latent periods and apparently many virus infections within the host.

A highly speculative model such as the one presented here to explain oncogenic transformation by leukosis viruses is a value primarily to suggest further studies. It is, therefore, important to find testable predictions made by the hypothesis. A cell neoplastically transformed due to the viral expression of host genes as described would presumably contain host genetic material expressed as though it were a viral gene, and probably physically associated with viral sequences. Many steps are required for a neoplastically initiated cell to produce a tumor, however, so even though the tumor might have originated as a cell containing a host-viral hybrid gene, the arrangement of this gene might be altered within the cells of the final tumor (due to selection against cells containing viral information during progression of the tumor). In order to demonstrate that a tumor resulted from virus "transduction" of host sequences it may not be possible, therefore, to look for gross evidence of retroviral infection. Instead, subtle observations such as duplication of host genetic sequences, association of these with non-host sequences, or the appearance of unexpected genetic material within the integration site of a retrovirus may be more telling. Unfortunately, it is not presently possible to predict which host genes might be involved in neoplastic transformation.

Whatever the role of retroviruses in neoplasia, it is apparent that the technique of microinjection coupled with viral genetics provides a powerful and unique tool for probing viral molecular biology. Of particular importance is the opportunity presented to study rare events obscured in traditional analyses. These studies along with those involving DNA tumor viruses and globin mRNA provide an idea of the potential of the technique of microinjection in future studies.

6. ACKNOWLEDGEMENTS

Thanks is expressed to H. Hanafusa for his review of this manuscript; and to Janet Hansen and Carola Martins for help in its preparation.

7. REFERENCES

1) STACEY, D.W. and ALLFREY, V.G. (1976). Microinjection studies of duck globin messenger RNA translation in human and avian cells. Cell, 9, 725.
2) STACEY , D.W. and ALLFREY, V.G. (1976). Evidence for the autophagy of microinjected proteins in HeLa cells. J. Cell Biol., 75, 807.
3) GRAESSMANN, A., GRAESSMANN, M. HOFFMANN, H., NIEBEL, J., BRANDNER, G. and MUELLER, N. (1976). Inhibition by interferon of SV40 tumor antigen formation in cells injected with SV40 cRNA transcribed *in vitro*. FEBS Lett., 39, 249.
4) GRAESSMANN, M., GRAESSMANN, A., NIEBEL, J., KOCH, H., FOGEL, M. and MUELLER, C. (1975). Experimental evidence that polyama-specific tumor antigen is a virus-coded protein. Nature, 258, 756.
5) GRAESSMANN, M. and GRAESSMANN, A. (1976). "Early" simian-virus-40-specific RNA contains information for tumor antigen formation and chromatin replication. Proc. Natl. Acad. Sci. U.S.A., 73, 366.
6) GRAESSMANN, A., GRAESSMANN, M. and MUELLER, C. (1976). Regulatory mechanism of simian virus 40 gene expression in permissive and nonpermissive cells. J. Virol., 17, 854.

7) VON DER HELM, K. and DUESBERG, P.H. (1975). Translation of Rous sarcoma virus RNA in a cell-free system from ascites Krebs II cells. Proc. Natl. Acad. Sci. U.S.A., 72, 614.

8) PATERSON, B.M., MARCIANI, D.J. and PAPAS, T.S. (1977). Cell-free synthesis of the precursor polypeptide for avian myeloblastosis virus DNA polymerase. Proc. Natl. Acad. Sci. U.S.A., 74, 4951.

9) HAYWARD, W.S. (1977). Size and genetic content of viral RNAs in avian oncornavirus-infected cells. J. Virol., 24, 47.

10) WEISS, S.R., VARMUS, H.E. and BISHOP, J.M. (1977). The size and genetic composition of virus-specific RNAs in the cytoplasm of cells producing avian sarcoma-leukosis viruses. Cell, 12, 983.

11) STACEY, D.W., ALLFREY, V.G. and HANAFUSA, H. (1977). Microinjection analysis of envelope-glycoprotein messenger activities of avian leukosis viral RNAs. Proc. Natl. Acad. Sci. U.S.A., 74, 1614.

12) STACEY, D.W. In press. Effect of microinjection upon cultured cells. In: Introduction of Macromolecules into Viable Mammalian Cells. (ed., R. Baserga).

13) STACEY, D.W. and HANAFUSA, H. (1978). Nuclear conversion of microinjected avian leukosis virion RNA into an envelope-glycoprotein messenger. Nature, 273, 779.

14) STACEY, D.W. and HANAFUSA, H. (1977). Microinjection analysis of the translational characteristics of avian oncornavirus RNAs. J. Cell Biol., 75, 400a.

15) STACEY, D.W. (1979). Messenger activity of virion RNA for avian leukosis viral envelope glycoprotein. J. Virol., 29, 949.

16) HSU, T.W., SABRAN, J.L., MARK, G.E., GUNTAKA, R.V. and TAYLOR, J.M. (1978). Analysis of unintegrated avian RNA tumor virus double-stranded DNA intermediates. J. Virol., 28, 810.

17) COLLET, M.S. and FARAS, A.J. (1976). Evidence for circularization of the avian oncornavirus genome during proviral DNA synthesis from studies of reverse transcription *in vitro*. Proc. Natl. Acad. Sci. U.S.A., 73, 1329.

18) COFFIN, J.M. (1979). Structure, replication, and recombination of retrovirus genomes: some unifying hypotheses. J. Gen. Virol. 42, 1.

19) STACEY, D.W. (1976). Microinjection studies in cultured cells: intracellular behavior of exogenous proteins and polyribosomal mRNA. Thesis: The Rockefeller University.

EXPRESSION OF RABBIT GLOBIN mRNA INJECTED INTO FUSED HeLa CELLS

G. Huez, C. Bruck, D. Portetelle* and
Y. Cleuter

Laboratoire de Chimie Biologique, Département de Biologie Moléculaire, Université Libre de Bruxelles, 67, rue des Chevaux, B-1640 Rhode St-Genèse et
**Chaire de Zootechnie, Faculté Agronomique de l'Etat, B-5800 Gembloux, Belgium*

1. INTRODUCTION

Introduction into a living cell of an isolated messenger RNA allows to answer many interesting questions concerning its translation as well as its stability (see article by Marbaix and Huez). So far the translation of a messenger RNA, upon its manual injection into somatic cells using glass capillaries, has been demonstrated by means of autoradiography (1) or immunofluorescence (2) of the recipient cells. As these detection methods present some limitations, it would be useful in some cases to use classical biochemical methods like gel electrophoresis (followed by autoradiography) to analyse the translation products of an injected mRNA. This implies that a relatively large amount of labelled proteins has to be extracted from the injected cells. This can, of course, be obtained by increasing the number of injected cells. The injection of a large number of cells (over one thousand) is, however, a tedious work. A better approach is to fuse the cells before injection as recently proposed by Graessmann *et al.* (3). By this way, giant cells are formed which can be injected very easily. The equivalent of one thousand of individual cells can indeed be injected in a matter of minutes.

In the present paper, we demonstrate that rabbit globin messenger RNA can be translated in such fused cells and furthermore, we show that the synthesis of globin can be detected using the classical technique of polyacrylamide gel electrophoresis.

2. MICROINJECTION OF GLOBIN mRNA INTO FUSED HeLa CELLS

Cells to be injected are grown on small fragments of glass slides (1 x 1 mm approx.). After fusion and injection, the pieces of glass carrying the cells are transferred into the wells of microtest plates. It is then possible to incubate the cells with a minimal amount of highly labelled medium. HeLa cells are fused in such a way that syncitia containing 25 to 50 nuclei are formed. In our hands, such cells have proven to stick more easily to the glass pieces we use for labelling purpose than the giant cells containing up to 500 nuclei as used by Graessmann *et al.* (3).

One can see on Fig. 1 that the injection of the fused HeLa cells with rabbit globin mRNA leads to the appearance of a labelled protein which migrates exactly at the position of the marker rabbit globin in gel electrophoresis. In control cells injected with water one observes but a faint band corresponding to an unidentified material which migrates in this region of the gel.

In order to more strongly prove that the protein made upon injection of globin mRNA is really rabbit globin, we submitted the cell extracts to an immunoprecipitation with an antibody directed against highly purified rabbit globin. The quality of this antibody was tested by immunoprecipitation of an extract of oocytes injected

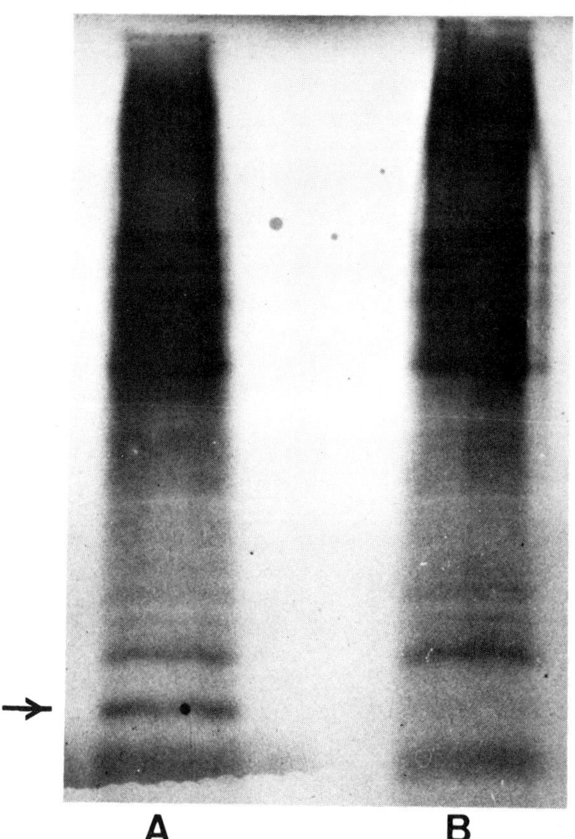

Fig. 1. *Fluorogram (after one week exposure) of SDS polyacrylamide gel electrophoresis of HeLa cells extracts (20% acrylamide gel).* Cell fusion was performed by a slight modification of the method described by Graessmann *et al.* (3) and our Ref. 4. Rabbit globin mRNA was prepared according to our method (5) and dissolved in water at a concentration of 1 mg/ml. Microinjections were performed using the technique of Graessmann *et al.* (1) under phase contrast microscope by means of glass microcapillaries. Only the cells sitting on the glass fragments were injected. 15-25 fused cells were injected with globin mRNA (lane A) or water (lane B). After injection, the small pieces of glass carrying the injected cells were transferred in a sterile way into the wells of a microtest plate (4). The slide fragments were then covered with 100 μl of histidine minus MEM medium. Labelled histidine (50 Ci/nmole) was added to 300 μCi/ml. The cells were incubated in such conditions for 8 hrs. Gel electrophoresis was performed according to Ref. 4.
The arrow shows the position of marker rabbit globin.

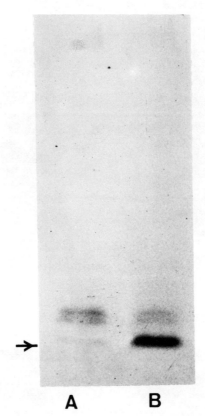

Fig. 2. *Fluorogram (after one week exposure) of SDS polyacrylamide gel electrophoresis of the immunoprecipitates obtained with anti-rabbit globin antibody from the same extracts of HeLa cells as in Fig. 1.* Lane A corresponds to cell injected with water. Lane B corresponds to cells injected with globin mRNA. The arrow shows the position of the globin marker. Immunoprecipitation and gel electrophoresis were performed according to Ref. 4.

with globin mRNA. In this case globin only is precipitated by the antibody (data not shown).

Fig. 2 gives the result of the immunoprecipitation of the extract of fused HeLa cells injected with either water or globin mRNA. In the latter extract one observed a strong radioactive band corresponding to globin which is not present into the control cells extract. One should note here that the faint background is due to some unspecific adsorption of proteins on the immunoprecipitate.

From the results presented here one can conclude that fused HeLa cells are perfectly able to translate rabbit globin mRNA. Moreover, using the labelling conditions described, the globin synthesized can be very easily detected by SDS gel electrophoresis followed by fluorography.

The present method is thus most suitable if one wants to study the translation on the stability of an isolated mRNA upon its introduction into a somatic cell.

3. ACKNOWLEDGEMENTS

We thank Professor A. Graessmann who helped one of us (G.H.) to learn his injection technique. We also thank Mr. R. Legas for excellent technical assistance. This work was made possible through the financial support of the "Fonds Cancérologique de la Caisse Générale d'Epargne et de Retraite" and the Belgian State Contract "Action Concertées". G.H. is Chercheur Qualifié, C.B. and D.P. are Aspirants of the "Fonds National de la Recherche Scientifique".

4. REFERENCES

1) GRAESSMANN, A. and GRAESSMANN, M. (1971). Über die Bildung von Melanin in Muskelzellen nach der Direkten Übertragung von RNA aus Harding-Passay-Melanomzellen. Hoppe-Seyler's. 2. Physiol. Chem., 352, 527.

2) STACEY, D.W. and ALLFREY, V.G. (1976). Microinjection studies of duck globin messenger RNA translation in human and avian cells. Cell, 9, 725.

3) GRAESSMANN, A, GRAESSMANN, M. and MUELLER, C (1979). Fused cells are suited for microinjection, Biochem. Biophys. Res. Commun., 88, 428.

4) HUEZ, G. BRUCK, C., PORTETELLE, D. and CLEUTER, Y. (1979). Translation of rabbit globin mRNA upon injection into fused HeLa cells. FEBS Lett., in press.

5) NOKIN, P., HUEZ, G. MARBAIX, G, BURNY, A. and CHANTRENNE, H. (1976). Molecular modifications associated with aging of globin mRNA *in vivo*. Eur. J. Biochem., 62, 509.

BIOLOGICAL ACTIVITY OF SIMIAN VIRUS 40 DNA FRAGMENTS AND T-ANTIGEN TESTED BY MICROINJECTION INTO TISSUE CULTURE CELLS

A. Graessmann, M. Graessmann and C. Mueller

Institut fuer Molekularbiologie und Biochemie
Freien Universitaet Berlin, Arnimallee 22
1 Berlin 33, West Germany

1. INTRODUCTION

The biological activity of macromolecules (DNA, RNA, protein) can be directly tested by microinjection into tissue culture cells (1, 2, 3). The transfer of the test material is performed with microglass capillaries under a phase contrast microscope at a 400 fold magnification. Technical details of the method have been described elsewhere (4, see also article by Celis, Kaltoft and Bravo). In this article, mapping of early Simian Virus 40 (SV40) specific functions and studies on the activity of purified SV40 T-antigen and T-antigen related proteins are used to demonstrate some aspects of the microinjection technique.

2. THE SV40 MODEL

SV40 is a small oncogenic DNA virus of the papova virus group. The virus transforms cells *in vitro* and induces tumor formation in animals (for review see 5). Since the oncogenic potency of SV40 is linked to the expression of the early viral genome-part, mapping of early SV40 specific functions is of certain interest. This genome region codes for two known proteins, the large T-antigen and the small t-antigen. The large T-antigen has a molecular weight of about 94 K Daltons and is encoded by two discontinuous DNA segments (map positions: 0.655-0.60; 0.533-0.172). The 17 K Dalton small t-antigen is coded for by DNA sequences between 0.655 and 0.53 (6, 7).

Biological studies revealed more than two early SV40 specific functions: (i) stimulation of cell DNA synthesis and T-antigenicity (8); (ii) helper function for adeno virus in monkey cells and U-antigenicity(5); (iii) induction of viral DNA replication (9); (iv) loss of actin cable structure (10); and (v) induction and maintenance of cell transformation (11, 12).

Our approach to further analyse these functions involves microinjection of SV40 DNA, DNA fragments, early SV40 RNA and purified T-antigens into different types of mammalian tissue culture cells.

(i) Stimulation of cell DNA synthesis and T-antigenicity

SV40 induces the synthesis of cellular DNA (8). The first experimental evidence that T-antigen is indeed a virus coded protein and that this protein induces cellular DNA synthesis was obtained by microinjection of early SV40 RNA. cRNA synthesized *in vitro* by *E. coli* DNA dependent RNA polymerase induced T-antigen formation after microinjection into monkey or mouse cells also when cellular RNA synthesis was blocked by actinomycin D. Furthermore, incorporation of [^{3}H]-thymidine was found in quiescent primary mouse kidney cells and TC7 cells after cRNA injection as in SV40 infected or SV40 DNA injected control cells. Similar results were obtained after inoculation of purified T-antigen molecules (2, 3, 13).

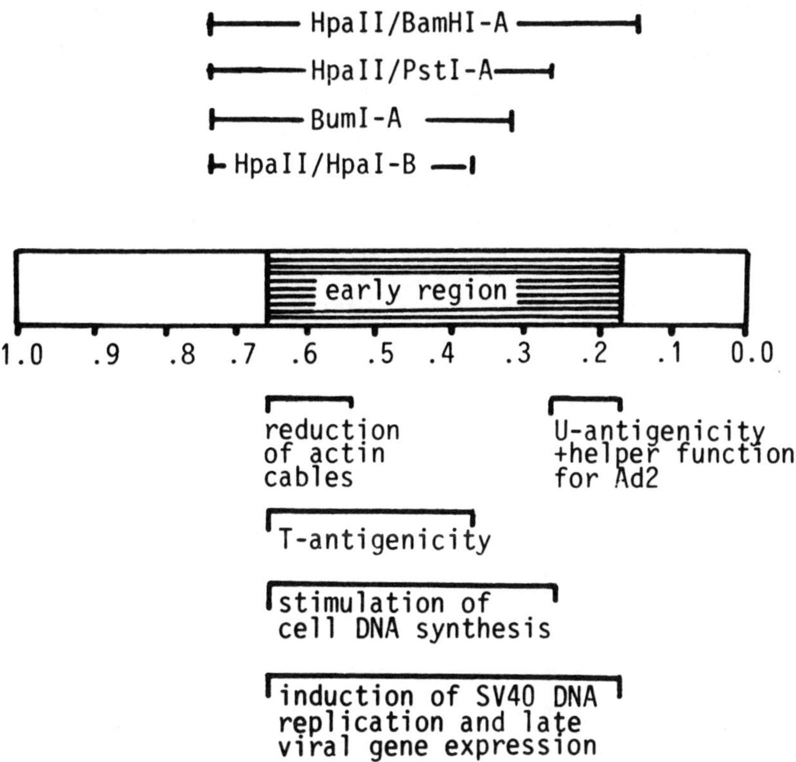

Fig. 1. *Assignment of SV40 DNA fragments and early viral functions to the physical map of the SV40 genome.*

In order to test which part of the early SV40 genome region is essential for this effect, SV40 DNA fragments of different sizes were microinjected into mouse kidney cells. The fragments used were obtained by digestion of SV40 DNA with restriction endonucleases (HpaI, HpaII, PstI, BamHI). The relevant cleavage sites of the restriction enzymes are shown in Fig. 1. The combination of immunofluorescence staining with autoradiography used in these studies, allows a direct correlation between T-antigen synthesis and DNA replication.

These experiments have proven that the information contained between map units 0.27-0.17 is not necessary to stimulate host cell DNA synthesis. Cells microinjected with the HpaII/Pst I A-DNA fragment (map position: 0.735-0.27) incorporated thymidine with the same efficiency as cells injected with full size SV40 DNA. DNA sequences between map position 0.655-0.375 are not sufficient to induce cell DNA synthesis. Cells microinjected with the HpaI/HpaII B fragment (0.735-0.375) stained positive for T-antigen but did not incorporate thymidine.

(ii) Helper function of SV40 for adeno virus in monkey cells and U-antigenicity

Monkey cells (e.g. TC7, CV1) are non-permissive for adeno virus (5). TC7 cells infected with adeno virus type 2 (50PFU/cell) synthesize hexon but not fiber protein (both are virus capsid proteins). Following coinfection with SV40 (10PFU/cell), fiber protein synthesis and virus maturation take place. This SV40 mediated effect is a large T-antigen function since microinjected purified large T-antigen (D2-protein, SV80-T-antigen) allows fiber formation and virus multiplication as SV40 virus (3). Experimental evidence that only the 50 C-terminal amino acids of the large T-antigen are involved in the helper function was obtained by microinjection of the SV40 DNA fragments and of the 23 K protein. The 23 K protein is a hybrid protein partly coded by the adeno fiber gene and partly by the SV40 A-gene (large T-antigen). The SV40 portion of this protein are 50 amino acids of the C-terminal part of large T-antigen. The adeno-helper activity is also mediated by the 23 K protein (3).

Intranuclear U-antigen synthesis is a further event associated with early SV40 gene expression (5). This antigenicity is part of the large T-antigen since anti U-serum immunoprecipitates purified T-antigen efficiently. SV40 DNA fragments lacking sequences downstream (map position 0.27) do not exert helper function for adeno virus (14).

These results implicate that U-antigenicity and helper function are closely related to the C-terminus of large T-antigen (Fig. 1).

(iii) Induction of SV40 DNA replication

SV40 DNA replication requires efficient synthesis of T-antigen in terms of quality and quantity (9, 15, 16). SV40 capsid protein synthesis (V-antigen) can be used as an indicator for viral DNA replication since expression of the late genome part occurs only after the onset of SV40 DNA replication (17). In our studies, complementation (V-antigen synthesis) of early temperature sensitive mutants (tsA) at the non-permissive temperature of 41.5^{0}C was used as a test system for viral DNA replication. So far, complementation of tsA7 or tsA58 virus with wild type early DNA fragments was only obtained with the HpaII/Bam HI A-fragment. This DNA fragment (0.735-0.16) contains the entire early coding region. The HpaII/Pst A-fragment which induced cell DNA synthesis failed to stimulate viral DNA replication (14). Induction of viral DNA replication depends not only on the quality but also on the quantity of T-antigen molecules synthesized per cell. The correlation between the amount of T-antigen molecules present per cell and the onset of viral DNA replication becomes obvious through double staining experiments using fluoresceine conjugated anti T-serum and rhodamine B conjugated anti V - serum (16).

The time course of intranuclear T-antigen accumulation in SV40 infected CV1 cells is shown in Fig. 2. In these experiments, intranuclear T-antigen concentration was measured in arbitrary units (AU) with a microscope fluorescence photometer. In order to test whether the onset of intranuclear V-antigen accumulation can be correlated to a threshold amount of T-antigen, T-antigen concentration in randomly chosen V-antigen positive cells was measured at different hrs

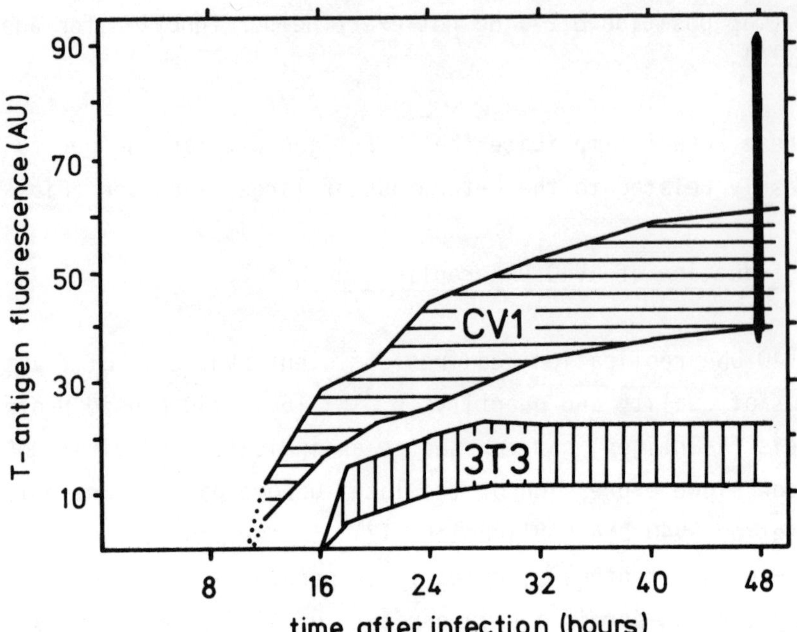

Fig. 2. *Time course of SV40 T-antigen accumulation.* Intranuclear T-antigen concentration was measured with a Zeiss fluorescence photometer 01 equipped with an operation and control unit, an electrically operated shutter, a light modulator and a digital printer XP2. Identical stained SV80 cells served as biological standard whose intranuclear T-antigen fluorescence was 13-27 AU. The black column at 48 hrs represent the T-antigen concentration in 3T3 cells microinjected with 2000-4000 SV40 DNA molecules.

after infection. Independent of the multiplicity of infection (100, 10, 1 PFU/cell), the minimal concentration of T-antigen in V-antigen positive cells was always 28 AU.

To learn how many T-antigen molecules are equivalent to 28 AU, purified T-antigen was microinjected at different concentrations into the nucleic of CV1 cells. Recipient cells were fixed and stained under similar conditions as for the above experiments. Using the direct immunofluorescence technique, the AU measured are linearly correlated to the amount of T-antigen molecules transferred per nucleus (Fig. 3). The threshold concentration of 28 AU is equivalent to 1-2 x 10^6 T-antigen molecules. This high amount of T-antigen molecules required for the onset of viral DNA replication implicates that its function is stoichiometric and not catalytic.

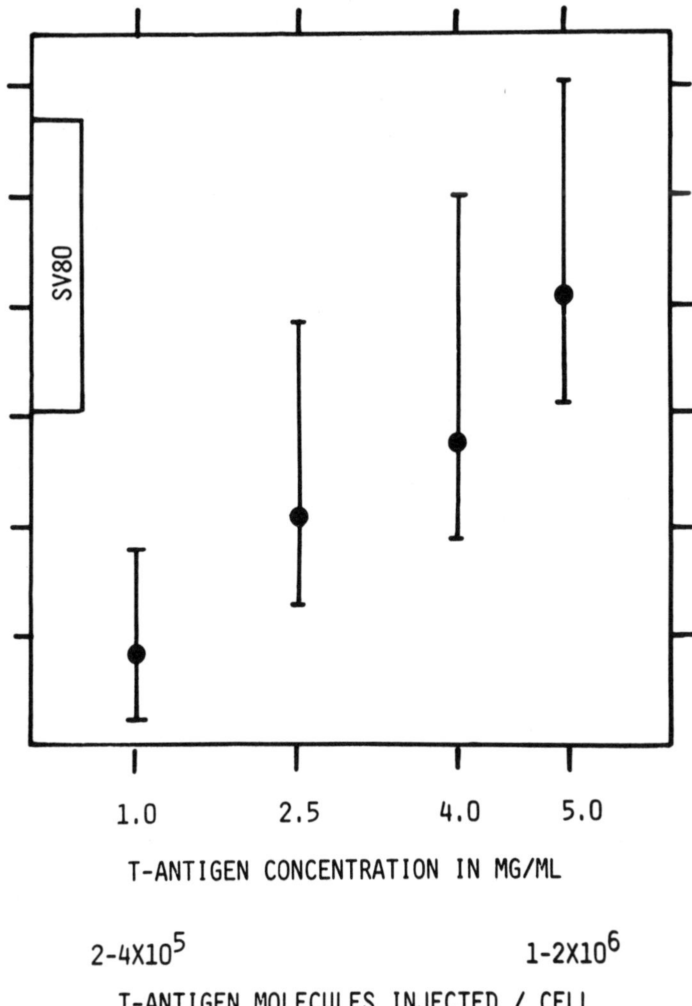

Fig. 3. *Correlation between AU and amount of T-antigen molecules.*

(iii) Late SV40 gene expression in non-permissive mouse cells

Mouse cells, infected by the conventional virus adsorption method are non-permissive for SV40. 3T3 cells (a permanent mouse cell line) infected with 500 PFU/cell synthesize T-antigen but viral DNA replication or capsid protein synthesis can not be demonstrated (5, 7). The T-antigen concentration of the infected 3T3 cells is always

Table 1. *SV40 T- and V-antigen formation in 3T3 cells microinjected with SV40 nucleic acids.*

Concentration of material injected		No. of injected DNA molecules per cell	% of injected cells positive for	
SV40 cRNA (μg/ml)	SV40 DNA I (μg/ml)		T-antigen	V-antigen
0	1000	2000 - 4000	100	38
0	100	200 - 400	100	4
0	10	20 - 40	100	0
500	0	0	72	0
500	10	20 - 40	100	50

Cells were fixed and stained 48 hrs or 24 hrs (cRNA experiments) after injection.

lower than in the permissive monkey cells (Fig. 2). However, mouse cells become permissive following microinjection of a high number of SV40 DNA form I molecules. The correlation between multiplicity of DNA injection and the number of cells synthesizing V-antigen is summarized in Table 1. Table 2 shows the virus yield at different hours after SV40 DNA injection in CV1 and 3T3 cells.

Late SV40 gene expression is also demonstrable after microinjection of early SV40 RNA together with a small number of SV40 DNA molecules or into virus infected 3T3 cells. The SV40 DNA injected mouse cells (2000-4000 DNA molecules/cell) synthesized significantly

Table 2. *Production of SV40 in 3T3 and TC7 cells microinjected with 2000-4000 DNAI molecules.*

Hours post injection	3T3 cells			TC7
	Cell number injected	Total Plaques	Plaques/ injected cell	Plaques/ injected cell
24	300	0	0	0
48	300	0	0	2×10^2
72	100	5×10^4	5×10^2	2×10^3
96	100	5×10^5	1×10^3	N.D.

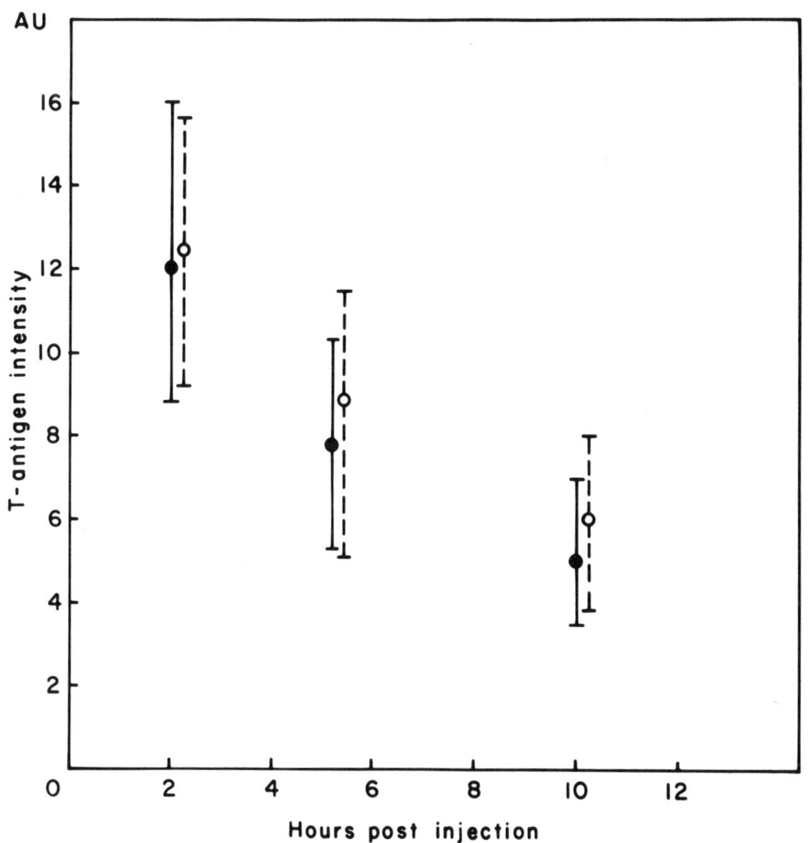

Fig. 4. *Turn over of T-antigen in CV1 and 3T3 cells microinjected with SV40 T-antigen. CV1 I----I; 3T3 I——I.*

higher amounts of T-antigen than cells infected by the conventional virus adsorption method (500 PFU/cell) (Fig. 2). The threshold concentration of T-antigen in V-antigen positive 3T3 cells was found to be about 52 AU.

It remains to be determined why SV40 DNA (or virus) injected but not infected 3T3 cells gain the T-antigen concentration required for late viral gene expression. SV40 T-antigen injection experiments indicate that this is not a question of a higher T-antigen turnover rate in 3T3 cells as shown in Fig. 4.

(iv) Loss of cytoplasmic actin cable structure

The loss of cytoplasmic actin cable structure is a common feature of many transformed cells (18). In order to test which part of the early SV40 genome region is required for this change, SV40 DNA form I, HpaI/HpaII B-fragment and purified T-antigen were microinjected into rat cells (rat 1, 19). Reduction of actin cables was observed after microinjection of the HpaI/HpaII B-fragment. About 80% of the T-antigen positive cells become actin cable negative after microinjection. The same proportion of actin negative cells was obtained after microinjection of SV40 DNA form I. In contrast purified large T-antigen (D2-protein or SV80 T-antigen) did not reduce this structure above the background (19).

This observation indicates that small t-antigen causes the change of the cytoskeleton. However, the HpaI/HpaII B fragment contains not only the coding region for small t-antigen but also additional sequences for the large T-antigen (a 30 K polypeptide). Therefore, it may be that this 30 K protein, related to large T-antigen acts coordinately with the small t-antigen.

(v) Induction and maintenance of cell transformation

The ultimate goal of the fragment injection experiments is to provide some clue of the early SV40 specific functions involved in the process of cell transformation. Experiments with tsA virus transformed cell lines revealed that continuous synthesis of large T-antigen is required for the maintenance of the transformed state (11, 12).

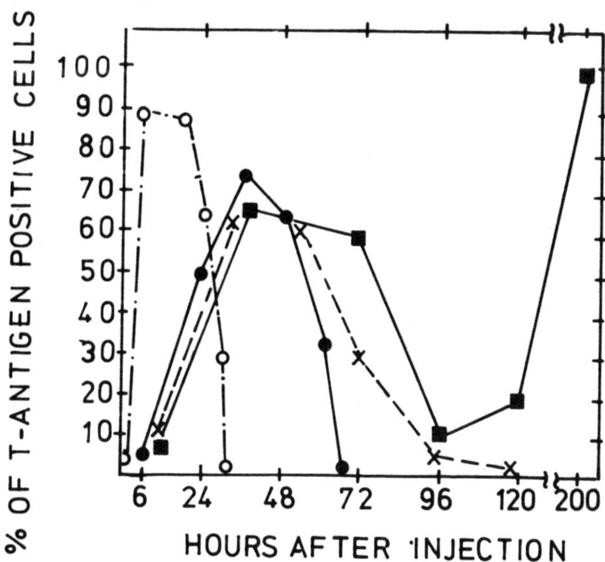

Fig. 5. *Time course of T-antigen synthesis in rat 1 cells microinjected with:*

● ——— ●	cRNA
O — · — · O	T-antigen
X ------- X	HpaII/Pst I A fragment
□ ——— □	HpaII/Bam HI A fragment

So far cell lines permanently positive for T-antigen were obtained only from permissive monkey cells and non-permissive rat 1 cells microinjected with DNA fragments containing the entire early information. These cells are maximally transformed (20). Cells microinjected with the HpaII/PstI A-fragment exhibited T-antigen synthesis only for 100-120 hrs after injection (Fig. 5).

This period of time is too short to test anchorage independent growth (in soft agar or methylcellulose) which is the most reliable *in vitro* test for tumorigenicity.

If the stabilisation of viral information (for example via enhanced integration of the viral DNA into the host DNA) transiently requires large T-antigen, permanently tumor antigen positive cell lines should be obtained by coinjection of the smaller early SV40 DNA fragments together with either early SV40 cRNA or purified large T-antigen.

3. ACKNOWLEDGEMENTS

We are grateful to Eva Guhl for skillful technical assistance. This work was supported by the Deutsche Forschungsgemeinschaft (Gr. 599/2, Gr. 384/7).

4. REFERENCES

1) GRAESSMANN, A. and GRAESSMANN, M. (1971). Ueber die Bildung von Melanin in Muskelzellen nach der direkten Uebertragung von RNA aus Harding-Passey-Melanomzellen. Hoppe-Seyler's Zeit. Physiol. Chem., 352, 527.

2) GRAESSMANN, M. and GRAESSMANN, A. (1976). Early simian virus 40 specific RNA contains information for tumor antigen formation and chromatin replication. Proc. Natl. Acad. Sci. USA., 73, 366.

3) TJIAN, R., FEY, G. and GRAESSMANN, A. (1978). Biological activity of purified simian virus 40 T-antigen proteins. Proc. Natl. Acad. Sci. U.S.A., 75, 1279.

4) GRAESSMANN, A., GRAESSMANN, M. and MUELLER, C. (1979). Microinjection of SV40 nucleic acids and SV40 T-antigen. Methods in Enzymology. (eds., L. Grossman, and K. Moldave). Academic Press, New York, Vol. 65. (in press).

5) TOOZE, J. (1973). The molecular biology of tumor viruses. Cold Spring Harbor Laboratory, Cold Spring Harbor, New York.

6) CRAWFORD, L.V., COLE, C.N., SMITH, A.E., TEGTMEYER, P., RUNDELL, K. and BERG, P. (1978). Organization and expression of early genes of simian virus 40. Proc. Natl. Acad. Sci. U.S.A., 75, 117.

7) PRIVES, C., GILBOA, E., REVEL, M. and WINOCCOUR, E. (1977). Cell-free translation of simian virus 40 early messenger RNA coding for viral T-antigen. Proc. Natl. Acad. Sci. U.S.A., 74, 457.

8) WEIL, R., SALOMON, C., MAY, E. and MAY, P. (1974). A simplifying concept in tumor virology: virus-specific "pleiotropic" effectors, Cold Spring Harbor Symp. Quant. Biol., 39, 381.

9) TEGTMEYER, P. (1972). Simian virus 40 deoxyribonucleic acid synthesis: the viral replicon. J. Virol., 10, 591.

10) RISSER, R. and POLLACK, R. (1974). A nonselective analysis of SV40 transformation of mouse 3T3 cells. Virology, 59, 477.

11) OSBORN, M. and WEBER, K. (1975). Simian virus 40 gene A function and maintenance of transformation. J. Virol., 15, 636.

12) TEGTMEYER, P. (1975). Function of simian virus 40 gene A in transforming infection. J. Virol., 8, 613

13) GRAESSMANN, A., GRAESSMANN, M., HOFFMANN, H:, NIEBEL, J., BRANDNER, G. and MUELLER, N. (1974). Inhibition by interferon of SV40 tumor antigen formation in cells injected with SV40 cRNA transcribed *in vitro*. FEBS Lett., 39, 249.

14) MUELLER, C., GRAESSMANN, A. and GRAESSMANN, M. (1978). Mapping of early SV40 specific functions by microinjection of different early viral DNA fragments. Cell, 15, 579.

15) GRAESSMANN, A., GRAESSMANN, M. and MUELLER, C. (1977). Regulatory function of simian virus 40 DNA replication for late viral gene expression. Proc. Natl. Acad. Sci. U.S.A., 74, 4831.

16) GRAESSMANN, A., GRAESSMANN, M., GUHL, E. and MUELLER, C. (1978). Quantitative correlation between simian virus 40 T-antigen synthesis and late viral gene expression in permissive and nonpermissive cells. J. Cell Biol., 77, R1.

17) GRAESSMANN, A., GRAESSMANN, M. and MUELLER, C. (1976). Regulatory mechanism of simian virus 40 gene expression in permissive and nonpermissive cells. J. Virol., 17, 854.

18) TOPP, W.C., RIFKIN, D., GRAESSMANN, A., CHANG, C.M. and SLEIGH, M.J. (1979). The role of early SV40 gene products in the maintenance of the transformed state. Hormons and Cell Culture. (eds., G. Sato and R. Ross). Cold Spring Harbor Laboratory, Cold Spring Harbor, New York. (in press).

19) GRAESSMANN, A., GRAESSMANN, M., TJIAN, R. and TOPP, W. (1979). Small SV40 t-antigen is necessary to induce the loss of actin cable structure. (Submitted for publication).

20) GRAESSMANN, M., GRAESSMANN, A. and MUELLER, C. (1979). SV40 DNA fragment transformed monkey cells and flat revertants synthesize large and small tumor antigens. Cold Spring Harbor Symp. Quant. Biol., 44 (in press).

ASPECTS OF CELL ARCHITECTURE AND LOCOMOTION

J.V. Small*, J.E. Celis# and G. Isenberg※

*Institute of Molecular Biology of the Austrian Academy of Sciences, 5020 Salzburg, Billrothstrasse 11, Austria; #Dept. of Chemistry, Aarhus University, 8000 Aarhus C, Denmark; ※Max-Planck-Institute for Psychiatrie, Munich, W. Germany

1. INTRODUCTION

Three morphologically and biochemically distinct filament types may be recognised in the cytoplasm of eukaryotic cells: actin filaments (or microfilaments), microtubules and 10nm filaments (Fig. 1) Although these filaments were recognised in many electron microscope studies of the last decade it is only relatively recently that their general and coextensive invasion of the cytosol has become apparent. From studies, primarily on cultured cells, by immunofluorescence microscopy and whole mount electron microscopy it has been shown that each filament type forms a characteristic and extensive network within the cell. Under specific conditions the membrane and soluble cellular components may be removed (for example with detergents) leaving the cell nucleus and the filament networks as the sole remaining components. Since the gross cell form is maintained in such preparations (Figs. 3 and 8), the filament systems together have been referred to as the "cytoskeleton", with the reservation, however, that the individual roles played by the filaments are not solely skeletal. In the present report we shall attempt to review briefly the current status of knowledge concerning the distributions and functions of the individual filament systems confining the survey in the main to cultured cells. Included in this discussion will be the possible mechanisms underlying cell locomotion and changes in the cytoskeleton associated with transformation. Finally, brief mention will also be made of the application of microinjection methods in probing the different functions of the components of the cytoskeleton.

2. COMPONENTS OF THE CYTOSKELETON

(i) Microtubules

As the first filament type to be recognised as an ubiquitous cell organelle the microtubule has received considerable attention (see reviews 1 and 2). Apart from being the primary components of the mitotic spindle microtubules occur in many other locations and have been attributed with both motile and shape determining functions.

→

Figures: unless otherwise stated the preparations depicted in the electron micrographs were obtained by Triton X-100 extraction and negative staining of cell monolayers according to (24).

Fig. 1. *Area intermediate between nucleus and cell edge in a mouse 3T3 cell showing the three filamentous components of the cytoplasm:* actin filaments occur in a stress fibre bundle on the left; elsewhere the 10nm filaments intermingle with the larger microtubules. Bar = 0.2 μ.

Fig. 2. *Mouse embryonal MO cell stained with antitubulin after the peroxidase-antiperoxidase method following the brief glytaraldehyde fixation procedure of De Mey et al. (9, 10).* Note the organisation of microtubules into well defined tracts expanding towards the actively spreading regions of the cell periphery. Micrograph kindly provided by Dr. J. De Mey.

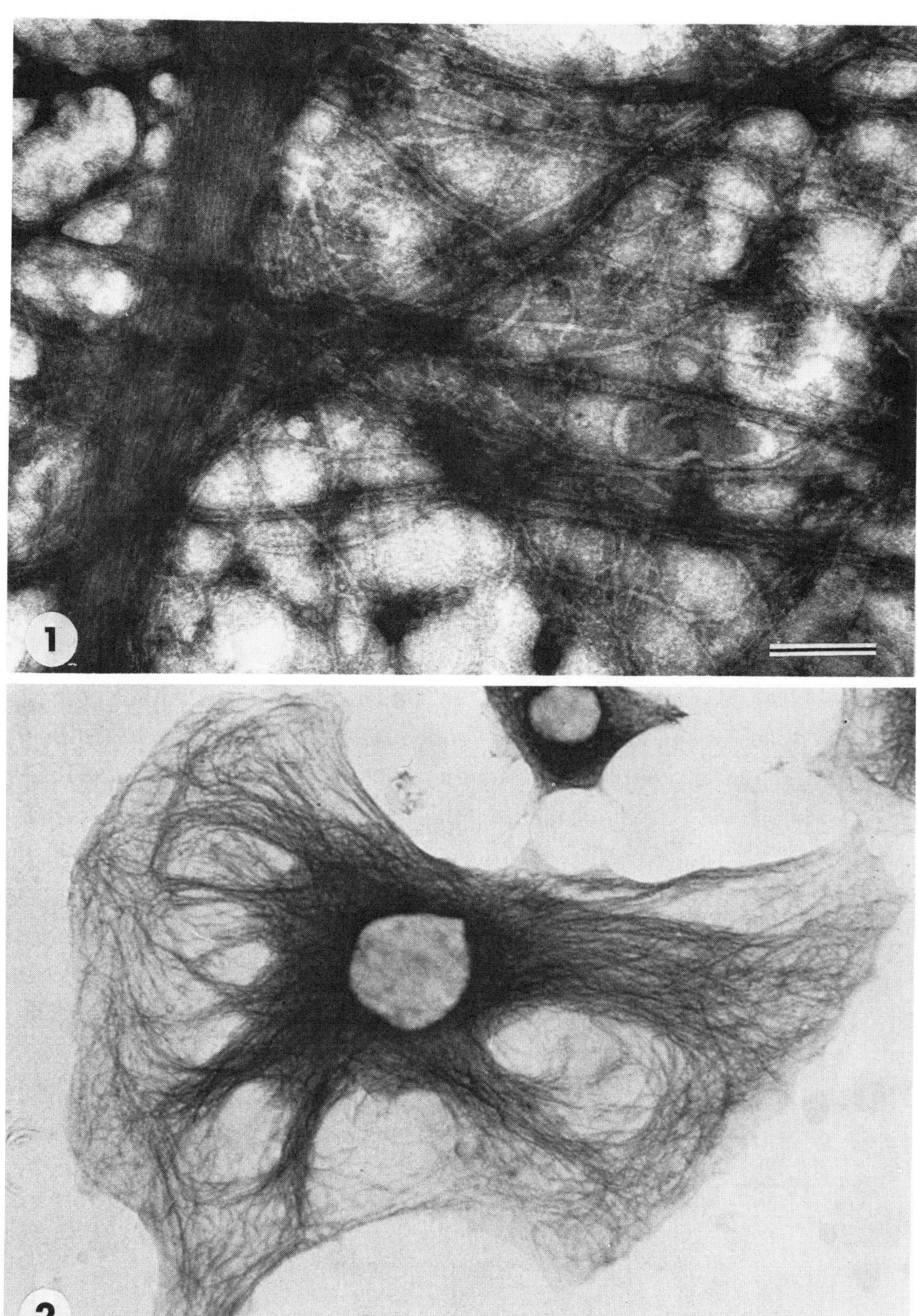
1
2

As components of cilia and flagella and other motile organelles of certain lower organisms, microtubules clearly function as elements of motility. In such situations they commonly show accessory "cross-bridge" structures which are taken as responsible for the production of the relative shearing movements between adjacent sets of microtubules. In the most well documented of these systems, the flagellum of the sea urchin sperm, the accessory structures have been shown to be composed of an ATPase, "dynein", which is different from muscle myosin but which, like the myosin head, probably undergoes a cyclic tilting process to produce movement (see 3). We may note that rather than being directly involved in the energy transduction process the microtubule here provides the flexible, structural framework of the motile organelle.

Numerous morphological studies have provided evidence for the involvement of microtubules also in the development and maintenance of cellular asymmetry. Evidence for this derives from the observation of the concomitant appearance of microtubule bundles with the development of an asymmetric form during differentiation, for example cell elongation (1, 2). Based on the effects of microtubule dissociating drugs, for example colchicine, a similar form determining function has been deduced for the microtubules of cultured cells. In this case, however, the effect of microtubules has been suggested as being indirect (4, 5). Following the dissociation of microtubules, cultured cells spread more or less equally in all directions, adopt an approximately circular profile and are incapable of net movement (4). On the reformation of microtubules in the absence of the drug the cells reacquire a specific polarity (4) and undergo net locomotion. Rather than being involved directly in the motile activity itself (see below) microtubules appear to act in determining the active (i.e. locomotory) and stable parts of the cytoplasm and in performing this function exert an indirect control on cell shape (4, 5).

Recent interest in the arrangement of microtubules in cultured cells has been stimulated by the availability of antibodies to tubulin, the protein subunit of microtubules (6-9). These studies have shown the presence in interphase cells of an extensive microtubule network concentrated around the cell nucleus and radiating in undulating strands towards the cell periphery. Unfortunately, the limitations set by the immunofluorescence method has in most cases precluded a detailed analysis of microtubule distribution. This has been primarily due to the poor preservation of microtubule organisation with the weak formaldehyde fixation required for subsequent antibody staining. To circumvent this problem De Brabander, De Mey and others (5, 9, 10) have utilised brief glutaraldehyde fixation under conditions for which the antibody reaction is still possible and the cell structures more faithfully preserved. A similar approach has been subsequently adopted by Weber and co-workers (11). Fig. 2 shows a mouse embryonal cell treated with antitubulin antibody and visualised after the peroxidase anti-peroxidase procedure according to De Mey *et al.* (1976). The microtubules can be seen to from large strands which radiate from the perinuclear region and extend towards the cell extensions. Other studies have shown that this network arises from the polar outgrowth of microtubules from one or two microtubule organising centres (2) situated in the centrosomal region (6, 8, 12).

Perhaps most interesting are the changes that occur when microtubules reform after drug treatment or when cells are newly seeded onto a substrate. Associated with the disruption of microtubules with the drug nocodazole (5) the mitochondria of mouse embryonal cells become concentrated around the cell nucleus. On removal of the drug radial microtubule bundles, or strands rapidly form and associated with their formation is an outward movement of mitochondria along the strands (De Mey, private communication). The same phenomenon has been detected in newly spreading endothelial cells (13) observed at different stages in whole mount preparations in the high voltage electron microscope (see also section 2(V)). Such movements which may be likened, for example to the radial transport of melanin granules along the microtubule tracts of pigment cells described earlier by Porter (1966) add further weight to the contention that microtubules serve an important function in the intracellular organisation of the cell organelles (see for example 5, 14). It is not unlikely that this fundamental function forms the basis of the effects that microtubules have on cell asymmetry, that we have already described.

(ii) Actin

The involvement of actin, in some way, in diverse cellular motile phenomena outside muscle contraction is now well documented. The first indication of the presence of actin (or more precisely actomyosin) in vertebrate non-muscle cells came from studies of blood platelets (15) which contain relatively high amounts of contractile proteins. Later, the presence of actin in other vertebrate cells was suggested from the identification of thin, actin-like filaments or "microfilaments" in thin sections of cultured fibroblasts in the electron miscroscope (16). Subsequently, the same filaments, seen in various tissues could be identified as actin from their specific interaction with heavy meromyosin (17) as recognised from the formation of the characteristic "arrowhead" complexes described by Huxley (18) for muscle actin.

Fig. 3. *Central region of well spread 3T3 cell showing general view of cytoskeleton.* Actin filaments are organised into prominent stress fibre bundles or sheaths. A few tracts of microtubules can be seen to radiate from the perinuclear zone. The 10nm filaments are mainly located in the dense patchy region surrounding the cell nucleus (see also Figs. 6 and 7). Bar, 5 μ.

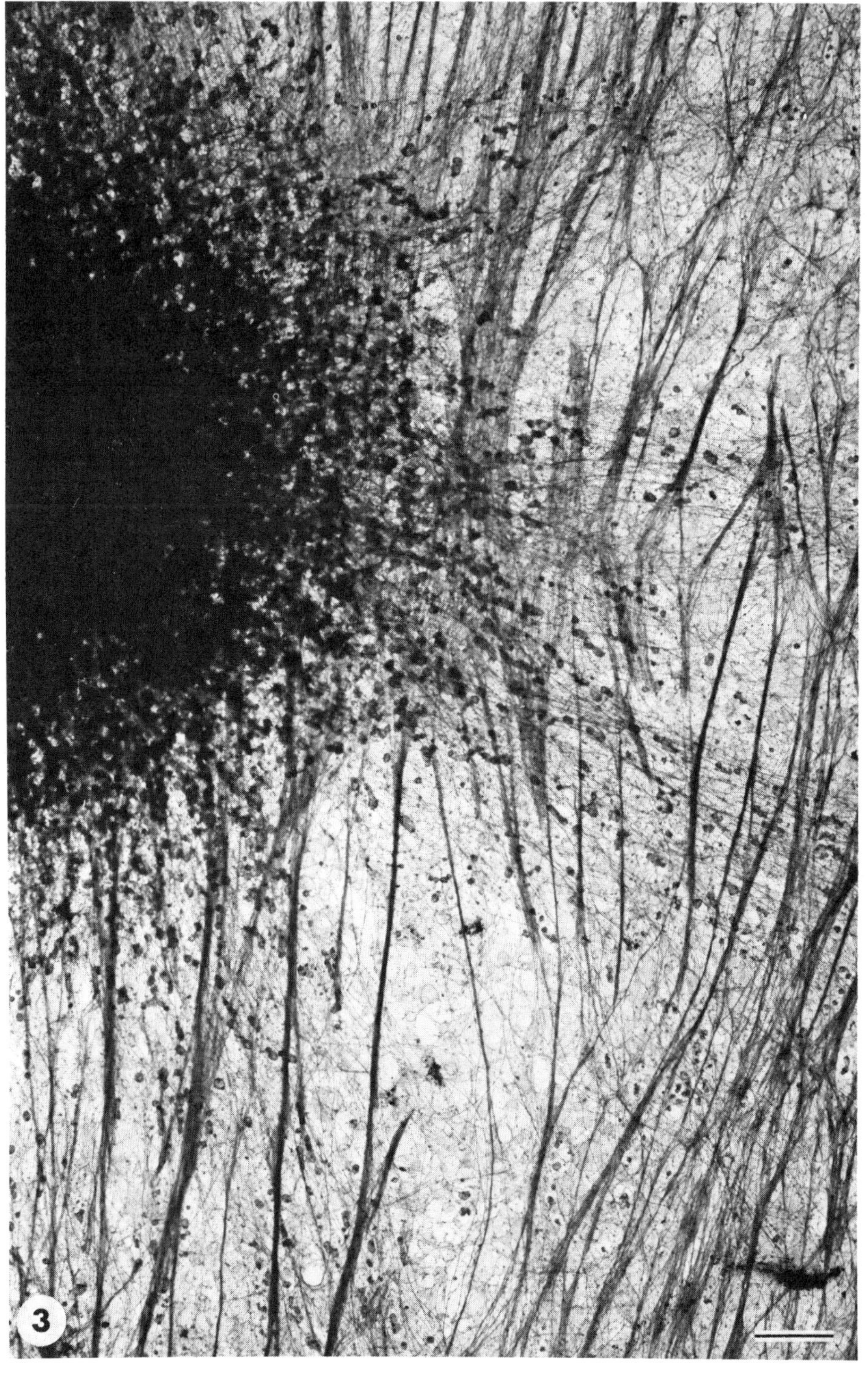
3

In cultured cells Buckley and Porter (1967) described two forms of thin filament organisation; linear bundles making up the so-called stress fibres visible in living cells in the light microscope and a submembranous filament mat or meshwork. Subsequently, Spooner, Wessels and Abercrombrie and their co-workers (19, 20) were able to relate the localisation of the meshwork filaments to the sites of cellular locomation and membrane ruffling. By the use of antibody methods (e.g., 21-23) and techniques to visualise the cytoskeletal components directly in the electron microscope (24) the different forms of actin are now more readily apparent (Figs. 1, 4, 8-11). Most striking, but not always typical, are the immunofluorescent images of well spread cultured cells showing the different patterns of organisation of the prominent stress fibres or sheaths of actin. Such bundles are composed of apparently continuous actin filaments (Fig. 4) and terminate at specific attachment sites on the cell membrane (see also below). A proportion of these sites has been shown to correspond to regions of temporary adhesion to the substrate (25-27); extracellularly, LETS protein appears to be involved at the adhesion site (28).

In addition to the stress fibres particular note should be made of the total delineation of the cell periphery by actin filaments. This delineation takes the form of concave actin bundles in those regions where the cell is free from the substrate (29) and actin meshworks in regions of active locomotion or membrane ruffling (Figs. 5, 8-10). In detergent-prepared cells the latter, leading edge regions (30) are particularly clear. These regions will be further dis-

Fig. 4. *Higher magnification view of a cytoplasmic region of a 3T3 cell such as depicted in Fig. 3.* Vertically running stress fibres composed of actin filaments are crossed by a diagonal tract of microtubules. A few randomly arranged 10nm filaments are also visible. Bar, 0.5 μ.

Fig. 5. *Concave edge of a well spread 3T3 cell showing delimiting bundle of actin filaments.* Bar, 1 μ.

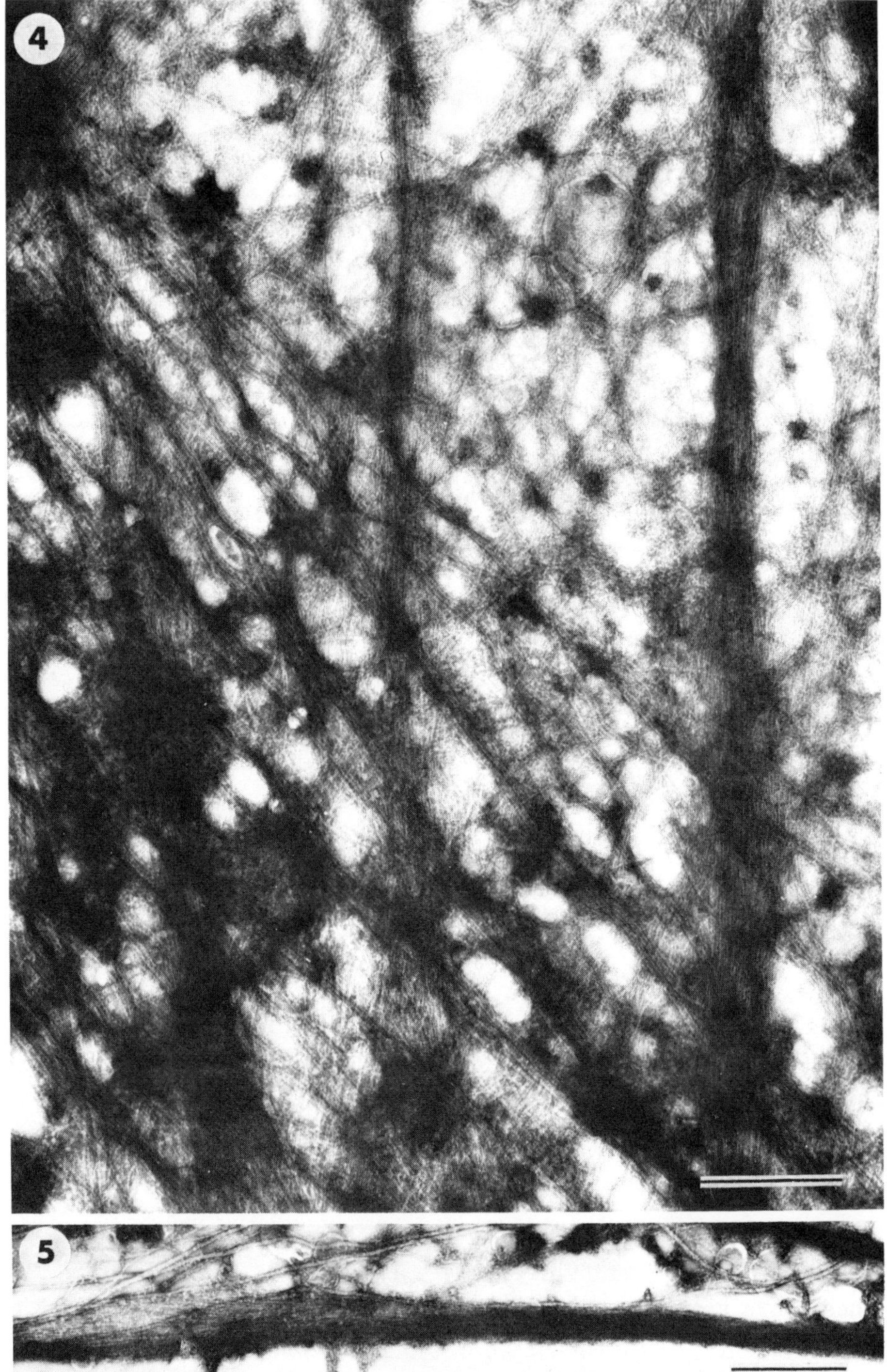
4
5

cussed in a later section when we consider the possible mechanisms underlying cell locomotion.

(iii) 10nm filaments

The last of the filament species to be recognised as a common component of vertebrate cells is the 10nm filament. Intermediate in diameter (about 10nm) between actin filaments and microtubules these filaments characteristically follow a meandering course and exhibit a smooth profile in thin sections or after negative staining (Fig. 7). On morphological grounds tonofilaments, neurofilaments and glial filaments, long recognised from early electron microscope studies (see for example 31) fall into the same filament class.

As components of other cells 10nm filaments were first observed in vertebrate smooth muscle (e.g. 31) where their orientation, approximately parallel to that of the myofilaments (see for example 32) facilitated their visualisation. Subsequently, the 10nm filament could be distinguished as a filament type distinct from actin filaments in various vertebrate cells (see review 33) including cells in culture (34). Of particular note in cultured cells was the accumulation of 10nm filaments into a juntanuclear cap (34) or prominent perinuclear bands (35) after treatment with microtubule disrupting agents such as colchicine or colcemid.

Using the more recently available antibodies against the filament protein the general organisation of the 10nm filament net has now been mapped in more detail in a variety of cultured cells (36-42). The filament network, although showing similarities to that described for microtubules does not in general extend as far towards the cell periphery. From the same studies some significant differences have been detected in the immunological cross reactivity of 10nm filaments in different cell types and more recently immunologically distinct 10nm filaments have been detected in the same cell (43).

The conclusion from these studies is that subclasses of 10nm filaments exist, although the exact number of these subclasses has yet to be settled. In discussing briefly these subclasses it is appropriate to begin from the standpoint of the noted differences between the filament proteins.

From electrophoretic analysis in the presence of sodium dodecyl sulphate neurofilaments and tonofilaments have been shown to exhibit very different polypeptide patterns as compared to other 10nm filament species: vertebrate neurofilaments show three bands with molecular weight values around 69,000, 150,000 and 200,000 (44) and tonofilaments from epidermal tissue four bands in the range 48-68,000 (45). On these grounds neurofilaments and tonofilaments (pre-keratin; see 45) can be considered as constituting two distinct subgroups. For the remaining 10nm filament types, found for example in muscle, glia, diverse fibroblasts and other cells of mesenchymal origin the biochemical differences seem to be rather slight. The filament proteins from these sources show the common property of resisting extraction in high salt and by non-ionic detergents, exhibit one or two polypeptides in the molecular weight range of 50-57,000 and on the data available show indistinguishable amino acid compositions (see 32, 46-48). Even though the immunological differences for example between the muscle-like and the fibroblast-like filaments are striking (42, 48, 49) it may be advisable to await further consolidation of the biochemical data before adopting further subdivisions of this class (40, 41, 45, 48).

As to the function of the 10nm filaments their primary role would appear to be a structural one. This has been indicated by experiments in which procedures have been employed to extract microtubules and actin leaving virtually the 10nm filaments as the sole filamentous components. Such experiments with isolated smooth muscle cells (32) and those of heart purkinje fibres (50), in which the filaments are abundant showed that the general cell form is still preserved by the remaining 10nm filament net. Similar experiments with cultured cells (Figs. 6 and 7) have indicated that the 10nm filaments perform an additional function in anchoring the nucleus within the cell (47, 51, 52). From the perinuclear accumulation of 10nm filaments that accompanies drug-induced microtubule disruption (see above) it may further be concluded that important interactions between these two filament types must, at least in cultured cells, play a role in the determination of cell form. The mutual and radial out-spreading of the two filament systems following drug removal may occur simply as a result of the mutual entanglement of the filaments or involve interfilament interactions via accessory proteins. An apparently close association of polyribosomes with the 10nm filament net also suggests that the 10nm filaments may provide a structural framework on which at least a proportion of the cell's protein synthesis takes place (37, 51). Clearly many areas remain to be explored.

The integrety of the 10nm filaments during the cell cycle appears to be rather stable, the filament monomer being undetectable in cultured cell extracts (39, 53). During cell division the filaments, organised in a perinuclear cage or ring, divide into two open baskets or horseshoe-shaped structures which follow and reform around the daughter nuclei (39, 54).

Figs. 6 and 7. *3T3 cell Triton cytoskeleton extracted further in solutions of high and low salt (51) and showing the remaining perinuclear 10nm filament net.* Bars, 10 and 0.2 μ, respectively.

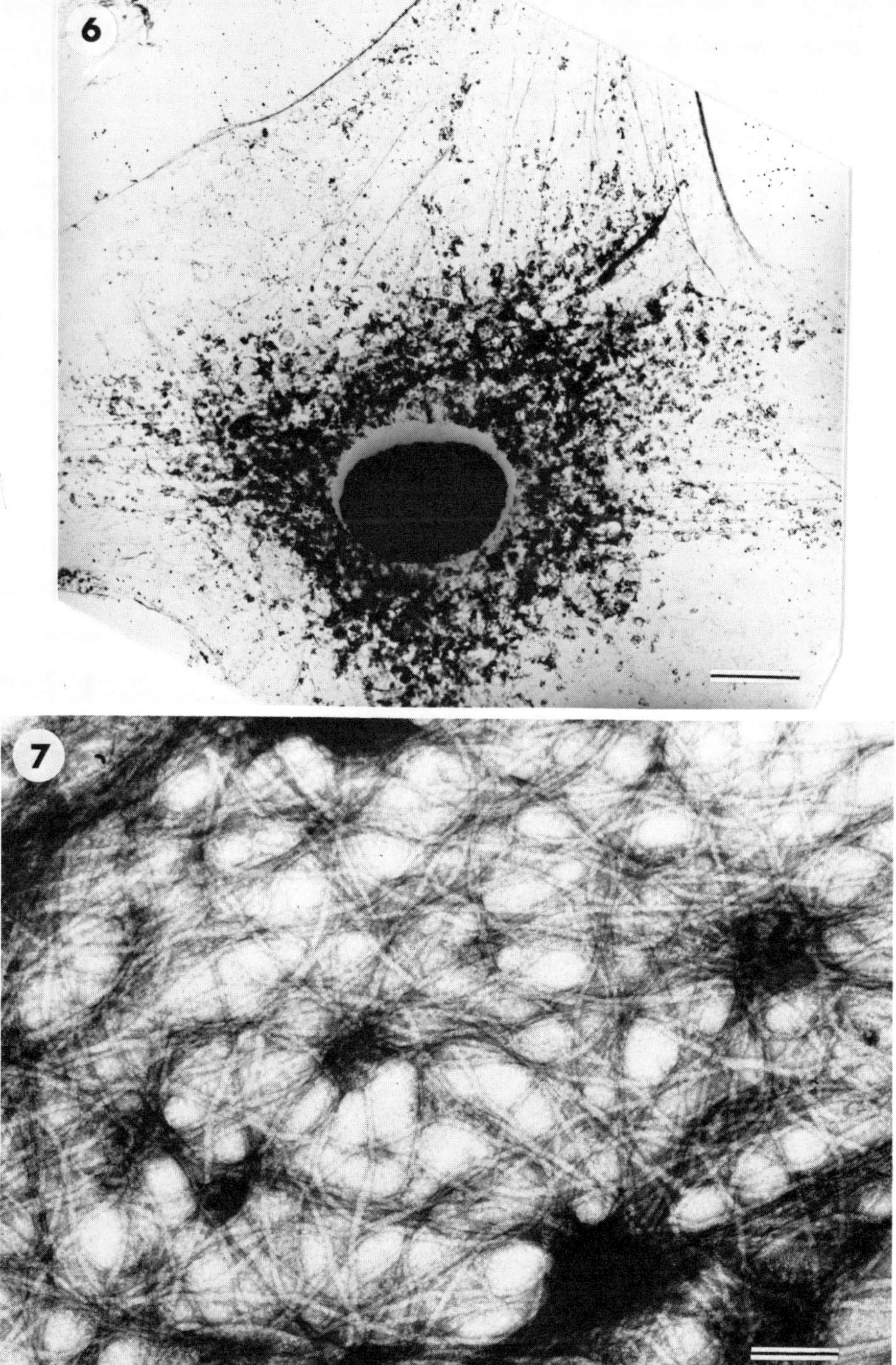
6
7

(iv) The accessory proteins

Together with the filamentous components described are additional proteins which have been localised on the filaments themselves by antibody methods or found to co-purify with the filament proteins. These proteins, which are currently receiving much attention probably play key roles *in vivo* in regulating filament assembly and organisation.

The so-called microtubule-associated proteins (MAPS:55) that have been characterised from preparations of brain tubulin fall into two main classes according to their molecular weight: the high molecular weight "HMW MAPS" (55, 56) of around 260-300,000 M.W. and the tau proteins (57) of 52-68,000 M.W. Separately, the τ proteins or the HMW MAPS are capable of initiating microtubule assembly (58) which occurs in both cases via the formation of tubulin "rings" (56, 57). As well as their apparent involvement in ring formation these proteins bind to and stabilise the microtubules against depolymerisation (59). Both stimulating factors (τ and MAP 2: - see 58) are heat stable and give either smooth microtubules in the case of τ and microtubules with side projections in the case of MAP 2 (58). While the existence of corresponding proteins in tissue other than brain has been questioned (60) apparently equivalent proteins have been isolated from microtubule preparations of various cultured cell lines (G. Wiche, private communication).

The search for components associated with actin in tissue culture cells has, for obvious reasons, invariably found its starting point in muscle tissue, notably vertebrate smooth muscle. From these studies, carried out mainly using antibody methods, the presence of all the protein components of the contractile apparatus of smooth muscle (see review 61) has now been established in various cultured, non-muscle cells. Without exception the different proteins, myosin, tropomyosin, filamin, α-actinin and a protein of around 130,000 M.W. have been localised on actin filaments. After formaldehyde fixation myosin, α-actinin and tropomyosin characteristically show a periodic distribution along the actin bundles or stress fibres found in well spread cells (62-64), the staining of myosin and tropomyosin alternating with that of α-actinin (64, 65). Although this has tempted comparison of the stress fibre with the sarcomere of vertebrate striated muscle (65) these filament bundles apparently play no direct role in cell locomotion (see also below). Alpha-actinin is also located close to the termini of the stress fibres where they approach the cell membrane (64) and more recent studies have established the presence of the 130,000 M.W. component even more closer to or at the membrane attachment site (66). In other studies the observed localisation of α-actinin suggests its involvement generally in the attachment of actin to the cell surface: it is found in the cleavage furrow of cells undergoing mitosis (67), at the tight junction and terminal web of intestinal epithelial cells (69, 71) and in association with secretory vesicles (71). The possible additional presence of the 130,000 M.W. protein in these locations awaits confirmation. Antibodies to filamin are apparently evenly distributed along the stress fibre bundles and diffusely arranged in other parts of the cytoplasm (72). Unfortunately, lesser attention has been given to the distribution of these actin binding proteins in the locomotory regions of cultured cells, in the leading lamella (Figs. 8 and section 3(i)). The data available does, however, indicate that filamin (72) α-actinin and the 130,000 M.W., protein are present at the leading edge (66) and, interestingly, that tropomyosin is absent (23). Whether or not myosin is present in this region has yet to be established. We shall return to this problem when discussing the possible mode of cell locomotion.

Although additional proteins have been found in preparations of the 10nm filaments obtained from cultured cells (46) their specific association with these filaments has not been established. Other studies have shown that polymerisation of the filament protein proceeds in the absence of any extra components (32, 73).

(v) The microtrabecular lattice

The pioneering studies of Porter and his co-workers has led in recent years to the development of techniques to visualise whole "unextracted" cultured cells in the high voltage electron microscope (74, 75). The preparative methods, involving chemical fixation and critical point drying have produced images which at relatively low magnification are very informative; the various organelles and filament systems are visible in their entirety and their interrelationships in space can be readily studied using stereo techniques. At the higher magnifications required to visualise smaller structures, however, the pictures are rather less easy to interpret, for example the distinction between single actin filaments and 10nm filaments is not readily apparent. Moreover, the protoplasm appears as an entangled net of fibres carrying ribosomes and encompassing organelles which at first glance would appear to be at least in part an artefact of the preparation. This network has, however, been taken as the likely form of the cytoplasmic ground substance *in vivo* and has been termed the microtrabecular lattice (74, 75). Taking an extreme view it may be claimed that this lattice is a product of the three filament networks in the cell which have been coagulated and covered during chemical fixation by components in the soluble phase. Such pessimism has prompted a recent and careful reappraisal of the techniques employed (76). These studies have indicated that the critical-point-dried preparations may be equivalent in their preservation to the normal embedded material viewed in ultrathin sections, the differences in appearance merely resulting from differences in electrom scattering of components of the lattice after plastic embedding. Whatever the final outcome the data serve to reemphasize the diffi-

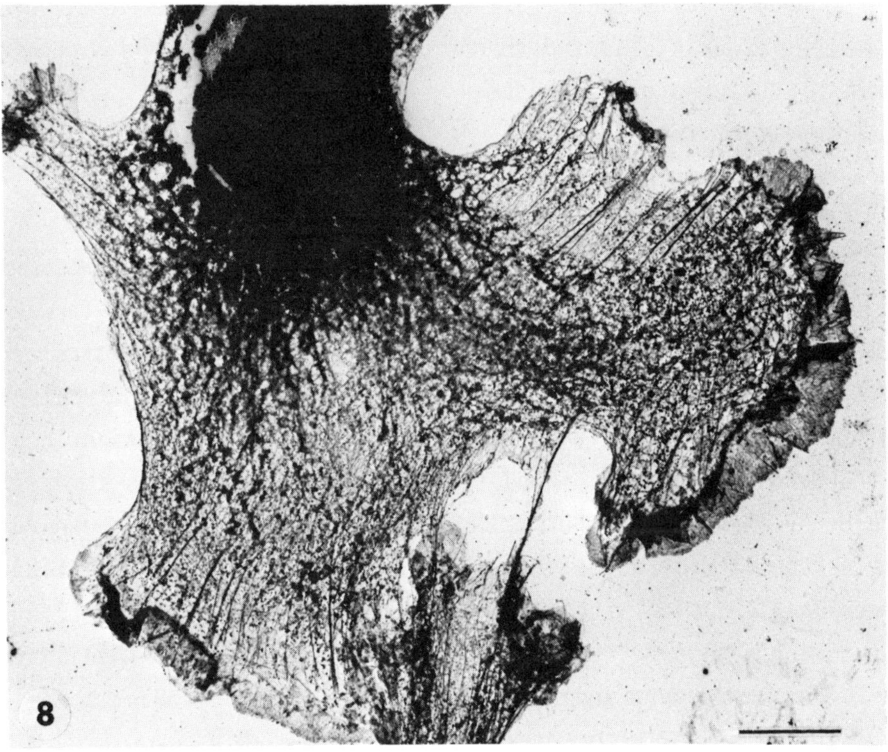

Fig. 8. *3T3 cell showing active locomotory activity and prominent leading lamellae.* Bar, 10 μ.

culties to preserve the cell protoplasm for microscopic analysis. We may only note that the delicate network of filaments seen at the leading edge after Triton extraction and negative staining (Figs. 9-11) is visible only as a disorganised lattice in the critical-point-dried preparations.

3. CELL LOCOMOTION AND CONTACT INHIBITION

(i) The leading lamellae

According, in 1970, to Abercrombie *et al.* (30) "the mechanism of locomotion of metazoan cells when they are crawling on a solid substrate can fairly be said to be wholly unknown". While today, almost a decade later the situation has little changed, some advances have been made in defining the structural details of the motile regions of cultured cells. In this section we shall briefly describe the results of these studies (24, 77, 78) and discuss their possible implications with regard to the mechanism of cell motility.

As a result of painstaking light microscope analysis Abercrombie and his co-workers defined the characteristics of the forward translocation of fibroblasts in culture (29, 30, 79). Particular attention was paid to the thin, advancing region of the cell referred to as the leading lamellae; such a region can be identified in Fig. 8. Forward movement was found to be discontinuous and to comprise phases of standstill, protrusion and withdrawal, "a slight and varying excess of protrusion over withdrawal accounting for the forward translocation" (30). The leading edge of the lamellae (the front 5 μ or so) could also be seen either to remain parallel to the substrate or to perform upward and backfolding movements to produce so-called "ruffles". The formation of ruffles was invariably associated with the phases of withdrawal of the leading lamellae.

Bearing these factors in mind we may turn to the detailed structure of the anterior edge of the leading lamellae. We have already noted the identification, in particular by Spooner *et al.* (19) of a meshwork of actin filaments in these regions. In cytoskeletons of cells prepared by Triton X-100 extraction of monolayer cultures grown on electron microscope grids (24) the organisation of the leading edge is more clear (Figs. 8-12). The leading edge is characterised by a broad band, up to a few microns wide, of thin actin filaments organised in an intricate diagonal meshwork. The filaments have been

⟶

Figs. 9 and 10. *Details of the leading edge of a hybrid C1 1D/CHO fibroblast (98).* The delicate meshwork shows diagonally arranged actin filaments, arranged singly or in bundles. Bars, 0.5 μ.

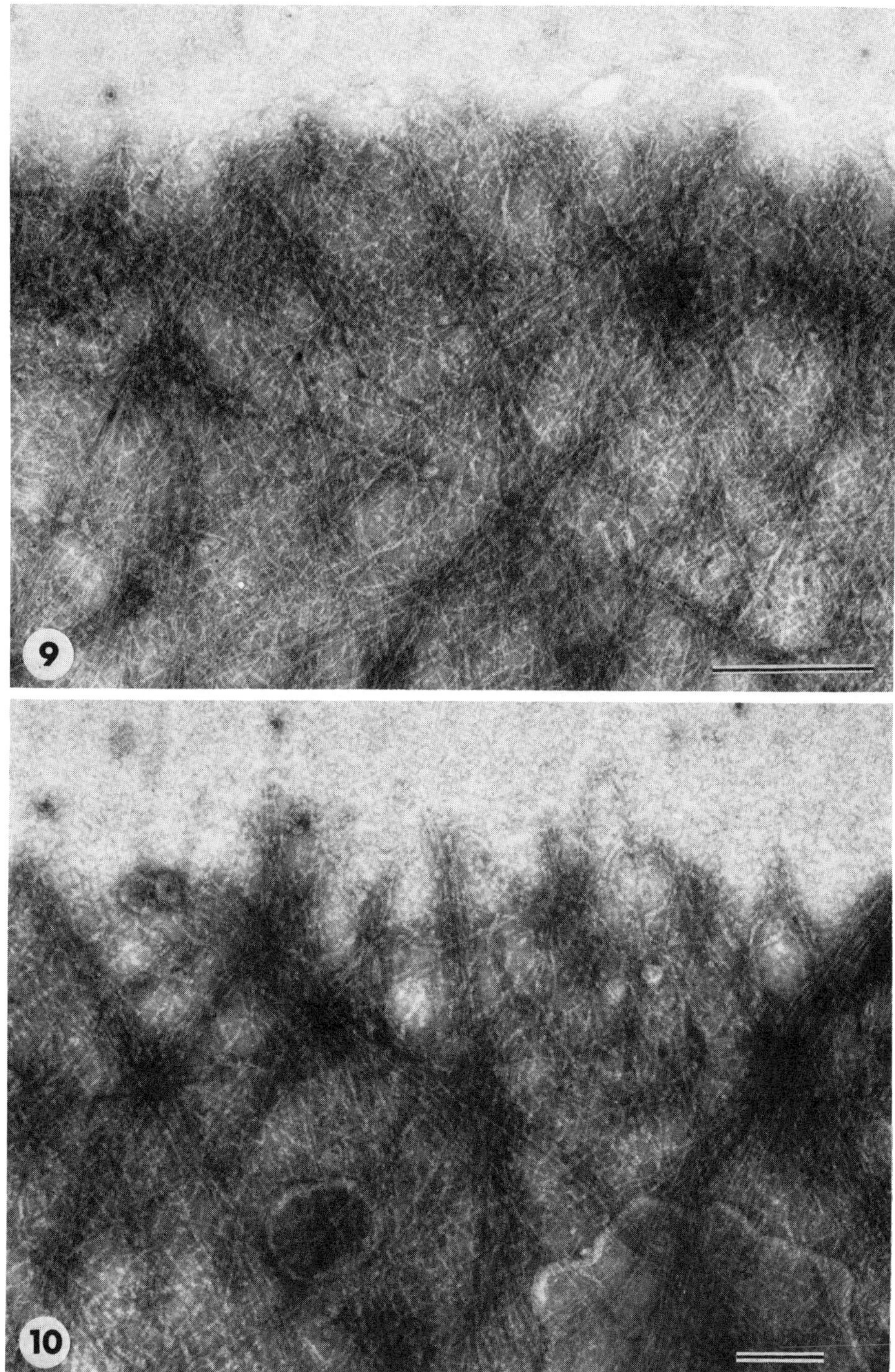
9
10

identified as actin from their decoration with myosin subfragment -1 (24) and staining with antibodies to actin (23). Embedded in this meshwork are also variable numbers of bundles of actin filaments which project to different extents from the anterior edge. As projecting structures these bundles are equivalent to the "microspikes" recognisable in the light microscope (see for example 4).

Of particular interest is the existence of clear transition stages between the diagonal meshwork and the filament bundles (Fig. 12). From the micrographs the bundles would appear to form by a collection of the ends of individual filaments or filament groups into foci at the anterior edge followed by an inwardly directed lateral aggregation. The presence of extra material at the foci as well as at the tips of the filament bundles (Fig. 12) would suggest that accessory proteins are involved in this transition. More recently the deduced temporal phases of this process have been confirmed in neuroblastoma cells treated with concanavalin A, under which conditions a gradual transition occurs between lamella showing only diagonal filaments to lamella containing numerous perpendicular bundles (78, 80). Bragina *et al.* (81) have also described the same process in cells undergoing spreading on the substrate.

This bundle formation is very closely analogous to the formation of filopodia in the lamella-shaped petaloids of the coelomocytes (or phagocytes) of echinoderms described earlier by Edds (82).

Fig. 11. *Leading edge region of a chick heart fibroblast showing filament bundles embedded in the diagonal meshwork.* Bar, 2 μ.

Fig. 12. *Stages in bundle formation.* a: Filaments of the diagonal meshwork begin to associate at foci at the cell periphery. b: bundles finally span the entire width of the meshwork (see also Fig. 11). c: extra material is seen to be associated at the tips of the microspikes. All from CHO/C11D cell hybrids (98). Bars, 0.3 μ.

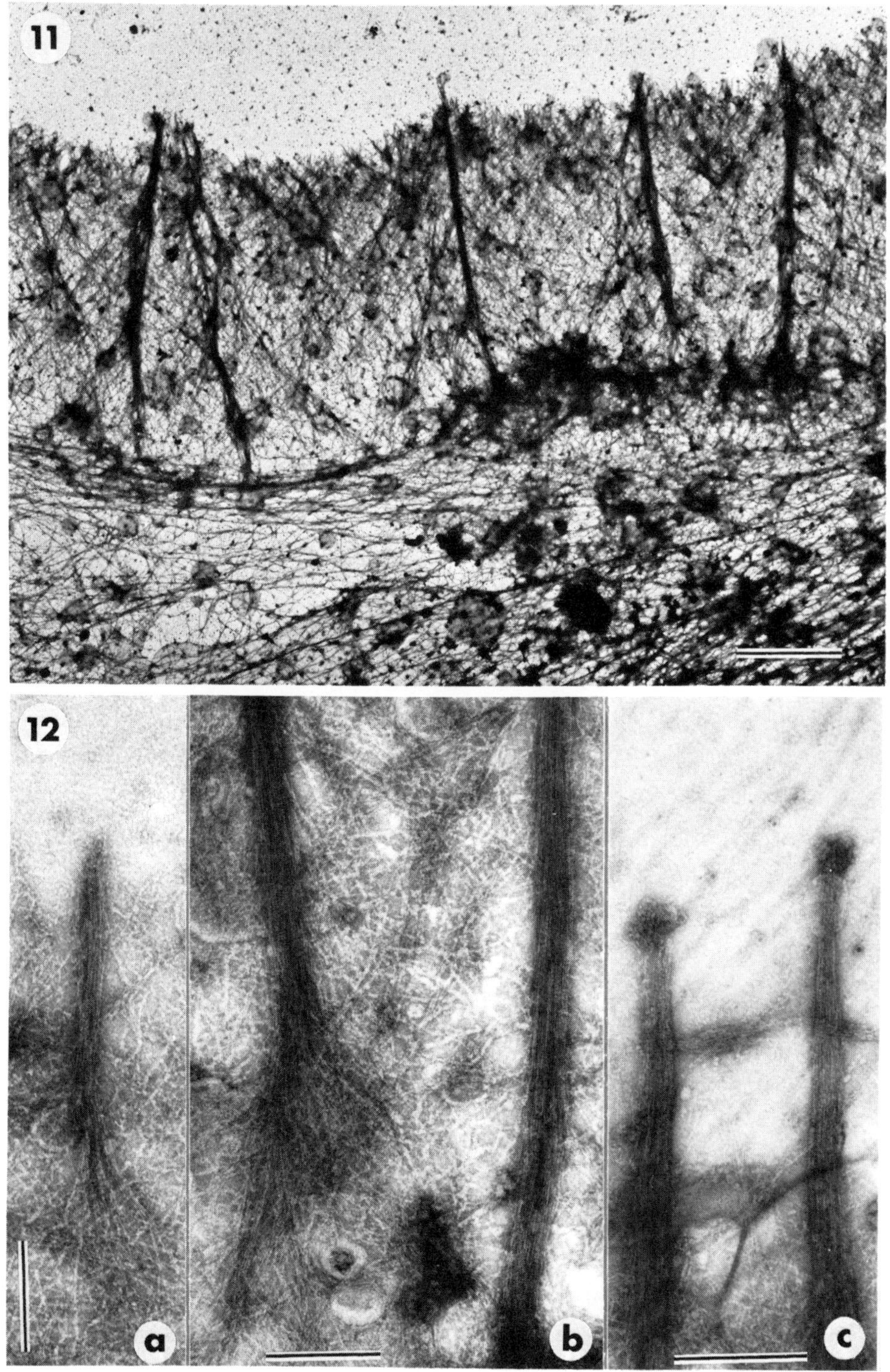
11
12
a
b
c

In this case an extra protein of M.W. around 58,000 termed "fascin" appears to be involved in the lateral aggregation of filaments into the filopodia (83).

With regard to vertebrate cells these structural data readily explain the basis of the oft described transition between lamella cytoplasm (or ruffling membrane) and microspikes (84) and retraction fibres (30) as well as the upward growth and concomitant narrowing of ruffles (29). Also the collapse of ruffles into the leading lamella which is associated with a thickening of the ruffle (79) is likely explained simply by a divergence of the filaments in the ruffle, automatically reducing its vertical height. Subsequently, the filaments are presumably depolymerised and recycled through the leading edge.

We may speculate that advancement of the leading edge involves a polymerisation of actin filaments, probably proceeding inwards from the cell membrane at specific initiation sites. The involvement of actin polymerisation in movement has earlier been demonstrated in the ejection of the axosomal process in echinoderm sperm (85). An inward polymerisation, bearing against the inner cytoskeleton would result in the outward growth of the leading edge. (We earlier suggested that polymerisation may proceed in a forward direction (77). It is difficult to imagine in this case, however, how a specific direction of polymerisation from presumably non-oriented intra-cellular sites may be determined. Also, in this event the aggregation of filaments into bundles may be expected to proceed from inside-out and not from the apical end inwards, as observed).

The general scheme of events underlying the different phases of withdrawal and protrusion of the leading edge is thus envisioned as involving a controlled polymerisation and depolymerisation of actin coupled with a dynamic rearrangement (divergence and convergence) of the filaments comprising the diagonal meshwork. That the movement is not continuously in the forward direction but fluctuates back and forth may be explained by the presence of a factor which limits the ultimate length of the actin filaments. In this respect it is interesting to note that the maximum breadth of the meshwork corresponds approximately to the recorded mean distance of protrusion of the leading edge (30).

(ii) Contact inhibition and underlapping

Contact inhibition of cell locomotion refers to the phenomenon by which cells adopt a non-random distribution in monolayer culture through a mutual resistance to cross over one another (see 86). Typically, when two cells come into collision involving the advancing lamella of one or both cells, movement ceases after a small degree of overlap occurs, the cells then retract and move away in different directions. The retraction phase is characterised by the formation of retraction fibres which correspond essentially to microspikes.

It is not the intention here to discuss this phenomenon in detail. It may only be noted that crossing of cells can occur when a leading lamella of one cell contacts the substrate free (29) and stable concave edges of another cell. Without exception the advancing lamella always passes beneath or "underlaps" the "stationary" neighbour cell (86, 87). The pronounced criss-crossing that occurs in cultures of transformed cells giving the impression that the cells "pile up" on each other is not due to the absence of contact inhibition. Rather, it reflects simply the presence in the less spread and normally more elongated transformed cells of a considerably higher incidence of substrate free edges, the area occupied by the leading lamellae being correspondingly smaller (4, 86, 88). The mutual contact of two lamellipodia of transformed cells results in the normal inhibition (88).

The mechanism of contact inhibition has yet to be defined. The involvement of a diffusable substance that passes between neighbour cells has been ruled unlikely by the observation that contact inhibition may occur between two lamellae arising from the same cell (89). We suggest that the primary effect of contact may be to inhibit actin polymerisation by blocking, for example, the initiation foci at the membrane. The existing meshwork would then coalesce into bundles (the retraction fibres) and subsequent locomotory activity, either locally (25) or elsewhere in the cell would effect release.

4. CYTOSKELETAL CHANGES ASSOCIATED WITH TRANSFORMATION

A common morphological characteristic of transformed cells is their inability to spread to the same extent on a solid substrate as their normal, untransformed counterparts (see 4). The area of lamella cytoplasm as already indicated, is much decreased as are the size of the leading and ruffling edges and the cells are consequently thicker.

Early studies by immunofluorescent microscopy suggested that the filaments in transformed cells may be in some way deranged since the networks characteristic of normal cells could not be visualised (90, 91). Subsequently, the failure to observe the filament nets was shown to be due mainly to the technical difficulties of resolving the filaments in these thicker cells in the light microscope (10, 92-94)and only relatively minor differences in filament arrangements at this level are now apparent. Actin filament bundles have been demonstrated in both virally and non-virally transformed cells (see for example 93-95) although in transformed cells they are generally thinner and sparser. Also, the microtubule (10, 92, 94), and 10nm filament networks (39, 41) are at least as extensive in transformed as in untransformed cells. Moreover, when transformed cells spread spontaneously or are induced to spread on a substrate the arrangement of filaments becomes indistinguishable from that of normal cells (96, 97).

Thus the changes in distribution of the cytoskeletal components and in particular the expression of prominent bundles or cables of actin may be attributed to changes in the degree of adhesion to the substrate (4, 96, 97), the factors regulating this adhesion being more substrate dependent in transformed, as compared to normal cells.

Using either colchicine binding activity (99) or a radioimmunoassay (100) the content of tubulin has been found to be invariable between normal 3T3 and transformed SV40 3T3 cells. The amount, about 2.5 - 4.0% of the total protein has been estimated to correspond to an intracellular concentration of about 2 mg/ml (100). Similar figures have been obtained (about 4% total protein) from the quantitation of spots obtained after two dimenstional gel electrophoresis of cells labelled with ^{35}S methionine (101). Under the conditions used for the preparations of the cytoskeletons described here (e.g. Fig. 8) about 50% of the tubulin is released by Triton for each of these two cell lines. For actin, the ratio of the Triton-soluble to the Triton-insoluble fraction is slightly higher in transformed cells (101), consistent with earlier findings (102). For normal cells about 30% of the actin is released by Triton whereas for transformed cells this figure exceeds 50% (101). Such differences may derive from the presence of abundant surface ruffles and microspikes on transformed cells (4) and which would be removed by the extraction procedure.

5. MICROINJECTION METHODS APPLIED TO STUDIES OF THE CYTOSKELETON

The application of microinjection methods to studies of the roles that cytoskeletal proteins play in structural support and motile phenomena has yet to be fully explored. Worth mentioning, however, are a few experiments which have already illustrated the usefulness of the microinjection technique in such investigations.

In probing for factors responsible for viral transformation the dissolutions of the stress fibres in a microinjected cell has been taken as one indication of the transition from a normal to a transformed-like state. Such changes have been reported following the injection of the cytoplasmic extract of virally transformed cells into normal cells (103) and, more recently with the injection of the DNA-fragment containing information for small t-antigen of the SV40 virus (104).

The injection of fluorescently-labelled cytoskeletal proteins promises to provide further insight into the motility, distribution and fate of these proteins within the cell. It has already been shown that rhodamine-labelled α-actinin can exchange with native α-actinin situated in the stress fibres of living fibroblasts (105) and the fate of fluorescently-labelled actin has also been followed after injection into amoeba (106).

More recently, evidence for the involvement of an actin-myosin system in the process of axoplasmic transport has been obtained from the injection into nerve cells of components which disturb the organisation of actin filaments (107). The injection of DNAase I and cytochalasin into the body of the giant "Retzius" nerve cells of the leech was found to block the transport of radioactively labelled protein down the axon (107). These same agents cause a depolymerization or disruption of actin filaments (see for example 108, 109). In addition, high concentrations of vanadate, at levels known to inhibit actomyosin ATPase blocked protein transport and some inhibition was also noted after the injection of filamin, a potent cross-linker of actin filaments (see 61).

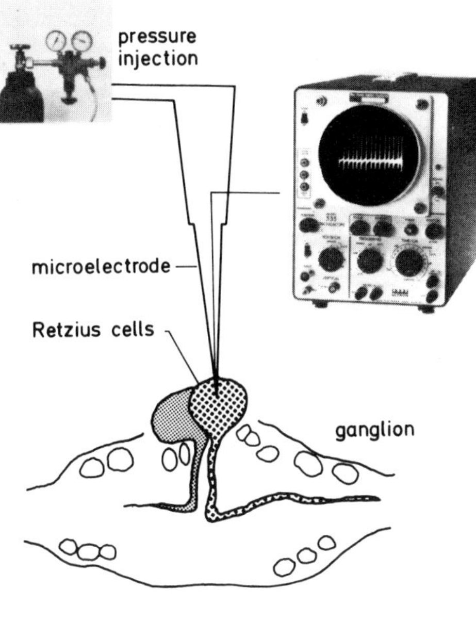

THF EFFECT OF INTRACELLULARLY INJECTED SUBSTANCES ON AXONAL TRANSPORT

SUBSTANCE	SOMAL GRAIN DENSITY	GRAIN DENSITY AT 70 μM AXONAL LENGTH AS % OF THE SOMAL VALUE	GRAIN DENSITY AT 300 μM AXONAL LENGTH AS % OF THE SOMAL VALUE
BLANK (^{3}H-GLYCINE ONLY)	100% (50-80 GR/100 μ^2)	80-90%	60-90%
VANADATE (LOW CONCENTRATION)	100% (80-120 GR/100 μ^2)	80-100%	60-100%
VANADATE (HIGH CONCENTRATION)	100% (70-80 GR/100 μ^2)	40-50%	0%
CYTOCHALASIN B IN DMSO	100% (70-80 GR/100 μ^2)	30-50% (AT 50 μM)	0%
DMSO	100% (30-40 GR/100 μ^2)	70-80%	40-60%
DNA-ASE I	100% (50-60 GR/100 μ^2)	20-40% (AT 60 μM)	0%
ACTIN-DNA-ASE I COMPLEX	100% (30-40 GR/100 μ^2)	70-80%	50-60%
S-1	100% (90-110 GR/100 μ^2)	90-100%	50-60%
ANTI α-ACTININ	100% (50-80 GR/100 μ^2)	90-100%	30-50%
FILAMIN	100% (85-100 GR/100 μ^2)	20-65%	0-25%

Fig. 13. *Microinjection methods applied to studies of axonal transport.* a. Schematic diagram of the experimental system. b. Table showing the effects of the injection of various substances which affect the actomyosin system, on axonal transport. The transport was monitored autoradiographically and is given as the grain density yielded by transported radioisotopes at different distances along the axon. (see 107 for details).

From these beginnings we may expect interesting developments in the further application of the microinjection method.

6. ACKNOWLEDGEMENTS

These studies were supported in part by grants (to J.V. Small) from the Volkswagen Foundation, the Muscular Dystrophy Association, the Austrian Science Research Council and the Austrian National Bank and (to J.E. Celis) from Euratom and the Danish Natural Science Research Council. We also thank Ms G. Langanger, Mr. P. Jertschin and Mrs. A. Celis for skilful technical assistance.

7. REFERENCES

1) PORTER, K.R. (1970). Cytoplasmic microtubules and their function. In: "Principles of Biomolecular Organisation" Ciba Fdn Symp. (eds., G.E.W. Wolstenholme and M. O'Connor), p. 308. London: Churchill.

2) ROBERTS, K. (1974). Cytoplasmic microtubules and their functions. Progr. in Biophys. and Molec. Biol., 28, 371.

3) SALE, W.S. and GIBBONS, I.R. (1979). Study of the mechanism of the dynein cross-bridge cycle in sea urchin sperm flagella. J. Cell Biol., 82. 291.

4) VASILIEV, J.M. and GELFAND, I.M. (1977). Mechanism of morphogenesis in cell cultures. Int. Rev. Cytol., 50, 159.

5) DE BRABANDER, M., DE MEY, J., VAN DE VEIRE, R., AERTS, F. and GEUENS, G. (1977). Microtubules in mammalian cell shape and surface modulation: an alternative hypothesis. Cell Biol. Int. Rep., 1, 453.

6) FULLER, G.M. and BRINKLEY, B.R. (1976). Structure and control of assembly of cytoplasmic microtubules in normal and transformed cells. J. Supramolec. Struct., 5, 497.

7) OSBORN, M. and WEBER, K. (1976). Tubulin-specific antibody and the expression of microtubules in 3T3 cells after attachment to a substratum. Expl. Cell Res., 103, 331.

8) FRANKEL, F.R. (1976). Organization and energy-dependent growth of microtubules in cells. Proc. Natl. Acad. Sci. USA, 73, 2798.

9) DE MEY, J., JONIAU, M., DE BRABANDER, M., MOENS, W. and GEUENS, G. (1976). Immunoperoxidase visualisation of microtubules and microtubular proteins. Nature, Lond., 264, 273.

10) DE MEY, J., JONIAU, M., DE BRABANDER, M., MOENS, W. and GEUENS, G. (1978). Evidence for unaltered structure and *in vivo* assembly of microtubules in transformed cells. Proc. Natl. Acad. Sci. USA, 75, 1339.

11) WEBER, K., RATHKE, P.C. and OSBORN, M. (1978). Cytoplasmic microtubular images in glutaraldehyde-fixed tissue culture cells by electron microscopy and by immunofluorescence microscopy. Proc. Natl. Acad. Sci. USA, 75, 1820.

12) OSBORN, M. and WEBER, K. (1976). Cytoplasmic microtubules in tissue culture cells appear to grow from an organising structure towards the plasma membrane. Proc. Natl. Acad. Sci. USA, 73, 867.

13) AUSPRUNK, D.H. and BERMAN, H.J. (1978). Spreading of vascular endothelial cells in culture: Spatial reorganisation of cytoplasmic fibers and organelles. Tiss. and Cell, 10, 707.

14) OLMSTED, J.V. and BORISY, G.G. (1973). Microtubules. Ann. Rev. Biochem., 42, 507.

15) BETTEX-GALLAND, M. and LUSCHER, E.F. (1959). Extraction of an actomyosin-like protein from human thrombocytes. Nature, 184, 276.

16) BUCKLEY, I.K. and PORTER, K.R. (1967). Cytoplasmic fibrils in living cultured cells: a light and electron microscope study. Protoplasma, 64, 349.

17) ISHIKAWA, H., BISCHOFF, R. and HOLTZER, H. (1969). Formation of arrowhead complexes with heavy meromyosin in a variety of cell types. J. Cell Biol., 43, 312.

18) HUXLEY, H.E. (1963). Electron microscope studies on the structure of natural and synthetic protein filaments from striated muscle. J. Molec. Biol. 7, 281.

19) SPOONER, B.S., YAMADA, K.M. and WESSELLS, N.K. (1971). Microfilaments and cell locomotion. J. Cell Biol., 49, 595.

20) ABERCROMBIE, M., HEAYSMAN, J.E.M. and PEGRUM, S.M. (1971). The locomotion of fibroblasts in culture. IV. Electron microscopy

of the leading lamella. Expl. Cell Res., 67, 359.

21) LAZARIDES, E. and WEBER, K. (1974). Actin antibody: the specific visualisation of actin filaments in non-muscle cells. Proc. Natl. Acad. Sci. USA, 71, 2268.

22) GOLDMAN, R.D., LAZARIDES, E., POLLACK, R. and WEBER, K. (1975). The distribution of actin in non-muscle cells. Expl. Cell Res., 90, 333.

23) LAZARIDES, E. (1976). Two general classes of cytoplasmic actin filaments in tissue culture cells: the role of tropomyosin. J. Supramolecular Struct., 5, 531.

24) SMALL, J.V. and CELIS, J.E. (1978). Filament arrangements in negatively stained cultured cells: the organisation of actin. Cytobiologie, 16, 308.

25) HEATH, J.P. and DUNN, G.A. (1978). Cell to substrate contacts of chick fibroblasts and their relation to the microfilament system. A correlated interference-reflexion and high-voltage electronmicroscope study. J. Cell Sci., 29, 197.

26) IZZARD, C.S. and LOCHNER, L.R. (1976). Cell-to-substrate contacts in living fibroblasts: an interference reflexion study with an evaluation of the technique. J. Cell Sci., 21, 129.

27) BADLEY, R.A., LLOYD, C.W., WOODS, A., CARRUTHERS, L., ALLCOCK, C. and REES, D.A. (1978). Mechanisms of cellular adhesion. Expl. Cell Res., 117, 231.

28) HYNES, R.O. and DESTREE, A.T. (1978). Relationships between fibronection (LETS protein) and actin. Cell, 15, 875.

29) HARRIS, A.K. (1973). Cell surface movements related to cell locomotion. In: "Locomotion of Tissue Cells" Ciba Found. Symp., 1972, Vol. 14, p. 3.

30) ABERCROMBIE, M., HEAYSMAN, J.E.M. and PEGRUM, S.M. (1970). The locomotion of fibroblasts in culture. I. Movements of the leading edge. Expl. Cell Res., 59, 393.

31) FAWCETT, C.W. (1966). An atlas of fine structure. The cell: its organelles and inclusions, Saunders Philadelphia.

32) SMALL, J.V. and SOBIESZEK, A. (1977). Studies on the function and composition of the 10 nm (100 Å) filaments of vertebrate smooth muscle. J. Cell Science, 23, 243.

33) ISHIKAWA, H. (1974). Arrowhead complexes in a variety of cell types. In: "Exploratory Concepts in Muscular Dystrophy". Vol. 2, (ed., A.T. Milhoret), p. 37, Amsterdam Excerpta Medica.

34) GOLDMAN, R.D. and KNIPE, D.M. (1973). Functions of cytoplasmic fibers in non-muscle cell motility. Cold Spring Harb. Symp., Quant. Biol., 37, 523.

35) CROOP, J. and HOLTZER, H. (1975). Response of myogenic and fibrogenic cells to cytochalasin B and to colcemid. I. Light microscope observations. J. Cell Biol., 65, 271.

36) KURKI, P., VIRTANEN, I., STENMAN, S. and LINDER, E. (1977). Human smooth muscle autoantibodies reacting with intermediate (100 Å) filaments. Nature, Lond., 268, 240.

37) OSBORN, M., FRANKE, W.W. and WEBER, K. (1977). Visualisation of a system of filaments 7-10 nm thick in cultured cells of an epithelioid line (PtK2) by immunofluorescence microscopy. Proc. Natl. Acad. Sci. USA, 74, 2490.

38) GORDON, W.E., BUSHNELL, A. and BURRIDGE, K. (1978). Characterisation of the intermediate (10 nm) filaments of cultured cells using an autoimmune rabbit antiserum. Cell, 13, 249.

39) HYNES, R.O. and DESTREE, A.T. (1978). 10 nm filaments in normal and transformed cells. Cell, 13, 151.

40) FRANKE, W.W., SCHMID, E., WEBER, K. and OSBORN, M. (1979). Intermediate-sized filaments of human endothelial cells. J. Cell Biol., 81, 570.

41) FRANKE, W.W., SCHMID, E., WEBER, K. and OSBORN, M. (1979). HeLa cells contain intermediate-sized filaments of the prekaratin type. Expl. Cell Res., 118, 95.

42) CAMPBELL, G.R., CHAMLEY-CAMPBELL, J., GRÖSCHEL STEWART, U., SMALL, J.V. and ANDERSEN, P. (1979). Antibody staining of 10 nm (100 Å) filaments in cultured smooth, cardiac and skeletal

muscle cells. J. Cell Sci., 37, 303.

43) FRANKE, W.E., SCHMID, E., BREITKREUTZ, D., LÜDER, M., BOUKAMP, P., FUSENIG, N.E., OSBORN, M. and WEBER, K. (1979). Simultaneous expression of two different types of intermediate sized filements in mouse keratinocytes proliferating *in vitro*. Differentiation, 14, 35.

44) SCHLAEPFER, W.W. and FREEMAN, L.A. (1978). Neurofilament proteins of rat peripheral nerve and spinal cord. J. Cell Biol., 78, 653.

45) FRANKE, W.W., SCHMID, E., OSBORN, M. and WEBER, K. (1978). The intermediate-sized filaments in rat kangaroo PtK2 cells. II. Structure and composition of isolated filaments. Cytobiologie, 17, 392.

46) STARGER, J.M., BROWN, W.E., GOLDMAN, A.E. and GOLDMAN, R.D. (1978). Biochemical and immunological analysis of rapidly purified 10 nm filaments from baby hamster kidney (BHK-21) cells. J. Cell Biol., 78, 93.

47) LEHTO, V.-P., VITANEN, I. and KURKI, P. (1978). Intermediate filaments anchor the nuclei in nuclear monolayers of cultured human fibroblasts. Nature, Lond., 272, 175.

48) FRANKE, W.W., SCHMID, E., OSBORN, M. and WEBER, K. (1978). Different intermediate-sized filaments distinguished by immunofluorescence microscopy. Proc. Natl. Acad. Sci. USA, 75, 5034.

49) BENNETT, G.S., FELLINI, S.A., CROOP, J.M., OTTO, J.J., BRYAN, J. and HOLTZER, H. (1978). Differences among 100 Å filament subunits from different cell types. Proc. Natl. Acad. Sci. USA, 75, 4364.

50) ERICKSSON, A. and THORNELL, L.E. (1979). Intermediate (skeletin) filaments in heart purkinje fibres. J. Cell Biol., 80, 231.

51) SMALL, J.V. and CELIS, J.E. (1978). Direct visualisation of the 10 nm (100 Å) -filement network in whole and enucleated cultured cells. J. Cell Sci., 31, 393.

52) TROTTER, J.A., FOERDER, B.A. and KELLER, J.M. (1978). Intra-

cellular fibres in cultured cells: analysis by scanning and transmission electron microscopy and by SDS-polyacrylamide gel electrophoresis. J. Cell Sci., 31, 369.

53) BRAVO, R. and CELIS, J.E., in preparation.

54) BLOSE, S.H., private communication.

55) SLOBODA, R.D., DETTLER, W.L. and ROSENBAUM, J.L. (1976). Microtubule-associated proteins and the stimulation of tubulin assembly *in vitro*. Biochemistry, 15, 4497.

56) MURPHY, D.B. and BORISY, G.G. (1975). Association of high molecular weight proteins with microtubules and their role in microtubule assembly *in vitro*. Proc. Natl. Acad. Sci. USA, 72, 2696.

57) WEINGARTEN, M.D., LOCKWOOD, A.H., HWO, S.-Y. and KIRSCHNER, M.W. (1975). A protein factor essential for microtubule assembly. Proc. Natl. Acad. Sci. USA, 72, 1858.

58) HERZOG, W. and WEBER, K. (1978). Fractionation of brain microtubule-associated proteins. Isolation of two different proteins which stimulate tubulin polymerisation *in vitro*. Eur. J. Biochem., 92, 1.

59) MURPHY, D.B., JOHNSON, K.A. and BORISY, G.G. (1977). Role of tubulin-associated proteins in microtubule nucleation and elongation. J. Mol. Biol., 117, 33.

60) NAGLE, B.W., DOENGES, K.H. and BRYAN, J. (1977). Assembly of tubulin from cultured cells and comparison with the neurotubulin model. Cell, 12, 573.

61) SMALL, J.V. and SOBIESZEK, A. (1979). The contractile apparatus of smooth muscle. Int. Rev. Cytol., in press.

62) WEBER, K. and GROESCHEL-STEWART, U. (1974). Antibody to myosin: the specific visualisation of myosin-containing filaments in non-muscle cells. Proc. Natl. Acad. Sci. USA, 71, 4561.

63) LAZARIDES, E. (1975). Tropomyosin antibody: the specific localisation of tropomyosin in non-muscle cells. J. Cell Biol., 65, 549.

64) LAZARIDES, E. and BURRIDGE, K. (1975). Alpha actinin: immunofluorescent localisation of a muscle structural protein in non-muscle cells. Cell, 6, 289.

65) GORDON, W.E. (1978). Immunofluorescent and ultrastructural studies of "sarcomeric" units in stress fibres of cultured non-muscles cells. Expl. Cell Res., 117, 253.

66) GEIGER, G. and SINGER, S.J., private communication.

67) FUJIWARA, K., PORTER, M.E. and POLLARD, T.D. (1978). Alpha-actinin localization in the cleavage furrow during cytokinesis. J. Cell Biol., 79, 268.

69) BRETSCHER, A. and WEBER, K. (1978). Localization of actin and microfilament-assocated proteins in the microvilli and terminal web of the intestinal brush border by immunofluorescence microscopy. J. Cell Biol., 79, 839.

70) CRAIG, S.W. and PARDO, J.E. (1970). Alpha-actinin localisation in the junctional complex of intestinal epithelial cells. J. Cell Biol., 80, 203.

71) JOCKUSCH, B.M., BURGER, M.M., DA PRADA, M., RICHARDS, J.G., CHAPONNIER, C. and GABBIANI, G. (1977). Alpha-actinin attached to membranes of secretory vesicles. Nature, Lond., 270, 628.

72) HEGGENESS, M.H., WANG, K. and SINGER, S.J. (1977). Intracellular distributions of mechanochemical proteins in cultured fibroblasts. Proc. Natl. Acad. Sci. USA, 74, 3883.

73) ZACKROFF, R.V. and GOLDMAN, R.D., private communication.

74) PORTER, K.R. (1976). Motility in cells. In: "Cell Motility" (eds., R. Goldman, T. Pollard and J. Rosenbaum). p. 1, Cold Spring Harb. Lab. 1976.

75) WOLOSEWICK, J.J. and PORTER, K.R. (1976). Stereo high-voltage electron microscopy of whole cells of human diploid line. Am. J. Anat., 147, 303.

76) WOLOSEWICK, J.J. and PORTER, K.R. (1979). Microtrabecular lattice of the cytoplasmic ground substance. Artefact or reality. J. Cell. Biol., 82, 114.

77) SMALL, J.V., ISENBERG, G. and CELIS, J.E. (1978). Polarity of actin at the leading edge of cultured cells. Nature, Lond., 272, 638.

78) SMALL, J.V. and ISENBERG, G., in preparation.

79) INGRAM, V.M. (1969). A side view of moving fibroblasts. Nature, Lond., 222, 641.

80) ISENBERG, G., SMALL, J.V. and KREUTZBERG, G. (1978). Correlation between actin polymerization and surface receptor segragation in neuroblastoma cells treated with concanavalin A. J. Neurocytol., 7, 649.

81) BRAGINA, E.E., VASILIEV, J.M. and GELFAND, I.M. (1976). Formation of bundles of microfilaments during spreading of fibroblasts on the substrate. Expl. Cell Res., 97, 241.

82) EDDS, K.T. (1977). Dynamic aspects of filopodial formation by reorganization of microfilaments. J. Cell Biol., 73, 479.

83) OTTO, J.J., Kane, R.E. and BRYAN, J. (1979). Formation of filopodia in coelomocytes: localisation of fascin, a 58,000 dalton actin cross-linking protein. Cell, 17, 285.

84) WESSELLS, N.K., SPOONER, B.S. and LUDUENA, M.A. (1973). Surface movements and microfilaments. In: "Locomotion of Tissue Culture Cells", Ciba Fdn Symp., 14, p. 53.

85) TILNEY, L.G. (1975). The role of actin in non-muscle cell motility. In: "Molecules and Cell Movement (eds., S. Inoue and R.E. Stephens), p. 339, Raven Press, New York.

86) ABERCROMBIE, M. (1970). Contact inhibition in tissue culture. *In vitro*, 6, 128.

87) BOYDE, A., GRAINGER, F. and JAMES, D.W. (1969). Scanning electron microscopic observations of chick embryo fibroblasts *in vitro*, with particular reference to the movement of cells under others. Z. Zellforsch., 94, 46.

88) BELL, P.B. (1977). Locomotory behaviour, contact inhibition, and pattern formation of 3T3 and polyoma virus-transformed 3T3 cells in culture. Expl. Cell Res., 110, 963.

89) EBENDAL, T. and HEATH, J.P. (1977). Self-contact inhibition of movement in cultured chick heart fibroblasts. Expl. Cell Res., 110, 469.

90) POLLACK, R., OSBORN, M. and WEBER, K. (1975). Patterns of organisation of actin and myosin in normal and transformed cultured cells. Proc. Natl. Acad. Sci. USA, 72, 994.

91) BRINKLEY, B., FULLER, G. and HIGHFIELD, D. (1975). Cytoplasmic microtubules in normal and transformed cells in culture: analysis by tubulin antibody immunofluorescence. Proc. Natl. Acad. Sci. USA, 72, 4981.

92) OSBORN, M. and WEBER, K. (1977). The display of microtubules in transformed cells. Cell, 12, 561.

93) GOLDMAN, R.D., YERNA, M. and SCHLOSS, J.A. (1976). Localisation and organisation of microfilaments and related proteins in normal and virus-transformed cells. J. Supramolecular Struct., 5, 155.

94) TUCKER, R.W., SANFORD, K.K. and FRANKEL, F.R. (1978). Tubulin and actin in paired non-neoplastic and spontaneously transformed neoplastic cell lines *in vitro*: fluorescent antibody studies. Cell, 13, 629.

95) CELIS, J.E., SMALL, J.V., ANDERSEN, P. and CELIS, A. (1978). Microfilament bundles in cultured cells. Correlation with anchorage independence and tumorigenicity in nude mice. Expl. Cell Res., 114, 335.

96) WILLINGHAM, M.C., YAMADA, K.M., YAMADA, S.S., POUYSSEGUR, J. and PASTAN, I. (1977). Microfilament bundles and cell shape are related to adhesiveness to substratum and are dissociable from growth control in cultured fibroblasts. Cell, 10, 375.

97) ALI, I.A., MAUTNER, V., LANZA, R. and HYNES, R.O. (1977). Restoration of normal morphology, adhesion and cytoskeleton in transformed cells by addition of a transformation-sensitive surface protein. Cell, 11, 115.

98) CELIS, J.E., SMALL, J.V., KALTOFT, K. and CELIS, A. (1979).

Microfilament bundles in transformed mouse CL1DX transformed CHO cell hybrids. Expl. Cell Res., 120, 79.

99) WICHE, G., LUNDBLAD, V.T. and COLE, R.D. (1977). Competence of soluble cell extracts as microtubule assembly systems. J. Biol. Chem., 252, 794.

100) HILLER, G. and WEBER, K. (1978). Radioimmunoassay for tubulin: a quantitative comparison of the tubulin content of different established tissue culture cells and tissues. Cell, 14, 795.

101) BRAVO, R. and CELIS, J.E. Gene expression in normal and virally-transformed 3T3B and BHK21 cells, submitted for publication.

102) FINE, R.E. and TAYLOR, L. (1976). Decreased actin and tubulin synthesis in 3T3 cells after transformation by SV40 virus. Expl. Cell Res., 102, 162.

103) MC CLAIN, D.A., MANESS, P.F. and EDELMAN, G.M. (1978). Assay for early cytoplasmic effects of the srC gene product of Rous sarcoma virus. Proc. Natl. Acad. Sci. USA, 75, 2750.

104) GRAESSMANN, A., GRAESSMANN, M. and MUELLER, C. This volume.

105) FERAMISCO, J.R. (1979). Microinjection of fluorescently labeled α-actinin into living fibroblasts. Proc. Natl. Acad. Sci. USA, 76, 3967.

106) TAYLOR, D.L. and WANG, Y.L. (1978). Molecular cytochemistry: incorporation of fluorescently labeled actin into cells. Proc. Natl. Acad. Sci. USA, 75, 857.

107) ISENBERG, G., SCHUBERT, P. and KREUTZBERG, G.W. (1979). Actin, a neuroplasmic constituent requisite for axonal transport. Proc. Natl. Acad. Sci. USA, in press.

RED CELL-MEDIATED MICROINJECTION STUDIES ON PROTEIN DEGRADATION

M. Rechsteiner

Department of Biology
University of Utah
Salt Lake City, Utah 84112, U.S.A.

1. INTRODUCTION

It has long been known that proteins are continually synthesized and degraded within animals (1). While there was once resistance to the idea that this represented protein turnover within cells (2), today there is considerable evidence that this is so (for reviews see 3-7). The physiological significance of protein turnover is not as firmly established. The early studies of Schimke on arginase (8) and Schimke *et al.* on tryptophan-pyrolase (9) clearly demonstrated that control of degradation could influence enzyme levels. Further support for the idea that selective protein degradation plays a regulatory role has been obtained by comparison of turnover rates for various proteins which has revealed that key metabolic enzymes usually turn over faster than structural proteins (6). Thus there is increasing evidence that this seemingly wasteful process plays a role in metabolic regulation.

During the past five years several structural features of proteins that influence their turnover have been elucidated. As a rule large, acidic proteins are degraded more rapidly than small, basic proteins (10-15). Except for a recently reported case (16), altered proteins, such as nonsense fragments, are degraded more rapidly than native proteins (17-21). In addition, the turnover of specific proteins has been shown to correlate with their susceptibility to proteases (22-24) and with their lipophilic affinity (25). Information has also accumulated on the effects of nutrition (26-29), growth rate (30-31), cellular aging (32, 33), and hormonal stimulation (34, 35) on overall rates of protein degradation.

A model for the turnover of plasma membrane proteins has recently emerged. It is proposed that portions of the plasma membrane form intracellular vesicles which subsequently fuse to lysosomes resulting in the degradation of membrane proteins. This model is based on the following experimental observations. Exposure of mouse L cells to latex beads resulted in large scale phagocytosis of the beads (36). If phagocytosis was induced in L cells after iodination of plasma membrane proteins, approximately 30% of the labeled surface membrane was soon found in phagolysosomes. There was no selectivity in the transfer of the iodinated membrane proteins, and most were rapidly degraded after formation of phagolysosomes (36). Studies with rat hepatoma cells under normal growth conditions have confirmed that, with the exception of certain glycoproteins, plasma membrane proteins are degraded at identical rates (37, 38). Electron microscopic autoradiography studies on the degradation of [^{125}I]-bungarotoxin bound to the acetylcholine receptor in chick muscle directly implicate lysosomes in the turnover of plasma membrane proteins (39). Under conditions permitting turnover, about 3.5% of the autoradiographic grains were associated with secondary lysosomes, of which 60% were labeled. At 4°C, where turnover was markedly inhibited, only 0.4% of the lysosomes were labeled. The degradation of [^{125}I]-epidermal growth factor has been shown to be similar to that observed for bungarotoxin (40).

In contrast to degradation of membrane proteins, the mechanism(s) for the turnover of soluble intracellular proteins remains unclear. The lack of detailed information has not prevented speculation, and a number of pathways have been advanced (Fig. 1). I will briefly review five proposed pathways.

2. TURNOVER OF SOLUBLE PROTEASES

A soluble ATP-dependent proteolytic system which degrades abnormal proteins has been described in reticulocytes (41). Whether such a system operates in cells where lysosomes are present has not been demonstrated.

3. MEMBRANE - BUT NOT LYSOSOME INVOLVEMENT IN TURNOVER

A general correspondence exists between *in vivo* degradation rates and the inactivation of soluble enzymes in liver extracts (22-24). Detailed examination of the inactivation of [^{3}H]-labeled phosphoenolpyruvate carboxykinase (PEP CK) in such a system revealed that PEP CK, stable in the cytosol, was inactivated when incubated with microsomal fractions (42). Denaturation and binding to microsomal membranes preceded any apparent proteolytic cleavage of the enzyme. It was proposed that either microsomal proteases or the subsequent transfer to lysosomes effected the eventual degradation of the enzyme. There is evidence for a similar sequence in the degradation of insulin. It has been postulated that insulin is cleaved into its A and B polypeptides by glutathione-insulin transhydrogenase bound to microsomal membranes. Soluble proteases are then thought to hydrolyze the individual peptide bonds in the A and B chains of insulin (43, 44).

4. AUTOPHAGY

A process similar to that proposed for plasma membrane turnover

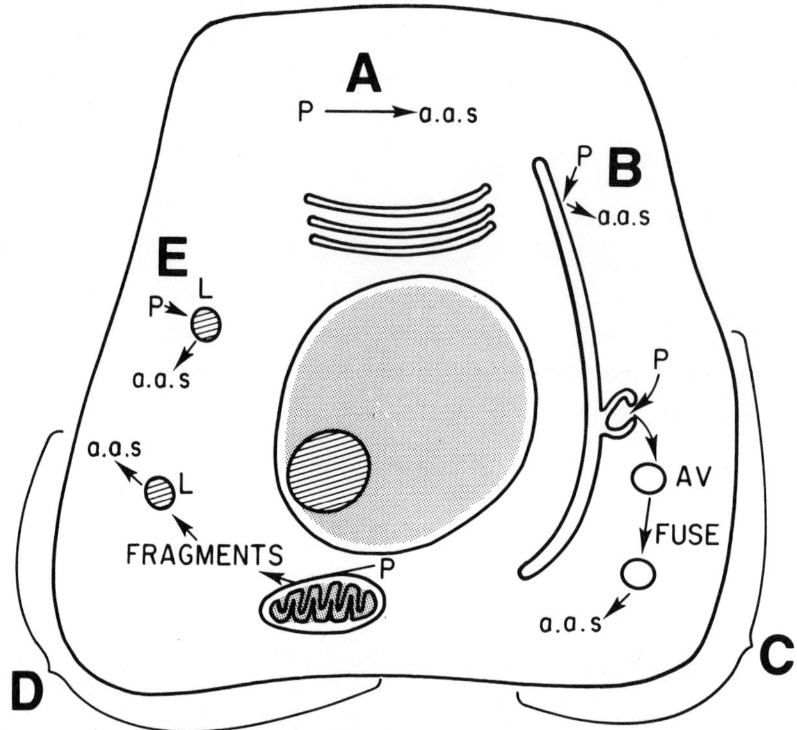

Fig. 1. *Conceivable pathways for the degradation of soluble, intracellular proteins.* A = Soluble proteases; B = Membrane-bound proteases; C = Autophagy; D = Group-specific proteases; E = Lysosomal uptake; P = Protein to be degraded; L = Lysosomes; AV = Autophagic vacuole; a.a. = Amino acids.

can explain turnover of internal membranes and organelles. Autophagy, first described in 1962 (45), is a process in which organelles or free cytosol are enclosed by membranes derived from the smooth endoplasmic reticulum (46). Autophagic vacuoles then fuse with lysosomes where the vesicle contents are degraded (47). The extent of autophagy is under the control of nutritional conditions and hormones. Particularly important are glucagon, which stimulates autophagy, and insulin which inhibits it (48, 49).

Simple models of autophagy do not easily explain the selective degradation of soluble proteins. However, the added assumption that an initial step in the turnover is adsorption of proteins onto the smooth endoplasmic reticulum membrane followed by autophagic vacuole formation is sufficient to explain most aspects of protein turnover. Injection of rhodamine-conjugated proteins into HeLa cells has provided direct evidence for autophagy of proteins (50). The injected proteins were observed to segregate from the bulk cytoplasm and collect in a lysosome-rich region near the nucleus. The rate of this process varied from protein to protein. However, as discussed in more detail below, our own injection studies indicate that the apparent autophagy of rhodamine-labeled proteins is a consequence of the fluorescent side groups.

5. GROUP-SPECIFIC PROTEASES

Katanuma and his colleagues (51, 52) have described a series of proteases which are specific for enzymes containing pyridoxal phosphate as cofactor. One such protease, present in a heavy mitochondrial fraction, has been shown to cleave ornithine aminotransferase at a specific site producing two discrete fragments of the original enzyme. Katanuma speculates that group-specific proteases are limiting in the degradation of enzymes containing pyridoxal phosphate and that cleaved enzymes or their fragments are subsequencly degraded within lysosomes. It should be mentioned that the idea of group-specific proteases is controversial. One enzyme isolated by Katanuma's group has been shown to cleave several proteins which do not have pyridoxal phosphate as a cofactor (53).

6. DIRECT UPTAKE OF SOLUBLE PROTEINS BY LYSOSOMES

The idea that lysosomes are involved in the degradation of soluble proteins enjoys considerable support. Their potential role in autophagy after selective adsorption of proteins onto smooth endoplasmic retculum membranes has just been described. Selective uptake of proteins directly by lysosomes (54-57) or bulk uptake of proteins into lysosomes coupled with selective release of proteins resistant to proteolysis (58), have also been proposed. Evidence to support the latter two hypotheses, mostly indirect, includes correlation of the rates of inactivation of specific enzymes by lysosomal proteases with the *in vivo* stabilities of the enzymes (24), correlation between the turnover rates of soluble proteins and adsorption of these proteins onto membranes in lysosomal fractions (55) and decreased protein turnover when protease inhibitors were transferred to cells via liposomes (59). More direct evidence that lysosomes may degrade soluble proteins is the recent report that tryptophan pyrolase accumulates in a lysosome fraction after exposure of liver cells to chloroquin (60).

It is not possible to choose with any confidence from among the above pathways. We do not know whether lysosomes are involved in the degradation of soluble proteins nor do we know the events that initiate degradation of a protein molecule. The rapid degradation of analog-containing proteins, the correlation of protein size and charge to turnover, and the effects of ligands on protein stability point to the general importance of protein conformation. However, the actual molecular events that designate a protein for destruction are poorly understood. Presumably an altered conformation, such as unfolding, triggers the destruction process. What follows is a matter for speculation. Protein modification, proteolytic cleavage, dissociation into subunits, or adsorption onto membranes could be important.

The paucity of detailed information on the mechanism for selective protein degradation is understandable in view of the difficulty associated with *in vitro* studies of the phenomenon. For example, if proteins or nucleic acids are digested within extracts, one must worry that the degradative enzymes were released from organelles during fractionation. On the other hand, if vesicle formation and fusion are normal steps in the degradative process, these will not continue after preparation of the extracts with current methods for cell fractionation.

The recent development of procedures for the large-scale microinjection of labeled proteins into cultured mammalian cells presents a new and powerful tool for studies on protein turnover (61-63). Microinjection permits studies using intact cells that are difficult, if not impossible, by traditional methods. Proteins can be modified and then injected into cells to discover those features of protein structure significant in determining degradation rates. More important, introduction of a specific iodinated protein into cells allows me to determine the half-life, location and size of the protein without confusion from other labeled proteins. The fact that iodotyrosine is not reutilized makes interpretation straightforward (64). Moreover, the availability of two isotopes of iodine permits one to follow two proteins or two pathways within the same cells. For example, modified and "native" forms of a protein can be separately labeled with ^{125}I and ^{131}I and co-injected into the same cells. Likewise, one can compare the fate of protein labeled with ^{125}I introduced into the cytosol by injection and the same protein labeled with ^{131}I taken up by pinocytosis. In the remainder of this paper I will review results from our initial microinjection studies on protein degradation. Experimental details for most of these studies can be found in Refs. 65-67.

7. THE DEGRADATION OF MICROINJECTED PROTEINS CONFORMS TO RULES ESTABLISHED FOR THE DEGRADATION OF INTRACELLULAR PROTEINS

When ^{125}I-labeled proteins were injected into HeLa cells, ^{125}I was lost from the injected cells at first-order rates with half-lives varying from 3 hrs for the trout, nonhistone chromosomal protein, HMGT, to 75 hrs for lactate dehydrogenase (see Fig. 2 and Table 1). Greater than 80% of the released ^{125}I chromatographed as iodotyrosine following injection of iodinated BSA, HMGT and IgG thereby firmly establishing degradation of these proteins (see Fig. 3a). [^{125}I]-iodotyrosine was not produced when [^{125}I]-BSA was added to the culture medium indicating that degradation of the injected proteins occurred at intracellular sites (Fig. 3b). Although iodotyrosine was not demonstrated after injection of ferritin, LDH or myoglobin, the loss of ^{125}I after injection of these proteins was first-order. Hence, it almost surely represents degradation.

[^{125}I]-BSA and [^{125}I]-ferritin conjugated with fluorescein were degraded more rapidly than their unmodified counterparts after injection into HeLa cells. A preparation of [^{125}I]-HMGT composed of dimers and trimers produced by abnormal disulfide linkages was rapidly degraded ($t_{\frac{1}{2}}$ = 3 hrs) whereas monomers of HMGT were more stable ($t_{\frac{1}{2}}$ = 30 hrs). The high turnover rate for dimers and trimers of HMGT represents an example of the rapid degradation of abnormal proteins.

Interesting comparisons can be made between the turnover of injected and normal cellular proteins. As mentioned in the Introduction large proteins are generally degraded faster than smaller proteins (10-12). Similar results were obtained with injected proteins. Excluding lactate dehydrogenase, the sequence myoglobin, (BSA, IgG) and ferritin describes both decreasing half-lives and increasing molecular weights. Also, in two separate experiments with each pro-

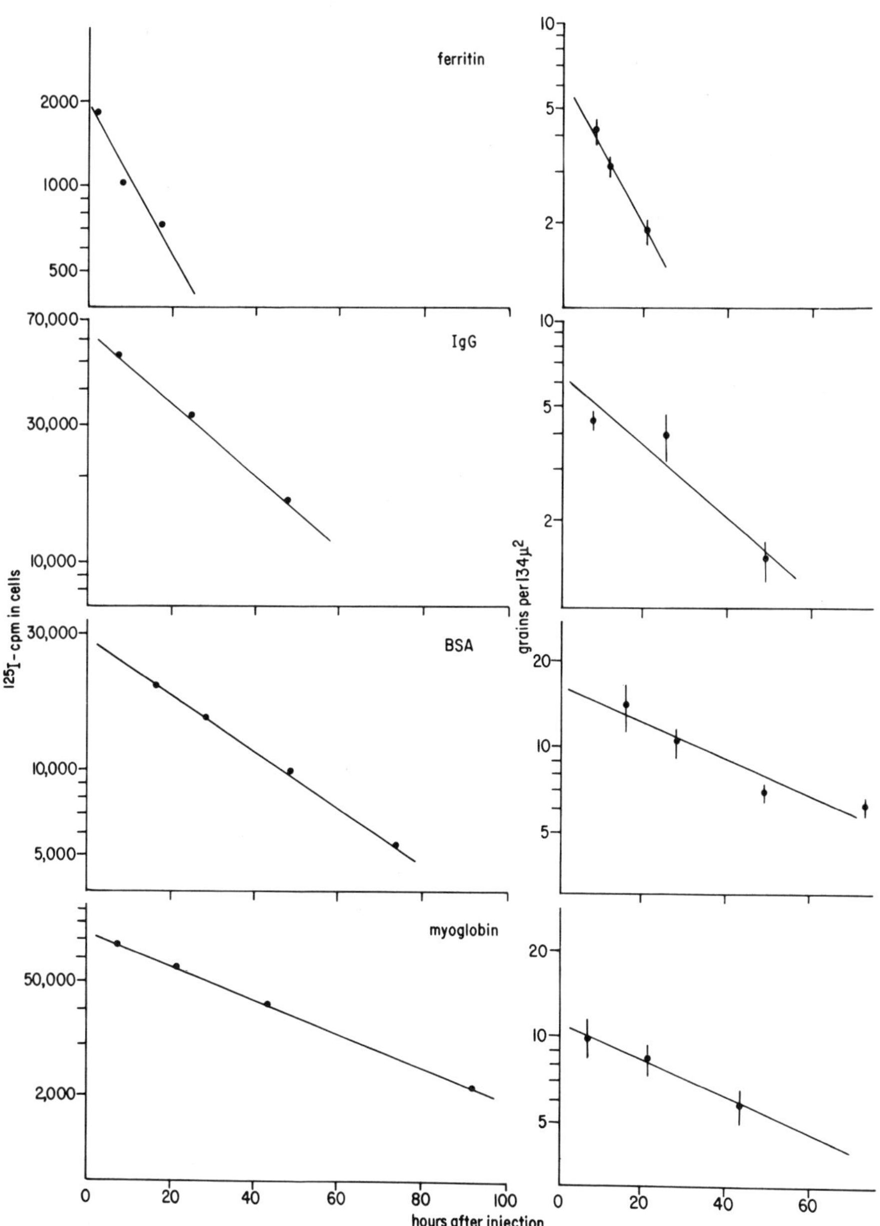

Fig. 2. *Loss of* ^{125}*I from HeLa cells after injection of* ^{125}*I-labeled proteins.* The panels on the left show the loss of ^{125}I from HeLa cells injected with the designated proteins as measured from ^{125}I in whole cells collected by trypsinization. The corresponding panels at the right show average grain densities over 25 labeled cells. Vertical bars denote standard errors of the mean.

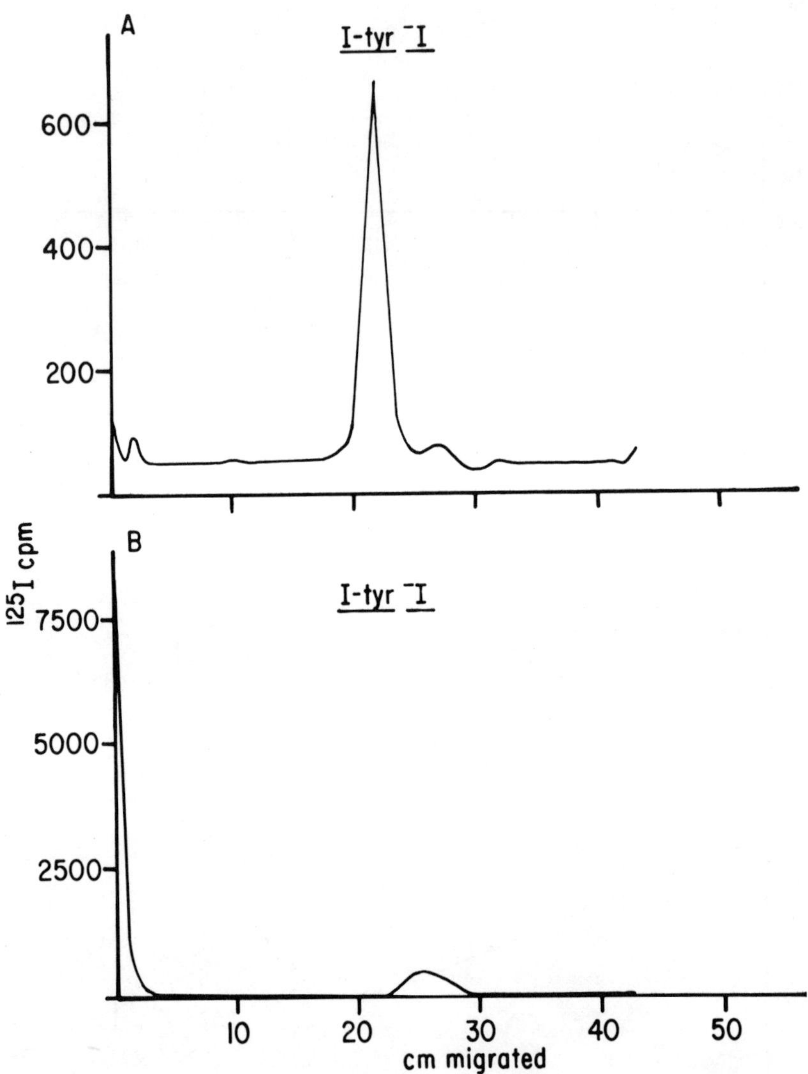

Fig. 3. *Chromatography of tissue culture media.* A. Chromatographic profile of ^{125}I released from HeLa cells injected with [^{125}I]-BSA. B. Chromotographic profile of culture medium containing [^{125}I]-BSA. The solid bars labeled I-tyr and I denote the chromatographic position of iodotyrosine and $^{-}$I, respectively.

Table 1. *Stability of iodinated proteins after injection into HeLa cells.*

Nuclear-Specific Proteins	Half-life (hrs)
Calf-Histone H4	3
Trout HMGT (monomer)	29
Duck HMGE	29
Calf-Histone H1	31
Calf HMG 1	65 - 100
Calf HMG 2	65 - 100
Cytoplasmic or Serum Proteins	**Half-life (hrs)**
Ferritin	11 - 19
Bovine Serum Albumin	14 - 34
Immunoglobulin G	21 - 25
Whale myoglobin	65
Pig lactate dehydrogenase 1	75
Pig lactate dehydrogenase 2	75
Abnormal Proteins	**Half-life (hrs)**
Trout HMG-T (dimers)	4
Fluoresceinated ferritin	7
Fluoresceinated BSA	10 - 12

tein, fluoresceinated-BSA and fluoresceinated-ferritin turned over more rapidly than their unmodified counterparts after injection into HeLa cells. These results and results with HMGT dimers accord well with observations that altered proteins are degraded more rapidly in animal cells (17-21).

(i) Injected proteins, unless altered or nuclear specific, remain distributed throughout the cytoplasm following injection

With the exception of one preparation of BSA heavily-conjugated with fluorescein, autoradiography failed to reveal perinuclear aggregation of those injected proteins which do not accumulate in the nucleus. Our results contrast to those obtained by microneedle injection of rhodamine-conjugated proteins (50). We believe that the conjugated fluorescent side groups lead to membrane association or aggregation of the injected proteins. Differences in the amounts of protein injected or the method of injection are alternative possibilities. Since perinuclear aggregation of ^{3}H-labeled, analog-containing proteins was not observed during their rapid degradation (Zavortink and Rechsteiner, unpublished), we believe that perinuclear aggregation does not normally occur during turnover of soluble, intracellular proteins. However, we cannot eliminate the possibility that transfer of proteins to a lysosome-rich, perinuclear region is a component in soluble protein turnover. Under normal physiological conditions, this transfer could well be rate limiting.

Proteins which are expected to bind to DNA rapidly accumulate in the nucleus following injection into HeLa cells. This is true for iodinated species of the high mobility chromosomal proteins, HMG1, HMG2 and trout HMG-T and also for histone H1. These proteins are degraded after injection, but their nuclear location does not permit one to determine whether they accumulate in a lysosome-rich perinuclear region prior to their degradation.

(ii) Proteolytic fragments of injected proteins are not detected during degradation

SDS-acrylamide electrophoresis was used to examine the size of iodinated proteins after injection into HeLa cells. Virtually all remaining [^{125}I]-HMG1 and [^{125}I]-HMG2 were intact following injection into bovine fibroblasts or HeLa cells. Similarly the remaining intracellular [^{125}I]-IgG or [^{125}I]-BSA was intact whenever examined (Fig. 4). The apparent differences in electrophoretic mobility between injected and uninjected [^{125}I]-BSA in Fig. 4 are presumed to result from ionic conditions in each tube gel since numerous electrophoretic analyses of mixtures of injected and uninjected [^{125}I]-BSA produced no evidence for two proteins of differing size. Recove-

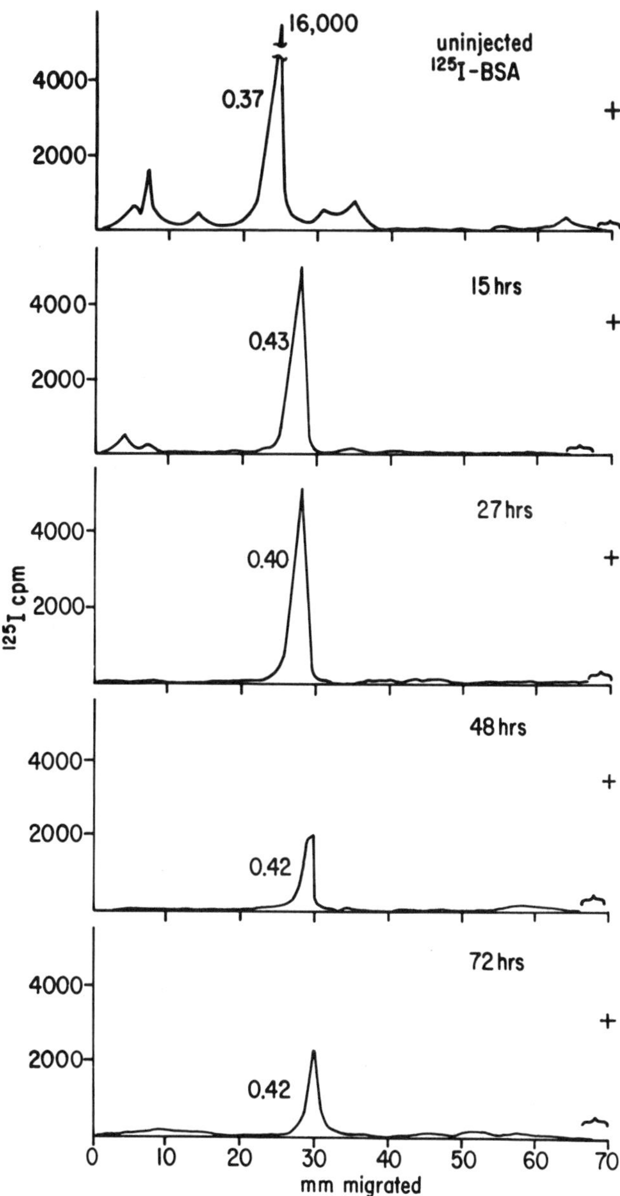

Fig. 4. *SDS-acrylamide electrophoresis of [^{125}I]-BSA after injection into HeLa cells.* HeLa cells were collected at various times after injection and cytoplasmic proteins were separated on 10% SDS-acrylamide gels. The numbers to the left of each peak denote the migration of [^{125}I]-BSA relative to bromphenol blue (brackets).

ry of ^{125}I during preparation of intracellular proteins for electrophoresis was greater than 95%, so it appears that virtually all injected HMG proteins, BSA or IgG were either intact or completely degraded. These results which confirm those of Wasserman *et al.* (68) argue against the existence of stable intermediates during protein degradation.

(iii) Diverse cell lines degrade microinjected BSA at similar rates

The half life of lactate dehydrogenase isozyme 5 varies from 1.6 days in rat heart to 31 days in rat skeletal muscle (69). It is not known whether this remarkable range in the stability of a specific protein reflects differences in the intracellular milieu or differences in the protein degradation systems of these tissues. The ability to microinject molecules from a single preparation of an iodinated protein into different cell lines permitted us to ask how similar the protein degradation systems are in diverse cell types.

[^{125}I]-BSA was injected into eight culture lines from 4 species. It can be seen in Fig. 5 that there was striking similarity in the rate of degradation of [^{125}I]-BSA in 6 cell lines, and less than a 2-fold difference in half-life among all cell lines. This suggests that protein degradation systems are similar from one cell line to another. The rat hepatoma line, FU5-5, and the mouse adrenal line, Y1, have been shown to express liver and adrenal functions *in vitro* (70, 71), so it is unlikely that similarity in the degradation of [^{125}I]-BSA reflects a common tissue culture phenotype among the cell lines injected.

(iv) Neither pepstatin, soybean trypsin inhibitor nor α-anitrypsin inhibits the degradation of injected [^{125}I]-BSA

A number of protease inhibitors have been identified and purified (72, 73). These inhibitors, which include small peptides, as well as plant and serum proteins, are often specific for a given class of proteinase. Since most of the protease inhibitors are relatively small molecules, we should be able to introduce them into cultured cells using red cell-mediated microinjection. We can then ask whether a specific protease inhibitor prevents or retards the degradation of a co-injected ^{125}I-labeled protein. In such a manner, we may identify a class, possibly even a specific protease, important in the degradation of soluble proteins in animal cells.

Although preliminary experiments with pepstatin, soybean trypsin inhibitor and α-antitrypsin have proved negative (Fig. 6), this approach nevertheless has considerable potential. If modifications such as adenylation, glycosylation, or phosphorylation serve to mark proteins for destruction, we may observe modified forms of ^{125}I-labeled proteins coinjected with protease inhibitors.

(v) <u>The Arrhenius plot for the degradation of microinjected [^{125}I]-BSA shows no transition between 7°C and 37°C</u>

Biochemical reactions can be investigated using temperature as a probe. A common analysis involves Arrhenius plots where the log of the rate vs. 1/T is often linear with a slope proportional to the activation energy of the reaction in question. In some phenomena involving membranes, one or more transitions in slope, often near 20°C, are observed, and these have been interpreted in terms of the fluidity of the lipids in the membrane (74-79).

If the degradation of soluble proteins requires membrane vesicle formation or translocation of the protein across a biological membrane one might observe a marked decrease in degradation below the transition temperature of the membrane phospholipids. The absence of a transition would provide circumstantial evidence for the non-involvement of membranes in protein degradation, although it

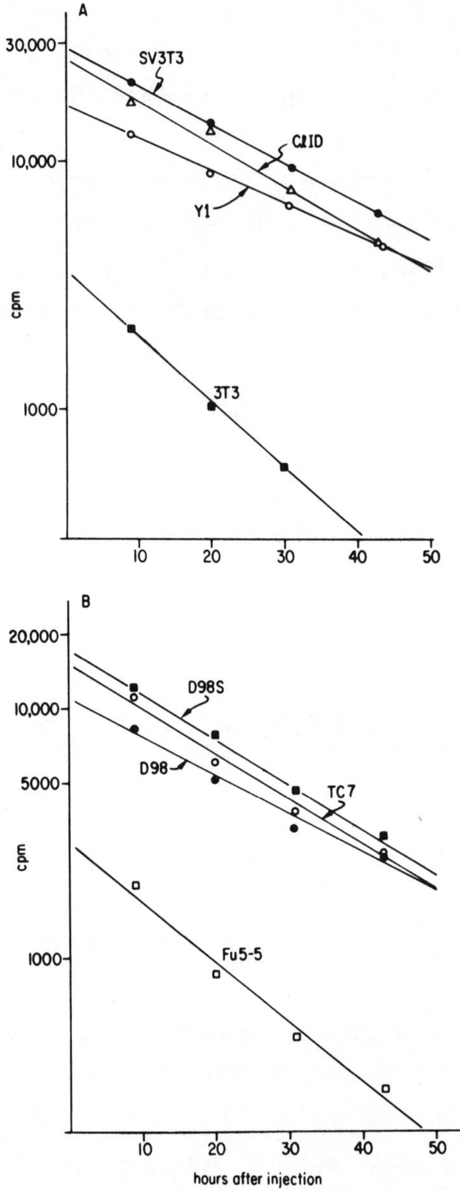

Fig. 5. *Degradation of [^{125}I]-BSA in eight mammalian cell lines.* A. The loss of ^{125}I from four mouse cell lines after injection of [^{125}I]-BSA was determined from the radioactivity remaining in whole cells collected at the times indicated. B. Data similar to those in A are presented for 4 additional cell lines of human, monkey and rat origin. The results are from experiments using a single preparation of [^{125}I]-BSA.

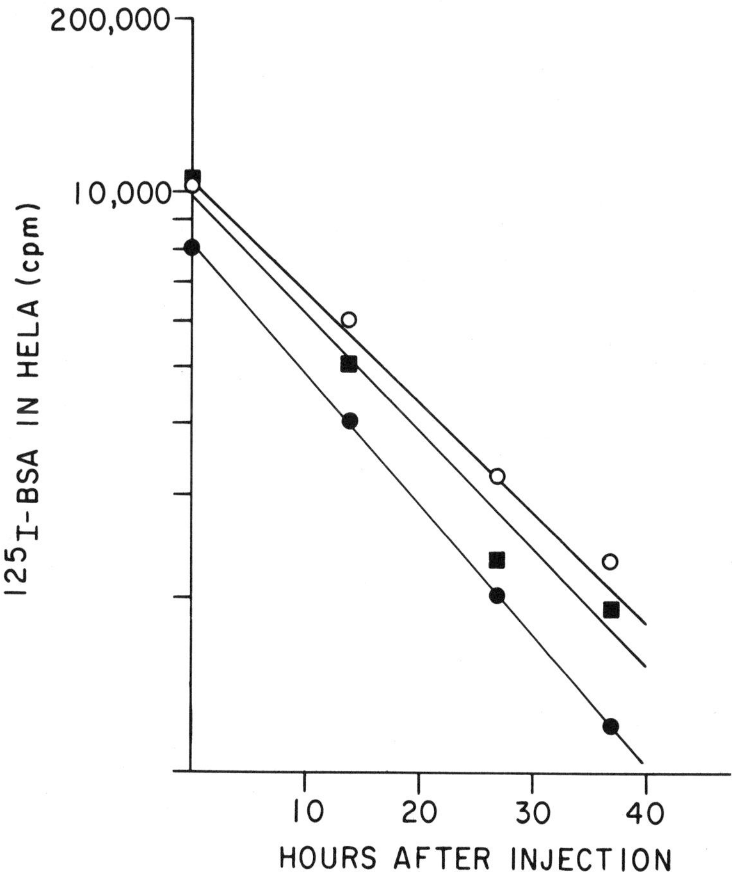

Fig. 6. *Degradation of [^{125}I]-BSA coinjected with protease inhibitors.* [^{125}I]-BSA was loaded into red cells in the presence of α-antitrypsin (25 mg per ml), soybean trypsin inhibitor (33 mg per ml) or pepstatin (a suspension at 10 mg per ml). These red cells were then fused to HeLa cells and the half-life of [^{125}I]-BSA was determined. ● = the stability of [^{125}I]-BSA injected with pepstatin; ■ = [^{125}I]-BSA injected with α-antitrypsin; O = [^{125}I]-BSA injected with soybean trypsin inhibitor.

should be noted that linear Arrhenius plots have been observed for some membrane phenomena, including pinocytosis (80-82).

In spite of the potential uncertainties inherent in this approach, the degradation of microinjected [^{125}I]-BSA was measured in HeLa cells maintained at various temperatures after injection. As shown in Fig. 7, there was no transition in the Arrhenius plot for [^{125}I]-BSA degradation, and the apparent activation energy for degradation was 26.5 Kcal per mole. The absence of a transition favors the non-involvement of membranes in the degradation of microinjected [^{125}I]-BSA. At the least we can conclude that membrane events similar to those which occur during pinocytosis rather than transport or membrane mixing are involved in the degradation of [^{125}I]-BSA, if indeed membranes are involved at all. The significance of 26 Kcal per mole for the activation energy for the degradation of [^{125}I]-BSA is unclear. It will be of interest to see whether this value is obtained with other proteins, since we can then assess what portion of the activation energy is contributed by the cellular machinery, and what portion reflects conformational changes in the protein being degraded.

8. FUTURE STUDIES

One of the central questions regarding the selective degradation of soluble cytoplasmic proteins is whether lysosomes play a role in the process. Red cell-mediated microinjection should allow us to answer this question. Our approach is based upon two previous observations. First, it has long been known that D-amino acid peptides are not hydrolyzed by cellular proteases (83) and second, it has recently been shown that sucrose covalently linked to low density lipoprotein (LDL) accumulates in lysosomes following pinocytosis and degradation of LDL (84). We will covalently attach small D-amino acid peptides that contain D-tyrosine to soluble carrier proteins

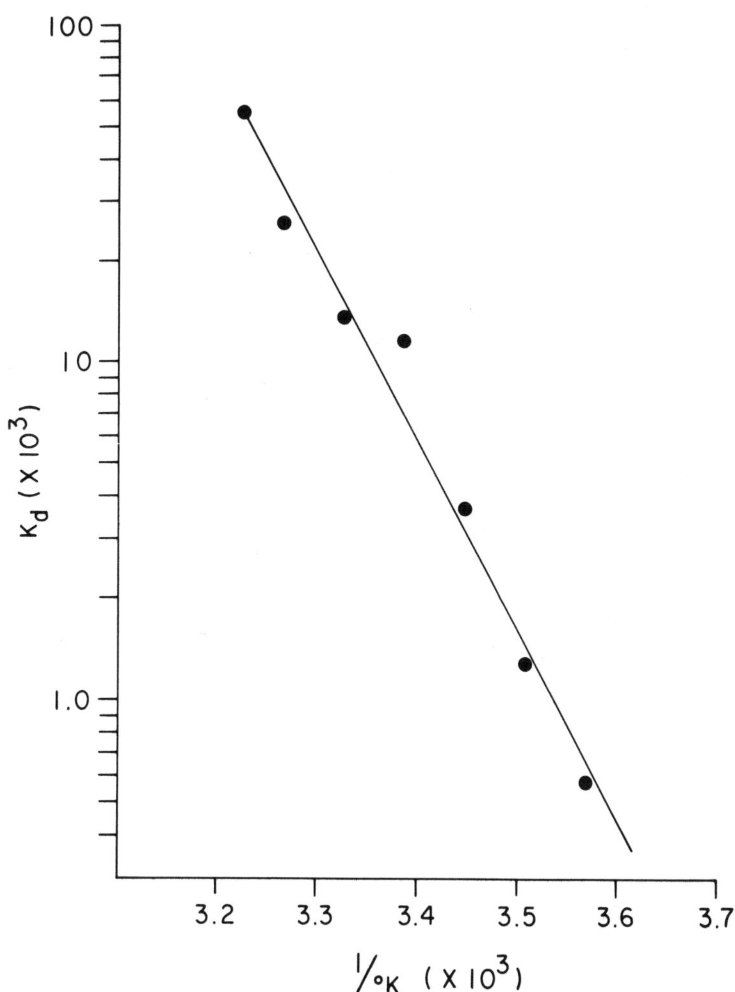

Fig. 7. *The effect of temperature on the rate of degradation of microinjected [^{125}I]-BSA.* After HeLa cells were injected with [^{125}I]-BSA, portions of the cells were then maintained at temperatures from 7°C to 37°C. The rate of degradation of [^{125}I]-BSA was determined for each temperature, and the data are presented as an Arrhenius plot.

and determine whether the non-degradable peptides accumulate within lysosomes or within the cytosol following the injection and degradation of the protein. Ehrenreich and Cohn (85) found that D-amino acid dipeptides accumulated within the lysosomes of macrophages so there is good reason to expect that D-amino acid conjugates will remain in lysosomes if the injected proteins are degraded there.

Another central question which remains unanswered has to do with the initial events in the degradation process. Specifically one would like to know whether there are biochemical reactions, such as adenylation, glycosylation, etc., which mark proteins for destruction. Or is the initial reaction a simple proteolytic cleavage? Co-injection of protease inhibitors and labeled proteins, though so far unsuccessful, remains an attractive approach to this problem. For if there are modifications prior to degradation, then modified forms of injected proteins may accumulate in the presence of protease inhibitors.

Finally, microinjection may allow us to isolate animal cells with altered abilities to degrade soluble proteins. It has been shown by Okada and his colleagues (86) that red cell-mediated injection of antibody to diphtheria toxin protected human KB cells when challenged with the toxin. We propose to select HeLa cells that slowly degrade rabbit IgG based on this observation. HeLa cells will be injected with antibodies to diphtheria toxin and challenged with lethal doses of the toxin at increasingly later times after injection. Rabbit IgG has a half-life of about one day in normal HeLa cells (see Table 1), and with cell division the intracellular concentration of anti-toxin IgG should be markedly diminished by 5-10 days after injection. In HeLa cells that slowly degrade IgG, however, IgG concentration is expected to remain higher and confer protection to toxin challenge for longer periods of time.

9. CONCLUSION

Red cell-mediated microinjection permits one to introduce significant quantities of macromolecules into cultured mammalian cells. In this article I have reviewed our initial studies on the degradation of microinjected proteins and outlined some future lines of research. I hope I have convinced the reader that microinjection will prove useful in determining the mechanism(s) by which soluble proteins are selectively degraded.

10. ACKNOWLEDGEMENTS

I would like to acknowledge the significant contributions of Michael Zavortink and Sean Bigelow to the studies presented here. I would also like to thank Maurine Vaughan for her excellent typing. This research was supported by USPHS Grant GM 24617.

11. REFERENCES

1) SCHOENHEIMER, R. and RITTENBERG, D. (1940). The study of intermediary metabolism of animals with the aid of isotopes. Physiol. Revs. Acta, 20, 218.

2) HOGNESS, D.S., COHN, M. and MONOD, J. (1955). Studies on the induced synthesis of β-galactosidase in *Escherichia coli*: The kinetics and mechanism of sulfur incorporation. Biochim. Biophys. Acta, 16, 99.

3) SCHIMKE, R.T. and DOYLE, D. (1970). Control of enzyme levels in animal tissues. Ann. Rev. Biochem., 39, 929.

4) GOLDBERG, A.L. and DICE, J.F. (1974). Intracellular protein degradation in mammalian and bacterial cells. Annu. Rev. Biochem., 43, 835.

5) SCHIMKE, R.T. (1975). Turnover of membrane proteins in animal cells. Methods in Membrane Biol., 5, 201.

6) GOLDBERG, A.L. and ST. JOHN, A.C. (1976). Intracellular protein degradation in mammalian and bacterial cells. Annu. Rev. Biochem., 45, 747.

7) BALLARD, F.J. (1977). Intracellular protein degradation. Essays in Biochem., 13, 1.

8) SCHIMKE, R.T. (1964). The importance of both synthesis and degradation in the control of arginase levels in rat liver. J. Biol. Chem., 239, 3808.

9) SCHIMKE, R.T, SWEENEY, E. and BERLIN, M. (1965). The roles of synthesis and degradation in the control of rat liver tryptophan pyrrolase. J. Biol. Chem., 240, 322.

10) GLASS, R.D. and Doyle, D. (1972). On the measurement of protein turnover in animal cells. J. Biol. Chem., 247, 5234.

11) DICE, J.F., DEHLINGER, P.J. and SCHIMKE, R.T. (1973). Studies on the correlation between size and relative rate of degradation of soluble proteins. J. Biol. Chem., 248, 4220.

12) DICE, J.F. and GOLDBERG, A.L. (1975). A statistical analysis of the relationship between degradation rates and molecular weights of proteins. Arch. Biochem. Biophys., 170, 213.

13) DICE, J.F. and GOLDBERG, A.L. (1975). Relationship between *in vivo* degradative rates and isoelectric points of proteins. Proc. Nat. Acad. Sci., 72, 3893.

14) DICE, J.F. and GOLDBERG, A.L. (1976). Structural properties of rat serum proteins which correlate with their degradative rates *in vivo*. Nature, 262, 514.

15) MOMANY, F., AGUANNO, J. and LARRABEE, A.R. (1976). Correlation of degradative rates of proteins with a parameter calculated from amino acid composition and subunit size. Proc. Nat. Acad. Sci, 73, 3093.

16) SIMON, L.D., TOMCZAK, K. and ST. JOHN, A.C. (1978). Bacteriophages inhibit degradation of abnormal proteins in *E. coli*. Nature, 275, 424.

17) CAPECCHI, M., CAPECCHI, N.E., HUGHES, S. and WAHL, G.M. (1974).

Selective degradation of abnormal proteins in mammalian tissue. Proc. Nat. Acad. Sci., 71, 4732.

18) KNOWLES, S.E., GUNN, J.M., HANSON, R.W. and BALLARD, F.J. (1975). Increased degradation rates of protein synthesized in hepatoma cells in the presence of amino acid analogues. Biochem. J., 146, 595.

19) PROUTY, W.F., KARNOVSKY, J.M. and GOLDBERG, A.L. (1975). Degradation of abnormal proteins in *Escherichia coli*. J. Biol. Chem., 250, 1112.

20) HENDIL, K.B. (1975). Degradation of abnormal proteins in HeLa cells. J. Cell. Physiol., 87, 289.

21) KNOWLES, S.E. and BALLARD, F.J. (1976). Selective control of the degradation of normal and aberrant proteins in Reuber H35 hepatoma cells. Biochem. J., 156, 609.

22) BALLARD, F.J., HOPGOOD, M., RESHEF, L. and HANSON, R. (1974). Degradation of phosphoenol pyruvate carboxykinase (guanosine triphosphate) *in vivo* and *in vitro*. Biochem. J., 144, 531.

23) HOPGOOD, M. and BALLARD, F.J. (1974). The relative stability of liver cytosol enzymes incubated *in vitro*. Biochem. J., 144, 371.

24) SEGAL, H.L., WINKLER, J.R. and MIYAGI, M. (1974). Relationship between degradation rates of proteins *in vivo* and their susceptibility to lysosomal proteases. J. Biol. Chem., 249, 6364.

25) SEGAL, H.L., ROTHSTEIN, D. and WINKLER, J. (1976). A correlation between turnover rates and lipophilic affinities of soluble rat liver proteins. Biochem. Biophys. Res. Commun., 73, 79.

26) POOLE, B. and WIBO, M. (1973). Protein degradation in cultured cells. J. Biol. Chem., 248, 6221.

27) WARBURTON, M.J. and POOLE, B. (1977). Effect of medium composition on protein degradation and DNA synthesis in rat embryo fibroblasts. Proc. Nat. Acad. Sci., 74, 2427.

28) LEE, G. T.-Y. and ENGELHARDT, D.L. (1977). Protein metabolism during growth of Vero cells. J. Cellul. Physiol., 92, 293.

29) HENDIL, K.B. (1977). Intracellular protein degradation in growing, in density inhibited, and in serum-restricted fibroblast cultures. J. Cellul. Physiol., 92, 353.

30) TANAKA, K. and ICHIHARA, A. (1977). Effect of the growth state on protein turnover in two lines of cultured BHK cells. J. Cellul. Physiol., 93, 407.

31) BRADLEY, M.O. (1977). Regulation of protein degradation in normal and transformed human cells. J. Biol. Chem., 252, 5310.

32) BRADLEY, M.O., DICE, J.F., HAYFLICK, L. and SCHIMKE, R.T. (1975). Protein alterations in aging W138 cells as determined by proteolytic susceptibility. Exp. Cell Res., 96, 103.

33) KAFTORY, A., HERSHKO, A. and FRY, M. (1978). Protein turnover in senescent cultured chick embryo fibroblasts. J. Cellul. Physiol., 94, 147.

34) RANNELS, D.E., KAO, R. and MORGAN, H.E. (1975). Effect of insulin on protein turnover in heart muscle. J. Biol. Chem., 250, 1694.

35) DEMARTINO, G.N. and GOLDBERG, A.L. (1978). Thyroid hormones control lysosomal enzyme activities in liver and skeletal muscle. Proc. Nat. Acad. Sci., 75, 1369.

36) HUBBARD, A. and COHN, Z. (1975). Externally disposed plasma membrane protein. J. Cell. Biol., 64, 461.

37) DOYLE, D., BAUMANN, H., ENGLAND, B., FRIEDMAN, E., HAU, E. and TWETO, J. (1978). Biogenesis of plasma membrane glycoproteins in hepatoma tissue culture cells. J. Biol. Chem., 253, 965.

38) BAUMANN, H. and DOYLE, D. (1978). Turnover of plasma membrane glycoproteins and glycolipids of hepatoma tissue culture cells. J. Biol. Chem., 253, 4408.

39) FAMBROUGH, D.M. and DEVREOTES, P.N. (1976). In: Biogenesis and Turnover of Membrane Macromolecules (ed., J.S. Cook) p. 121. Development of chemical excitability in skeletal muscle. Raven Press, New York.

40) GORDEN, P., CARPENTER, J.L., COHEN, S. and ORCI, L. (1978). Epidermal growth factor: morphological demonstration of bind-

ing, internalization and lysosomal association in human fibroblasts. Proc. Nat. Acad. Sci., 25, 5025.

41) ETLINGER, J.D. and GOLDBERG, A.L. (1977). A soluble ATP-dependent proteolytic system responsible for the degradation of abnormal proteins in reticulocytes. Proc. Nat. Acad. Sci., 74, 54.

42) BALLARD, F.J. and HOPGOOD, M. (1976). Inactivation of phosphoenolpyruvate carboxykinase (GTP) by liver extracts. Biochem. J., 154, 717.

43) VARANDANI, P.T. (1973). Unmasking of glutathione-insulin transhydrogenase in rat liver microsomal membrane. Biochim. Biophys. Acta, 304, 642.

44) ANSORGE, S., BOKLEY, P., KIRSCHKE, H., LANGNER, J., WIEDEWANDERS, B. and HANSON, H. (1973). Metabolism of insulin and glycagon. 32, 27.

45) ASHFORD, T.P. and PORTER, K.R. (1962). Cytoplasmic components in hepatic cell lysosomes. J. Cell. Biol., 12, 198.

46) NOVIKOFF, A.B. and SHIN, W.-Y. (1978). Endoplasmic reticulum and autophagy in rat hepatocytes. Proc. Nat. Acad. Sci., 75, 5039.

47) HOLTZMAN, E. (1976). Lysosomes: A survey. Springer Verlag, New York.

48) PFEIFER, U. (1978). Inhibition by insulin of the formation of autophagic vacuoles in rat liver. J. Cell. Biol., 78, 152.

49) DICE, J.F., WALKER, C.D., BYRNE, B. and CARDILL, A. (1978). General characteristics of protein degradation in diabetes and starvation. Proc. Nat. Acad. Sci., 75, 2093.

50) STACEY, D.W. and ALLFREY, V.G. (1977). Evidence for the autophagy of microinjected proteins in HeLa cells. J. Cell. Biol., 75, 807.

51) BANNO, Y., SHIOTANI, T., TOWATARI, T., YOSKIKAWA, D., KATSUNUMA, T., AFTING, E.-G. and KATUNUMA, N. (1975). Studies of new intracellular proteases in various organs of rat. Eur. J. Biochem., 52, 59.

52) KATUNUMA, N., KOMINAMI, E., BANNO, Y., KITO, K., AOKI, Y. and URATA, G. (1976). Concept on mechanism and regulation of intracellular eznyme degradation in mammalian tissues. Adv. Reviews Enzyme Regul., 14, 325.

53) HAAS, R., HEINRICH, P.C., TESCH, R. and WITT, I. (1978). Cleavage specificity of the serine proteinase from the rat liver mitochondria. Biochem., Biophys. Res. Commun., 85, 1039.

54) DEAN, R.T. (1975). Concerning a possible mechanism for selective capture of cytoplasmic proteins by lysosomes. Biochem. Biophys. Res. Commun., 67, 604.

55) DEAN, R.T. (1975). Lysosomal enzymes as agents of turnover of soluble cytoplasmic proteins. Eur. J. Biochem., 58, 9.

56) LLOYD, J.B. (1978). The role of lysosomes in turnover of cytoplasmic exogenous proteins. J. Biochem. Soc. Trans., 6, 500.

57) NEELY, A.N. and MORTIMORE, G.E. (1974). Localization of products of endogenous proteolysis in lysosomes of perfused rat liver. Biochem. Biophys. Res. Commun., 59, 680.

58) HAIDER, M. and SEGAL, H.L. (1972). Some characteristics of the alanine aminotransferase and arginase inactivating system of lysosomes. Arch. of Biochemistry and Biophys., 148, 228.

59) DEAN, R.T. (1975). Direct evidence of lysosomes in degradation of intracellular proteins. Nature, 257, 414.

60) RUDEK, D., DIEN, P. and SCHNEIDER, D.L. (1978). Identification of tryptophan pyrrolase in liver lysosomes after treatment of rats with hydrocortisone and chloroquine. Biochem. Biophys. Res. Commun., 82, 342.

61) FURUSAWA, M., NISHIMURA, T., YAMAIZUMI, M. and OKADA, Y. (1974). Injection of foreign substances into single cells by cell fusion. Nature, 249, 449.

62) SCHLEGEL, R. and RECHSTEINER, M. (1975). Microinjection of thymidine kinase and bovine serum albumin into mammalian cells by fusion with red blood cells. Cell, 5, 371.

63) LOYTER, A., ZAKAI, N. and KULKA, R. (1975). "Ultramicroinjec-

tion" of macromolecules or small particles into animal cells. J. Cell. Biol., 66, 292.

64) RYSER, H. J.-P. (1963). Comparison of the incorporation of tyrosine and its iodinated analogs into the proteins of Ehrlich ascites tumor cells and rat liver slices. Biochem. Biophys. Acta, 78, 759.

65) SCHLEGEL, R.A., IVERSON, P. and RECHSTEINER, M. (1978). The turnover of tRNAs microinjected into animal cells. Nucl. Acid. Res., 5, 3715.

66) RECHSTEINER, M. (1978). Red cell-mediated microinjection. Nat. Cancer Inst. Monogr., 48, 57.

67) ZAVORTINK, M., THACHER, T. and RECHSTEINER, M. (1979). Degradation of proteins microinjected into cultured mammalian cells. J. Cellul. Physiol., 100, 175.

68) WASSERMAN, M., KULKA, R.G. and LOYTER, A. (1977). Degradation and localization of IgG injected into friend erythroleukemia cells by fusion with erythrocyte ghosts. FEBS Lett., 83, 48.

69) FRITZ, P.J., VESELL, E.S., WHITE, E.L. and PRUITT, K.M. (1969). The roles of synthesis and degradation in determining tissue concentrations of lactate dehydrogenase 5. Proc. Nat. Acad. Sci., 62, 558.

70) DESCHATRETTE, J. and WEISS, M.C. (1975). Extinction of liver-specific functions in hybrids between differentiated and dedifferentiated rat hepatoma cells. Som. Cell. Gen., 1, 279.

71) GARDNER, D.A., SATO, G.H. and KAPLAN, N.O. (1972). Pyridine nucleotides in normal and nicotinamide depleted adrenal tumor cell cultures. Dev. Biol., 28, 84.

72) AOYAGI, T. and UMEZAWA, H. (1975). Proteases and biological control (eds, E. Reich, D.B. Rifkin and E. Shaw). Cold Spring Harbor Laboratory Press, p. 429.

73) SCHNEBLI, H.P. (1975). Proteases and biological control (eds, E. Reich, D.B. Rifkin and E. Shaw). Cold Spring Harbor Laboratory Press, p. 785.

74) OVERATH, P., SCHAIRER, H.U. and STOFFEL, W. (1974). Correlation of *in vivo* and *in vitro* phase transitions of membrane lipids in *Escherichia coli*. Proc. Nat. Acad. Sci., 67, 606.

75) WILSON, G. and FOX, C.F. (1971). Biogenesis of microbial transport systems: evidence for coupled incorporation of newly synthesized lipids and proteins into membrane. J. Mol. Biol., 55, 49.

76) LAGUNOFF, D. and WAN, H. (1974). Temperature dependence of most cell histamine secretion. J. Cell. Biol., 61, 809.

77) PETIT, V. and EDIDIN, M. (1974). Lateral phase separation of lipids in plasma membranes: effect of temperature on the mobility of membrane antigens. Science, 184, 1183.

78) PLAGEMANN, P.G.W. and RICHEY, D.P. (1974). Transport of nucleosides, nucleic acid bases, choline and glucose by animal cells in culture. Biochim. Biophys. Acta., 344, 263.

79) WISNIESKI, B.J., PARKES, J.G. HUANG, Y.O. and FOX, C.F. (1974). Physical and physiological evidence for two phase transitions in cytoplasmic membranes of animal cells. Proc. Nat. Acad. Sci., 71, 4381.

80) STEINMAN, R.M., SILVER, J.M. and COHN, Z.A. (1974). Pinocytosis in fibroblasts. J. Cell. Biol., 63, 949.

81) MAHONEY, E.M., HAMILL, A.L., SCOTT, W.A. and COHN, Z.A. (1977). Response of endocytosis to altered fatty acyl composition of macrophage phospholipids. Proc. Nat. Acad. Sci., 74, 4895.

82) SANDVIG, K. and OLSNES, S. (1979). Effect of temperature on the uptake, excretion and degradation of abrin and ricin by HeLa cells. Exp. Cell. Res., 121, 15.

83) BERGMANN, M. and FRUTON, J.S. (1941). The specificity of proteinases. Adv. in Enzymol., 1, 63.

84) PITTMAN, R.C. and STEINBERG, D. (1978). A new approach for assessing cumulative lysosomal degradation of proteins or other macromolecules. Biochem. Biophys. Res. Commun., 81, 1254.

85) EHRENREICH, B.A. and COHN, Z.A. (1969). The fate of peptides

pinocytosed by macrophages *in vitro*. J. Exp. Med., 129, 227.

86) YAMAIZUMI, M., UCHIDA, Y., OKADA, Y. and FURUSAWA, M. (1978). Neutralization of diphtheria toxin in living cells by microinjection of antifragment A contained within resealed erythrocyte ghosts. Cell, 13, 227.

TRANSFER OF FUNCTIONAL COMPONENTS INTO PLASMA MEMBRANE OF LIVING CELLS: A NEW TOOL IN MEMBRANE RESEARCH

A. Loyter, D.J. Volsky, M. Beigel,
H. Ginsburg and Z.I. Cabantchik

Department of Biological Sciences
Institute of Life Sciences
The Hebrew University of Jerusalem
Jerusalem, Israel

1. INTRODUCTION

It is known for years that cells are endowed with a periplasmic structure, the plasma membrane, which served both as an insulating surface and as a medium of communication between the external and internal cell world. Due to its intrinsic structural properties and to specific mechanisms, the cell membrane gives selective admittance to particular agents while excluding many others. These properties although important for controlling the cellular milieu, have limited on the other hand, the access to the intracellular apparatus of probes and therapeutic agents. This restricted, in the past, the scope of studies of genetic and membrane engineering as well as chemical therapy.

With the advent of methods for membrane fusion (1, 2), it became possible to deliver otherwise impermeant agents into the cytosol of recipient cells (3-5) and thus pave new routes for studying a variety of biological processes. While in our laboratory (3-6) as well as in several others (4, 5), we emphasized the use of resealed erythrocyte ghosts as a vehicle for entrapping macromolecules and deliver them into cells via *Sendai* virus mediated cell fusion, others have used liposomes for gaining access to the cell interior (7).

Methods for membrane fusion, however, might also serve as a means for introducing molecules into plasma membranes, and thus help to elucidate the relationship between particular membrane function and the relevant membrane components. For instance the transfer of functional agents such as enzymes, transporters, immunoglobulins, hormones and virus receptors into membranes of living cells lacking the function provide an excellent tool for probing biological system and for medical research.

In recent studies, fusion of membranes were instrumental for demonstrating the functional coupling between a catacholamine receptor residing in one cell membrane and adenylate cyclase residing in receptor deficient cell membrane (8). These studies showed that individual components originally present in different membranes can intermix after fusion and yield new functional complexes (8). In other studies (9), liposomes containing cytochrome oxidase were used as a carrier for introducing the enzyme into membrane of human red blood cells. However, very few studies have hitherto shown the insertion of functionally and structurally defined components into membranes of living cells.

We shall attempt to describe here the present status of *in vivo* implantation of membrane polypeptide by means of viral mediated fusion as well as access their possible use for physiological means. We shall refer to two main implantation approaches according to the model system and the respective vehicles used for inserting the components into plasma membranes of living eucaryotic cells. In the first case we have used the membranes of the human red blood cell

(RBC) as the donor of membrane polypeptides and associated function, the Friend erythroleukemic cell (FELC) as the recipient cell system and intact *Sendai* virus as the fusogenic agent (10, 11). In the second case we made use of the fact that the *Sendai* virus envelopes (VE) are fused with membranes of living cells such as FELC and become integrated in their plasma membranes without affecting cell viability (2, 12). We therefore develop techniques for: (A) isolating membrane proteins (MP) and incorporate them into reconstituted VE and, (B) implanting the VE containing MP into cells such as FELC (13, 14).

We shall provide structural and functional evidence for the implantation of the anion transport system of human red blood cell membranes, which have been associated with a particular RBC membrane polypeptide of 100,000 daltons commonly referred to as band 3 (B_3) (15, 16) into FELC. The FELC were chosen as recipient cells on the basis that they are demonstrably deficient in the anion transport classically associated with red blood cell membranes (10, 11, 17). We shall demonstrate that FELC which acquired band 3 polypeptides by fusion either with RBC in the presence of *Sendai* virus or with the fusogenic band 3-virus enveloped (B_3-VE) hybrid vesicles acquired a high anion transport capacity. Since anion transport is, by its nature, a trans-membrane property, the results would indicate the successful fusion-medicated integration of exogenous membrane polypeptide into plasma membrane of living cells.

2. TRANSFER OF RBC MEMBRANE COMPONENTS INTO PLASMA MEMBRANES OF LIVING CELLS

A simple useful model for studying the integration of protein into plasma membranes of living eucaryotic cells makes use of the human RBC as a membrane donor, FELC as a membrane acceptor and *Sendai* virus as an agent for accomplishing fusion between the donor and acceptor membranes. The structural and functional marker of integral erythrocyte membrane protein was band 3 whose association with anion transport in the RBC (particularly transmembranal Cl^--exchange) has been well documented and extensively reviewed (15, 16). The rationale of our approach was based on the idea that fusion should lead to the integration of the erythrocyte membrane components (i.e., band 3) into FELC membranes with the concomitant appearance of a fast component of Cl^--exchange otherwise absent in FELC (10, 11, 17). We have first observed that after fusion with RBC, the plasma membranes of FELC showed by electron microscopic techniques, antigenic determinants of RBC origin widely spread out and exposed on their external surface (11). However, in order to ascertain that the above exposure denoted the presence of genuine integrated rather than adsorbed RBC membrane protein, we subjected the fused cells to more vigorous tests. These consisted of functional assays aimed at elucidating whether a transmembrane anion exchange capacity with properties similar to those of RBC was acquired and maintained by FELC after fusion. We have first establisehd, in line with previous studies (15), that Cl^--exchange at 0^oC was a fast process across RBC but demonstrably slow across FELC. In contrast $SO_4^=$-exchange (at 37^oC) was considerably faster in FELC than in RBC (11). In addition, both Cl^- and $SO_4^=$ exchange were fully inhibited by non-penetrating probes such as 4,4'-di-isothiocyano-stilbene-2-2'-disulfonic acid (DIDS) and the 4,4'-dinitro analog (DNDS) in RBC but only poorly in FELC (11). These various properties, summarized in Table 1, were used in order to test the alleged integration of band 3 in FELC after fusion with RBC. We observed that the latter indeed displayed a fast component of Cl^--exchange at 0^oC which showed high susceptibility to either DIDS or DNDS. Since neither a fast Cl^--exchange properties nor significant susceptibility to the above inhibitors was observed in unfused FELC the results were in line with the aformentioned claim of band 3 integration in FELC. Various quantitative tests of sulfate exchange across RBC, FELC, mixture of RBC and FELC and RBC-fused-FELC indicated that the observed anion flexes took place only in RBC-fused-FELC (11). These tests were based on the fact that $^{35}SO_4^{=}$ fastly exited from FELC even in the presence of inhibitors but was fully retained in RBC under the same conditions (Ref. 11 and Table 1). Therefore, any sulfate retention in a given suspension of RBC-fused-FELC served as a measure of the presence of sealed RBC membranes. In our observations only trace amounts of (^{35}S) were retained by the fused FELC, (11), thus eliminating the possibility that erythrocytes adsorbed to FELC contributed to the fast Cl^--exchange displayed by RBC-fused-FELC.

Table 1. *Stimulation of Cl^- transport across membranes of FELC fused with intact RBC.*

System	Cl^--exchange	$SO_4^{=}$-exchange
RBC	Fast at 0^oC ($t\frac{1}{2}$ = 0.38 min)	Slow at 0^oC and 37^oC ($t\frac{1}{2}$ at 37^oC = 20 min)
DIDS or DNDS treated RBC	Fully inhibited	Fully inhibited
FELC	Very slow at 0^oC ($t\frac{1}{2}$ = 38 min)	Relatively high at 37^oC ($t\frac{1}{2}$ = 2 min)
DIDS or DNDS treated FELC	Poorly inhibited	Poorly inhibited
FELC fused with RBC	Appearance of a fast component, completely inhibited by DIDS ($t\frac{1}{2}$ of 0^oC = 1-4 min depending on the fusion yield)	
FELC fused with DIDS treated RBC	The fast component of CL^--exchange is completely inhibited	

All experimental conditions as described in Ref. 11.

3. IMPLANTATION OF ISOLATED BAND 3 PROTEIN INTO PLASMA MEMBRANES OF FELC BY RECONSTITUTED ENVELOPES OF SENDAI VIRUS

The infection of cells by enveloped viruses such as *Sendai* virus is comprised of two main steps (2, 19): (A) The binding of the virus to the cell surface, and (B) The fusion of the viral envelope with the plasma membrane of the recipient cell with the concomitant injection of the viral nucleocapsid into the cell interior. Since as part of the fusion process, the viral envelope becomes integrated into the cell plasma membranes, we explored the possibility of using it for incorporating defined membrane components (MP), first by incorporating proteins into the viral envelope, and subsequently used the viral envelope (VE) as a vehicle for inserting the relevant component into the recipient cell membrane (13, 14). The method for isolation of pure and fusogenic viral envelopes was described elsewhere (20). Briefly, it consisted of Triton X-100 extraction of intact viruses which yielded a detergent soluble fraction comprised of viral envelope glycoproteins. Upon removal of the detergent by dialysis, we observed the appearance of vesicles of viral envelopes which displayed characteristic viral spikes (20). These vesicles were demonstrably fusogenic towards cells such as FELC as monitored by microscopic methods (20).

The implantation of defined functional membrane protein, band 3 (B_3) into FELC was accomplished in two major steps: (Ref. 14 and Fig. 1). First, functional B_3 was isolated in Triton X-100 according to previously developed techniques (15, 18) and it was mixed with detergent solution of viral envelopes (Fig. 1). Upon removal of the detergent by co-dialysis of the above mixture, vesicles containing the aforementioned proteins formed spontaneously (Ref. 14 and Fig. 1). That a substantial proportion of the vesicles were of hybrid nature, i.e., containing band 3 as well as viral envelope glycoproteins were verified by various immunological tests. These showed the precipitation of only [^{3}H]-DIDS labelled band 3 by anti-viral antibodies added to VE coreconstituted with [^{3}H] DIDS-labelled band 3 (B_3-VE hybrids) but not of isolated [^{3}H]-labelled band 3. In the second step (see Fig. 1), the hybrids B_3-VE vesicle preparation were added to FELC which were then examined for binding of vesicles at 4°C and for the integration of the B_3-VE polypeptides after 37°C incubation (Fig. 1). In line with our previous observation with intact RBC (see above), we obtained first structural data for the alleged incorporation of isolated band 3 as well as of viral envelope glycoproteins into the FELC membranes (14). Similar to our previous

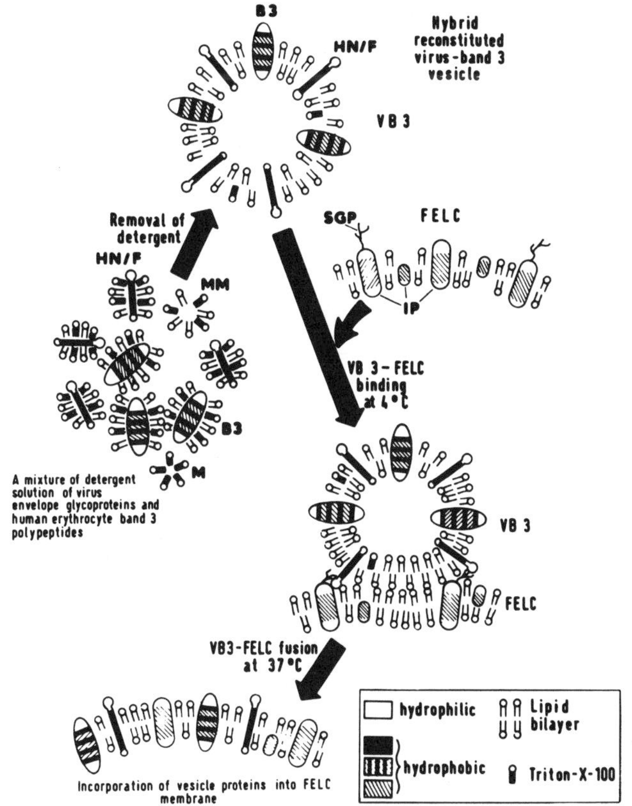

Fig. 1. *Schematic representation of the membrane protein implantation method.* In the scheme we have incorporated ideas regarding the mechanism of solubilization of membranes by detergents and the

reassembly of membrane components upon removal of detergent (20). HF/F = agglutinin-neuraminidase or fusion glycoprotein of *Sendai* virus envelope; B3 = human erythrocyte band 3 polypeptide; M = detergent micelle; MM = mixed membrane phospholipid-detergent micelle; FELC = Friend erythroleukemic cells; SGP = sialoglycoprotein; IP = integral membrane protein.

work with RBC, we subjected also the FELC which were incubated with various preparations of vesicles to a series of Cl^- transport tests aimed to detect the incorporation of functional band 3 polypeptides. The results obtained with these preparations are depicted in Table 2.

Table 2. *The appearance of Cl^- exchange transport system in FELC fused with B_3-VE hybrid vesicles.*

FELC incubated with:	Rate constant (K) of Cl^- ingress (sec^{-1}) x 10^2 measured at 0^oC
None	0.03
B_3 (4^oC)	0.05
B_3 37^oC)	0.06
VE (37^oC)	0.07
Hybrid B_3-VE (4^oC)	0.05
Hybrid B_3-VE (37^oC)	5.5
Hybrid DIDS-B_3-VE	0.05
Hybrid B_3-VE (37^oC) + Antiviral antibody	0.05

Adapted from Ref. 14. RBC displayed at 0^oC a K = 3 sec^{-1} x 10^2. For experimental conditions, see Refs. 14 and 20.

They indicate that a specific fast Cl^--exchange component, operative at 0^oC in RBC, was acquired by FELC only after binding and fusion of B_3-VE hybrid vesicles. Since the above component was fully inhibited by pretreating B_3 vesicles with DIDS, a covalent and specific inhibitor of anion exchange (15), our results indicate that Cl^--exchange capacity acquired by FELC after fusion with B_3-VE vesicles was of a specific functional nature. Our quantitative estimation (14) indicates that ca. 30% of all FELC acquired functional band 3 polypeptides by fusion with B_3-VE vesicles. For this fraction of the cell population, the rate constant of Cl^--exchange was ca. two-fold higher than exhibited by RBC (Table 2). Taking into consideration the fact that the density of B_3 polypeptides was smaller in B_3-VE fused FELC than in RBC and that the FELC have at least a two-fold smaller surface to volume ratio than the RBC, the above difference in transport rate constant clearly underscores the high transmembrane functional activity of B_3 incorporated into FELC. Furthermore, it is conveivable that the FELC plasma membrane provided a much more favourable matrix for harboring B_3 polypeptides and for expresssing Cl^--exchange than the RBC membrane. This might have resulted from the respective lipid composition and plasticity of the membranes, factors which are likely to affect membrane protein structure and function.

4. CONCLUSIONS

The present work describes the insertion of functional membrane protein into plasma membrane of living eucaryotic cells via *Sendai* virus mediated cell fusion and via fusion of viral envelopes co-reconstituted with membrane proteins. While both methods made use of the fusogenic properties of the *Sendai* virus envelope, they differ operationally in the sense that the first uses intact viruses and intact membranes as the respective vesicles and donors of proteins, whereas the second uses isolated viral envelopes as carrier and donors of the membrane proteins. With both methods FELC served as the recipient cell for harboring the implanted proteins in their plasma membranes. Both methods offer various advantages in that (1) they are conservative of the isolated functional protein; (2) they lead to massive fusion (i.e., implantation) without affecting cell viability; and (3) they lead to the implantation of a new membrane property in a living cell. It is also reasonable to assume that these methods should be applicable to other cell lines inasmuch as a large variety of cells are susceptible to *Sendai* virus fusion. However, it is still premature to predict whether any given cell might provide to an implanted protein the appropriate milieu for expressing its function.

Beside the intrinsic merit of the above methods in studies of basic membrane phenomena, it is expected that they will provide a useful tool for implantation of receptors, hormones, viruses, lectins, etc. into membranes of cells otherwise lacking these receptors. The present described methods are also expected to be instrumental for cellular therapeutic at the membrane level and for bioengineering systems at the cellular level.

5. ACKNOWLEDGEMENTS

This work was supported by grants from the National Council for Research and Development, Jerusalem, Israel, the G.F.F. Munich, Federal Republic of Germany (to A.L.) and the USA-Israel Binational Science Foundation (to Z.I.C.).

6. REFERENCES

1) POSTE, G. and ALLISON, A.C. (1973). Membrane fusion. Biochem. Biophys. Acta, 300, 421.
2) POSTE, G. and PASTERNAK, C.A. (1978). Virus induced cell fusion. In: Cell Surface Reviews (eds. G. Poste and G.L. Nicolson) Vol. 5, p. 305, North Holland Publishing Co., Amsterdam.
3) LOYTER, A., ZAKAI, N. and KULKA, R.G. (1975). Ultramicroinjection of macromolecules or small particles into animal cells. A new technique based on virus induced cell fusion. J. Cell Biol. 66, 292.

4) SCHEGEL, R.A. and RECHSTEINER, M. (1978). Red cell-mediated microinjection of macromolecules into mammalian cells. In: Methods in Cell Biology (ed., D.M. Prescott), Vol. XX, p. 341. Academic Press, New York.

5) FURUSAWA, M, YAMAIZUMI, M., NISHIMURA, T., UCHIDA, T. and OKADA, Y. (1976). Use of erythrocyte ghosts for injection of substances into animal cells by cell fusion. In: Methods in Cell Biology (ed., D.M. Prescott), Vol. XIV p. 73, Academic Press, New York.

6) WASSERMAN, M., ZAKAI, N., LOYTER, A. and KULKA, R.G. (1976). A quantitative study of ultramicroinjection of macromolecules into animal cells. Cell, 7, 551.

7) POSTE, G., PAPAHADJOPOULOS, D. and VAIL, W.J. (1976). Lipid vesicles as carriers for introducing biologically active materials into cells. In: Methods in Cell Biology (ed., D.M. Prescott), Vol. XIV, p. 33, Academic Press, New York.

8) SCHRAMM, M., ORLY, J., EIMERL, S. and KORNER, M. (1977). Coupling of hormone receptors to adenylate cyclase of different cells by cell fusion. Nature, 268, 310.

9) EYTAN, A.E. and BROZA, R. (1979). Israel J. Med. Sci., 15,66 (Abstract).

10) BEIGEL, M, GINSBURG, H: CABANTCHIK, Z.I. KULKA, R.G. and LOYTER, A. (1979). Incorporation of human erythrocyte Cl^--exchange system into Friend cells by virus-induced cell fusion. Israel J. Med. Sci., 15, 68 (Abstract).

11) BEIGEL, M., VOLSKY, D.J., GINSBURG, H, CABANTCHIK, Z.I. and LOYTER, A. (1979). Functional incorporation of the human erythrocyte chloride exchange system into plasma membranes of Friend erythroleukemic cells by *Sendai* virus induced cell fusion. Exp. Cell Res., submitted for publication.

12) OKADA, Y., KIM, J., MAEDA, Y. and KOSEKI, I. (1974). Specific movement of cell membranes fused with HVJ (*Sendai* virus). Proc. Natl. Acad. Sci. U.S.A., 71, 2043.

13) VOLSKY, D.J. LOYTER, A. (1979). The use of *Sendai* virus envelopes as a vehicle for transferring isolated erythrocyte membrane proteins into plasma membrane of Friend erythroleukemic cells. Israel J. Med. Sci., in press.

14) VOLSKY, D,J., CABANTCHIK, Z.I., BEIGEL, M. and LOYTER, A. (1979). Implantation of the isolated human erythrocyte anion channel into plasma membrane of Friend erythroleukemic cells by the use of *Sendai* virus envelopes. Proc. Natl. Acad. Sci. U.S.A., in press

15) CABANTCHIK, Z.I., KNAUF, P.A. and ROTHSTEIN, A. (1978). The anion transport system of the red blook cell. The role of membrane protein evaluated by the use of probes. Biochim. Biophysis. Acta, 515, 239.

16) ROTHSTEIN, A. (1978). The functional role of band 3 protein of the red blood cell. In: Molecular Specialization and Symmetry in Membrane Function (ed., A.K. Solomon and M. Karnosky), p. 128, Harvard Book in Biophysics., Number 2, Cambridge, Mass.

17) HARPER, P., MACDOUGALL, A. and KNAUF, P.A. (1977). Fed. Proc. 36, 564 (Abstract).

18) GERRITSEN, W.J., VERKLEY, A.J. ZWALL, R.F.A. and VAN DEENEN, L.L.M. (1978). Freeze-fracture appearance and disposition of band 3 protein from the human erythrocyte membrane in lipid vesicles. Eur. J. Biochem., 85, 255.

19) ROTH, R. and KLENK, H.D. (1977). Structure and assembly of viral envelopes. In: Cell Surface Reviews (ed., G. Poste and G.L. Nicolson), Vol. 2, p. 47, North Holland Publishing Co., Amsterdam.

20) VOLSKY, D.J. and LOYTER, A. (1978). An efficient method for reassembly of fusogenic *Sendai* virus envelopes after stabilization of intact virions with Triton X-100. FEBS Letters, 92, 190.

LIPOSOMES AS MACROMOLECULAR CARRIERS FOR THE INTRODUCTION OF RNA AND DNA INTO CELLS

D. Papahadjopoulos*, T. Wilson# and R. Taber※

**Cancer Research Institute, UC San Francisco Medical Center, San Francisco, CA 94143, U.S.A.*

#*Department of Physiology and Biophysics, CMDNJ-Rutgers Medical School, Piscataway, New Jersey 08854, U.S.A.*

※*Department of Viral Oncology and Experimental Pathology, Roswell Park Memorial Institute, Buffalo, New York 14263, U.S.A.*

1. INTRODUCTION

Liposomes are vesicles composed of one or more lipid bilayers completely surrounding an internal aqueous space. They are usually composed of phospholipids either in pure form or in combination with other amphipathic molecules such as sterols, long chain bases or acids. The structure of liposomes varies from large (0.5 to 5μ) multilamellar vesicles (1) to small (~300Å) unilamellar vesicles (2, 3) or to unilamellar vesicles of intermediate size (4-6).

The main features of liposomes that have made them important as macromolecular carriers are the following: Their characteristic morphology, where a relatively impermeable membrane completely encloses an aqueous space; and their ability to encapsulate various solutes present in the aqueous phase during their formation. The concept behind the use of liposomes as carriers of drugs and macromolecules is related to an expected protection of the encapsulated molecules in the extracellular medium, as well as to an increased uptake into cells by mechanisms that are not normally available for these molecules. Some of these expectations have been verified through studies in various laboratories during the last few years. Such studies have shown that liposome encapsulation can enhance the uptake of the encapsulated substances into cells, and it can increase their pharmacological efficacy. A critical evaluation of the early literature indicates reasons for both optimism and caution in relation to the future use of liposomes as macromolecular carriers. The simplicity of the initial concept can lead to an underestimate of the technical difficulties of liposome preparation, and the biological complexities in relation to the mechanism of interaction of liposomes with various cells. Several recent reviews have discussed these early results in considerable detail (7-13).

2. METHODOLOGY OF LIPOSOME PREPARATION

An informal agreement was reached during a recent conference on the use of a three letter acronym to designate the type of liposome such as multilamellar vesicles (MLV) or small unilamellar vesicles (SUV) or large unilamellar vesicles (LUV) with the chemical composition in parenthesis after the acronym (14, p. 367). The term liposome is therefore to be used as a generic name to include all types of artificial vesicles composed of phospholipids and other amphipathic lipids.

The original preparation of Bangham *et al.* (1) consisting of multilamellar vesicles (MLV), has been very useful in defining many membrane properties and was the basis for the development (2) of the sonicated unilamellar vesicles (SUV). However, both preparations show a relatively low volume of entrapped aqueous space per mole of lipid and restricted ability to encapsulate large macromolecules. The ethanol injection method (15, 16) produces vesicles of about the same size as SUV with the same shortcomings. The ether infusion technique (5) produces large unilamellar vesicles with high captured volume per mole of lipid, but the efficiency of encapsulation is relatively low. Several other techniques for preparing LUV liposomes of varying size have been described and reviewed recently (17). Most of our work with viral RNA has used the LUV produced by Ca^{2+} fusion (4), which has proven valuable for encapsulating polio virus (18) and purified viral RNA (19). A new method (REV) which was developed for the efficient encapsulation of macromolecules (6) has been used recently in our laboratory for the encapsulation and cellular delivery of DNA. The most recent methodological improvement involves the production of liposomes of well-defined size distribution by extrusion of MLV or LUV through a nucleopore polycarbonate membrane (20). Table 1 summarizes the relative properties of various liposome preparations developed in our laboratory.

3. INTERACTION OF LIPOSOMES WITH CELLS *IN VITRO*

The mechanism of interaction of lipid vesicles with cells in culture has been studied in detail during the last few years in several laboratories, and the results were reviewed recently (12, 21). The evidence has been obtained with various types of vesicles and cells under varying conditions, and it therefore seems contradictory in several cases. There is general agreement, however, that liposomes are taken up quite efficiently by cells in culture, that the process of uptake is temperature dependent, but in most cases it does not require metabolic energy, and that at least part of the vesicle contents are incorporated along with the lipids. In cases where the uptake has been quantitated, it appears that several million SUV liposomes per cell can be incorporated within a few hours

Table 1. *Comparison of various liposome preparations.*

Properties	MLV	SUV	LUV#	REV
Diameter* (microns)	0.2-10	0.02-0.05	0.2-1.0	0.2-1.0
Encapsulation⌑ Efficiency (%)	5-15	0.5-1.0	5-15	35-65
Captured⌑ Volume (μl/mg)	4	0.5	9	14

Vesicles preparations were composed of PG/PC/Chol (1/4/5 mole ratios) prepared at 66 μmoles/ml in phosphate buffered saline.
#Prepared from PS/Chol (1/1) by fusion of SUV with Ca^{2+}, followed by EDTA.
*Diameter range was based on EM observation by negative stain and freeze fracture.
⌑Encapsulation efficiency and captured volume were obtained with radioactive sucrose as marker.
MLV: Multilamellar vesicles. SUV: Small unilamellar vesicles. LUV: Large unilamelar vesicles. REV: Vesicles prepared by Reverse Phase Evaporation.

without overt cytotoxic effects (22). Concerning the mechanism of uptake, the evidence indicates that it could involve any of the following: fusion with the plasma membrane (22, 23-29) endocytosis (24, 29, 30) adsorption to the cell surface (31, 32) or molecular exchange (23, 33). The predominance of any of these mechanisms is controlled by the chemistry and physical properties of the liposomes and perhaps by the cell type and the state of the cell. Since the evidence for most of the mechanism of uptake is indirect and the contribution of each type of uptake is very difficult to quantitate, most conclusions that have been drawn up-to-now should be considered at best only qualitative statements. There is clearly need for further work in this area, especially in developing quantitative assays for estimating the extent of fusion and distinguishing it from classical endocytosis or adsorption followed by molecular exchange at the cell surface.

4. INFECTIVITY OF LIPOSOME-ENCAPSULATED POLIOVIRUS RNA

The infectivity of encapsulated poliovirus RNA was measured by two types of plaque assays (19). The first, a direct plaque assay, involved the exposure of cell monolayers to RNA leprations with subsequent washing, incubation and staining to indicate plaque formation. Encapsulated RNA formed about 5 x 10^3 pfu/ng RNA applied while free RNA, either alone or mixed with preformed vesicles, showed little or no biological activity. Free RNA with DEAE Dextran/DMSO also showed very low infectivity (3.0 - 10 pfu/ng) probably due in part to the cytotoxicity of this treatment for the monolayer cells in our assays; even when relatively short incubations (10-15 min) were used, significant cytotoxic effects and cell detachment were observed.

Infectious center assays were also used to measure the infectivity of the RNA preparation (19). These assays were performed by incubating suspension cells with RNA samples, separating the cells by centrifugation and applying them in an agarose overlay on monolayer cells. The results are shown in Table 2. Encapsulated RNA formed 1-2 x 10^4 pfu/ng under optimal conditions while RNA in DEAE Dextran/DMSO yielded approximately 5 x 10^2 pfu/ng. Furthermore, >90% of the cells were sensitive to infection by encapsulated RNA while even at high RNA concentration only 50-60% of the DEAE Dextran/DMSO-treated cells were infected. Free RNA, either in the absence or the presence of vesicles, had no significant biological activity, and encapsulated RNA incubated in the absence of cells did not form plaques in this assay. No significant differences in the efficiency of infection of HeLa and L cells were found using either encapsulated RNA or the DEAE Dextran/DMSO method (19).

Table 2 also shows the enhanced infectivity of encapsulated samples after treatment with pancreatic RNAse. In the presence of

Table 2. *Infectivity of liposome-encapsulated poliovirus RNA*

RNA treatment	ngrams RNA/ 10^6 cells	Infectious centers 10^6 cells	Infectious centers/ngram RNA
a) RNA in liposomes	5.0×10^0	4.0×10^4	8.0×10^3
	5.0×10^1	8.0×10^5	1.6×10^4
	1.1×10^2	9.0×10^5	8.2×10^3
b) RNA in liposomes +RNAse	4.6×10^0	8.5×10^5	1.8×10^5
	4.6×10^1	9.5×10^5	2.1×10^4
	1.0×10^2	9.0×10^5	9.0×10^3
c) Free RNA +DEAE Dextran DMSO	1.0×10^2	5.0×10^4	5.0×10^2
	1.0×10^3	4.5×10^5	4.5×10^2
	1.0×10^4	6.0×10^5	6.0×10^1
d) Free RNA	1.0×10^4	0	-
	5.0×10^4	0	-
e) Free RNA + liposomes	1.0×10^3	0	-
	1.0×10^4	2	2.0×10^{-4}

a, b) Encapsulated RNA (6.3×10^{-1} ng/nmole) was prepared from 2×10^4 nmoles PS/Ca^{2+} cochleate cylinders and 1.25×10^5 ng RNA. After washing, a fraction of the vesicle preparation was removed and treated with 10 ng RNAse/nmole lipid. Inocula were diluted in EMEM (spinner salts). c) RNA samples were diluted in EMEM (spinner salts) + DEAE Dextran/DMSO). d) RNA samples were diluted in EMEM (spinner salts). e) LUV(PS) were added to RNA dilutions in EMEM (spinner salts); final concentration: 10^3 ng/RNA/nmole lipid.
 From Wilson *et al.*, 1979.

RNAse, the titer of a sample was consistently found to be 10-50 fold greater than in the absence of the enzyme. The mechanism responsible for this enhancement is not presently understood, but it is possible that the neutralization of the negatively charged surface of the vesicle by the positive charges of RNAse may in part be responsible for an increase in cell-associated vesicle material (19).

Although encapsulation in lipid vesicles significantly increases the efficiency of transfection with poliovirus RNA, the infectious titer of pure RNA in vesicles (1 pfu/10^4 genome equivalents) is considerably lower than that of the intact virus preparation from which the nucleic acid is extracted (1 pfu/2.0 x 10^2 genome equivalents). In order to test whether this was a consequence of the efficiency of delivery in this system (e.g., the number of vesicles introducing their contents in an infectious form) or the ability of the RNA to initiate an infection once it has entered the cell, LUV containing a wide range of concentrations were prepared. The biological activity of these preparations was measured by infectious center assays; the results are shown in Fig. 1. Poliovirus RNA concentration $\geq$ 1 ng/nmole lipid gave virtually identical titers at all dilutions. A linear decrease in the specific infectivity of the vesicles was observed when the concentration of encapsulated RNA was less than 1 ng/nmole. We made a rough calculation (19) that a LUV preparation containing 1 nmole lipid and 1 ng RNA should have an average of 1 RNA molecule/vesicle. The data in Fig. 1 indicate that when the ratio of encapsulated RNA lipid was > 1 ng/nmole, specific infectivity of the vesicle preparation was independent of RNA concentration inside the vesicles; where RNA was present at < 1 ng/nmole, a linear relationship between the RNA/lipid ratio and specific infectivity was observed. These results are consistent with the conclusion (34) that infection can be initiated by a single molecule of poliovirus RNA and suggests that the entry of the molecule into the cell (possibly involving fusion of the liposome with the cell membrane) is a limiting step in establishing an infection.

5. QUANTITATION OF EFFECTIVE DELIVERY OF LIPOSOMAL RNA

In order to determine the relationship between the concentration of applied vesicle material, the number of cell-associated vesicles and the effective delivery of encapsulated macromolecules, we incubated radioactively labelled LUV(PS) containing poliovirus RNA with cells and subsequently measured the cell-associated lipid

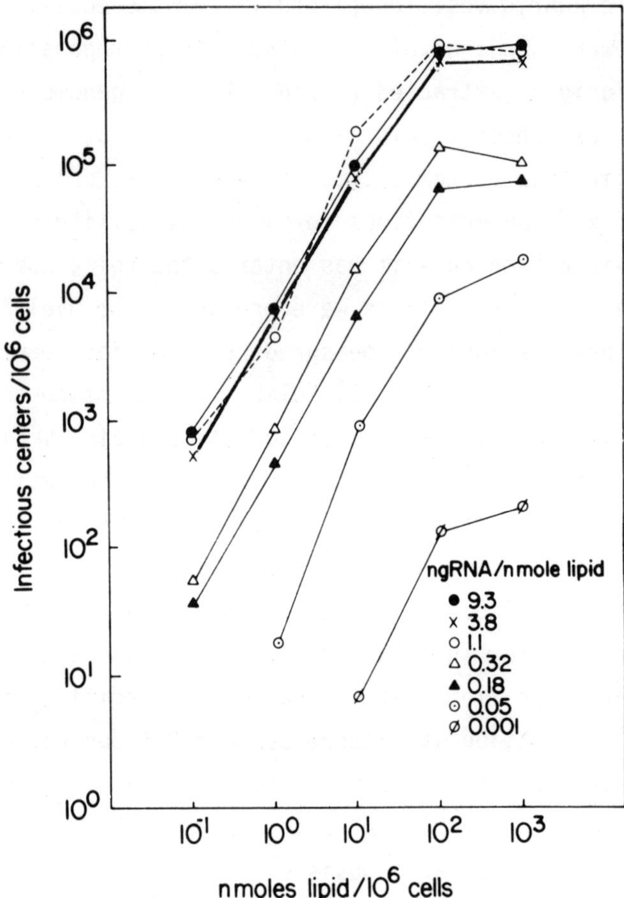

Fig. 1. *Infectivity of different concentrations of encapsulated poliovirus RNA*. Liposomes, LUV(PS) were prepared in the presence of mixtures of ^{32}P-labelled (10^8 cpm/ngram) and unlabelled RNA at a range of concentrations (5×10^1 - 10^5 ng/nmole lipid). Vesicles were washed and the infectivity of the different preparations was measured by infectious center assays. Ratios of ng RNA/nmole of lipid as indicated on figure.
Copyright with MIT Press. From Wilson *et al.*, 1979.

radioactivity and the formation of poliovirus infectious centers. We had previously determined that the levels of cell-associated vesicles and the delivery of encapsulated RNA were constant over a

30-180 min range of incubation times (unpublished results); thus all experiments were conducted within this time period. Representative results are given in Table 3. When incubation mixtures contained 10^{-1}-10^{2} nmoles lipid/10^{6} cells, an approximately linear relationship between associated vesicle material and applied vesicle concentration was observed; at lipid concentrations > 10^{2} nmoles/10^{6} cells it appeared that a smaller fraction of the applied lipid was associated with the cells. In experiments similar to those shown in Table 3 we have studied the relationship between vesicle-mediated delivery, as measured by the infectivity of the encapsulated poliovirus RNA, and cell-associated vesicle concentration. A linear correlation between the efficiency of infectious center formation with cell-associated vesicles was observed in the lower range of lipid concentrations. Higher doses of vesicles (e.g. > 10^{2} nmoles lipid applied/10^{6} cells or > 5 x 10^{0} nmoles associated/10^{6} cells) did not yield increased titers, suggesting that at high vesicle/cell ratios (>10^{4} LUV(PS)/cell) the liposomes were saturating the available sites on the cell surface. As discussed earlier, the specific infectivity of a vesicle preparation was also dependent upon the concentration of RNA in the vesicles.

Analogous experiments were performed utilizing LUV in which a radioactive marker, poly A - oligo (^{32}P)dT, was coencapsulated with poliovirus RNA, allowing us to measure vesicle mediated association and delivery of the entrapped nucleic acid. Results in Table 3 also relate infectivity to the amounts of cell-associated RNA. When incubation mixtures contained large amounts of vesicle-entrapped RNA (>10^{2} ng/10^{6} cells applied or > 10^{0} ng/10^{6} cells associated) the assay system was saturated; that is, essentially all the cells were infected. At lower RNA concentrations the actual titer was measurable, and these results indicate that effective delivery is, for the most part, a function of the amount of RNA that is specifically associated with the cells. This relationship does not hold true when

Table 3. *Quantitation of effective delivery of liposomal RNA.*

	Amount Applied (per 10^6 cells)		Amount Assoc. (per 10^6 cells)		Infectivity[¤] (cell-assoc.)
	nmole lipid	ng RNA	nmole lipid(I,II) ng RNA (III-VI)		pfu/nmol lip.(I,II) pfu/ng RNA (III-VI)
I.	4.9×10^{2}	(5.0×10^{2})	6.6×10^{0}	(1.3)*	6.1×10^{4}
	9.9×10^{1}	(1.0×10^{2})	3.6×10^{0}	(3.6)	1.7×10^{5}
	9.9×10^{0}	(1.0×10^{1})	4.2×10^{-1}	(4.2)	1.2×10^{5}
	9.9×10^{-1}	(1.0×10^{0})	4.1×10^{-2}	(4.1)	1.9×10^{5}
II.	3.9×10^{2}	(5.0×10^{1})	1.1×10^{1}	(2.8)	5.5×10^{4}
	3.9×10^{1}	(5.0×10^{0})	4.5×10^{0}	(11.5)	1.1×10^{4}
	3.9×10^{0}	(5.0×10^{-1})	7.8×10^{-1}	(20.0)	5.1×10^{3}
	3.9×10^{-1}	(5.0×10^{-2})	4.1×10^{-2}	(10.6)	7.3×10^{3}
III.	(3.5×10^{2})	3.6×10^{3}	9.5×10^{0}	(0.26)	9.5×10^{4}
	(7.0×10^{1})	7.2×10^{2}	5.2×10^{0}	(0.72)	1.8×10^{5}
	(7.0×10^{0})	7.2×10^{1}	1.3×10^{0}	(1.8)	3.8×10^{4}
IV.	(5.0×10^{2})	6.5×10^{1}	4.4×10^{-1}	(0.68)	1.1×10^{5}
	(5.0×10^{1})	6.5×10^{0}	2.0×10^{-1}	(3.0)	1.3×10^{5}
	(5.0×10^{0})	6.5×10^{-1}	4.0×10^{-2}	(6.2)	5.0×10^{4}
V.	(7.0×10^{2})	5.0×10^{3}	3.0×10^{0}	(0.08)	0
	(7.0×10^{1})	5.0×10^{2}	3.5×10^{-1}	(0.07)	0
VI.	0	1.0×10^{4}	8.1×10^{2}	(8.1)	3.7×10^{-3}
	0	1.0×10^{3}	9.3×10^{1}	(9.3)	0

Experiments I and II were conducted with labeled lipid, ^{3}H-DPPC. The amounts of RNA in parenthesis were estimated from parallel experiments with ^{3}H-PolyA-oligo (^{32}P)dT. Experiments III and IV were conducted with ^{3}H-PolyA-oligo (^{32}P)dT coencapsulated with polio RNA as a marker. The amounts of lipid in parenthesis are estimates from parallel experiments with ^{3}H-DPPC. Experiment V was conducted with preparations of pre-formed vesicles and free RNA added to the cells. The amount of cell-associated RNA was determined with radioactive marker as above. Experiment VI was conducted as V above, except that vesicles were omitted from the incubation. Infectivity was determined by infectious center assays. *Numbers in parenthesis in this column represent fraction of applied material that becomes cell-associated, expressed as percent. ¤Calculations of infectivity are based on the amounts of lipid (I,II) or RNA (III-VI) which were found to be associated with cells.

the concentration of the vesicles exceeds the above mentioned saturation level of 10^4 LUV(PS)/cell: the relative efficiencies of both vesicle-mediated association and effective delivery of the entrapped material are reduced when high concentrations of LUV(PS) are applied to cells.

A comparison of experiments I and II with III in Table 2 reveals a discrepancy between the measurements of cell-associated vesicle material using lipid and encapsulated markers: approximately 10 times more labelled lipid than encapsulated nucleic acid was associated with the cells. Two simple explanations could account for this discrepancy. Either lipid exchange between vesicles and cells could give an artificially high estimate of vesicle association, because labelled lipid has been transferred to the cells, or cell-induced leakage of encapsulated material from the vesicles could reduce the measurable cell-associated nucleic acid relative to vesicle lipid. In order to distinguish between these two possibilities, a re-exposure experiment was done. LUV containing poliovirus RNA and either labelled lipid or encapsulated label were incubated with cells under standard conditions, the cells were removed by centrifugation and the supernatants containing free vesicles were incubated with fresh cells; cell-associated vesicle material and effective delivery were measured after both the primary and secondary incubations. When the association was measured as a function of lipid label there was no significant difference between the fraction of cell-associated vesicles in the primary and secondary exposures. However, experiments using LUV with encapsulated label gave considerably different results. There was a notable decrease in the level of association of the applied RNA upon re-exposure to cells. More significantly the specific infectivity of the vesicles, in terms of applied lipid concentration, applied RNA concentration or cell-associated lipid, was reduced more than 10 fold. On the other hand, the cell-associated RNA was equally infectious in both sets of assays. Incubation of vesicles under similar conditions in the absence of cells did not noticeably affect either the level of association or the efficiency of delivery upon subsequent interaction with cells. These results suggest that interaction with cells induces a destabilization of LUV(PS), with a concomitant increase in vesicle permeability and loss of encapsulated material. This is in reasonable agreement with recently observed effects of cells on the leakage of carboxyfluorescein from vesicles (35).

6. DISCUSSION AND CONCLUSIONS

Vesicle-mediated delivery of macromolecules into cells offers several advantages over other methods of bypassing the plasma membrane permeability barrier: special skills or equipment are not required (as for microinjection), vesicles do not significantly alter cellular metabolism or permeability (in contrast to osmotic shock or polycation treatment) and large scale experiments are easily executed. LUV are considerably more versatile than vesicles produced by mechanical dispersion or sonication because the vesicles have a large interior aqueous volume, they entrap various macromolecules efficiently, and are easily separated from unencapsulated material (36). Furthermore, the LUV(PS) we have used can encapsulate biological material without subjecting it to the rigors of sonication, detergent treatment, organic solvents or extremes of temperature or pH. Having demonstrated that LUV(PS) can encapsulate poliovirus RNA and introduce it into cells (19) we have attempted to quantitate the LUV(PS)-mediated delivery of nucleic acids.

Our results indicate that after incubation with cells approximately 10% of the vesicle lipid marker became cell-associated; under the same conditions only about 1% of the entrapped nucleic acid was cell-associated (Table 3). When vesicle preparations were exposed to 2 sets of cells in succession after the same fraction of vesicle lipid was cell-associated with each batch while there was a significant decrease in the cell-associated fraction of nucleic acid during the secondary exposure. These and other data suggest that interaction with cells increases the permeability of LUV(PS). Leakage of encapsulated material upon exposure to cells can account for the disparity between the levels of cell-associated vesicle lipid and nucleic acid. More recent experiments indicate that the cell-induced increase in permeability can be greatly reduced by the incorporation of cholesterol (1:1 mole ratio) during the formation of the LUV (Fraley and Papahadjopoulos, unpublished observation).

Several interesting conclusions can be drawn from the data on the infectivity of encapsulated RNA. When the concentration of encapsulated RNA exceeded 1 ng/nmole lipid (e.g. an average of > 1 molecule/vesicle) the specific infectivity of the RNA was reduced. This result is consistent with our earlier observation that vesicle-mediated RNA infection exhibits one-hit kinetics and that infection may be initiated by a single molecule (19). The second, and rather obvious, conclusion is that the efficiency of vesicle-mediated delivery is a function of the amount of cell-associated entrapped material (rather than a cell-associated lipid) and that vesicles can only deliver nucleic acid trapped within the vesicle lumen. A sizable fraction of the cell-associated RNA may well remain in vesicles adsorbed to the surface of the cell or enter the cell via a pathway that does not result in cytoplasmic delivery because only about 0.1% (or 2-5% in the presence of RNAse) of the cell-associated RNA was infectious in our assays. Maximum levels of effective delivery in our system were obtained when the lipid/cell ratio was 10^1-10^2 nmoles/10^6 cells. Under these conditions 5-10% of the vesicle lipid (1-5 nmoles/10^6 cells or 0.2-1.0 x 10^3 LUV(PS)/cell) and 0.5-3% of the encapsulated material associate stably with the cells. Under the same conditions we observe titers of 1-2 x 10^5 pfu/ng cell-associated RNA. Given that 1 ng of poliovirus RNA contains approximately 2 x 10^8 molecules, we calculate that about 0.1% of the cell-associated RNA is infectious, or that approximately 1000 cell-associated RNA molecules are needed to initiate an infection. In the presence of RNAse, the same calculations indicate that approximately 100 RNA molecules per cell are needed for infection. These figures are comparable to those found for whole virus if one assumes one infectious unit per 2 x 10^2 genome equivalents (19) and > 90% binding of the virions to cells (37).

A clear interpretation of the mechanism of vesicle-mediated delivery in our system is difficult because the amount of cell-associated material is much greater than the amount functionally delivered. Nevertheless, our results do allow us to conclude that LUV(PS) are delivering the RNA by a mechanism that bypasses the plasma membrane barrier rather than simply increasing the permeability of the cells to macromolecules. It is not possible at this time to conclude with certainty whether vesicle contents enter the cell via a fusion event between the vesicle and a cellular membrane, via endocytosis and cytoplasmic release or by some as yet undefined mechanism. We feel that it is likely that a fusion event at some level may be an essential step in the intracellular release of vesicle contents.

Although cytoplasmic delivery does not appear to be a major component of cell-vesicle interactions, LUV(PS) are very useful vehicles for the introduction of nucleic acids into cells. They deliver RNA to cells considerably more efficiently than chemical techniques (19) and allow the study of intracellular events under relatively normal conditions (38, 39). They are easily prepared and stored (36) and should prove a valuable tool in many areas of investigation. Finally, they can encapsulate intact DNA molecules quite efficiently. The cellular incorporation of encapsulated DNA is currently under active investigation in our laboratory.

7. ACKNOWLEDGEMENTS

This work was supported by the following grants from NIH: CA-18527, GM18921 (to D.P.), CA-16705, AI-14042 (to R.T.).

8. REFERENCES

1) BANGHAM, A.D., STANDISH, M.M. and WATKINS, J.C. (1965). Diffusion of univalent ions across the lamellae of swollen phospholipids. J. Mol. Biol., 13, 238.

2) PAPAHADJOPOULOS, D. and MILLER, N. (1967). Phospholipid model membranes. I. Structural characteristics of hydrated liquid crystals. Biochim. Biophys. Acta, 135, 624.

3) HUANG, C.H. (1969). Studies on phosphatidylcholine vesicles. Formation and physical characteristics. Biochem., 8, 344.

4) PAPAHADJOPOULOS, D., VAIL, W.J., JACOBSON, K. and POSTE, G. (1975). Cochleate lipid cylinders: Formation by fusion of unilamellar lipid vesicles. Biochim. Biophys. Acta, 394, 483.

5) DEAMER, D. and BANGHAM, A.D. (1976). Large volume liposomes by an ether evaporization method. Biochim. Biophys. Acta, 443, 629.

6) SZOKA, F. and PAPAHADJOPOULOS, D. (1978). A new procedure for preparation of liposomes with large internal aqueous space and high capture, by reverse phase evaporation (REV). Proc. Natl. Acad. Sci. USA, 75, 4194.

7) PAPAHADJOPOULOS, D. and KIMELBERG, H.K. (1973). Phospholipid vesicles (liposomes) as models for biological membranes. In: Progress in Surface Science (ed. S.G. Davison), 4, 141, Pergamon Press.

8) BANGHAM, A.D., HILL, M.W. and MILLER, N.G.A. (1974). Preparation and use of liposomes as models of biological membranes. In: Methods in Membrane Biology (ed., E.D. Korn), 1, 1, Ch. 1, Plenum Press.

9) GREGORIADIS, G. (1976). The carrier potential of liposomes in

biology and medicine, New Eng. Journ. Med., 295, 704, 705.

10) POSTE, G., PAPAHADJOPOULOS, D. and VAIL, W.J. (1976). Lipid vesicles as carriers for introducing biologically active materials into cells. In: Methods in Cell Biology (ed., D.M. Prescott), 14, 33, Academic Press, New York.

11) TYRELL, D.A., HEATH, T.D., COLLEY, C.M. and RYMAN, B.E. (1976). New aspects of liposomes. Biochim. Biophys. Acta, 457, 259.

12) PAGANO, R.E. and WEINSTEIN, J.N. (1978). Interactions of phospholipid vesicles with mammalian cells. Ann. Rev. Biophys. Bioengin., 7, 435.

13) KIMBELBERG, H.K. and MAYHEW, E. (1979). Properties and biological effects of liposomes and their uses in pharmacology and toxicology. Crit. Revs. Toxicol., 6, 25.

14) PAPAHADJOPOULOS, D. (1978). Liposomes and their uses in biology and medicine. Ann. N.Y. Acad. Sci., 308, 1.

15) BATZRI, S. and KORN, E.D. (1973). Single bilayer liposomes prepared without sonication. Biochim. Biophys. Acta, 298, 1015.

16) KREMER, J.M.H., ESKER, J., PATHMAMANOHARAN, C. and WIERSEMA, P.H. (1977). Vesicles of variable diameter prepared by a modified injection method. Biochem., 16, 3932.

17) SZOKA, F. and PAPAHADJOPOULOS, D. (1980). Comparative properties and methods of preparation of lipid vesicles (liposomes). Ann. Rev. Biophys. Bioengin., in press.

18) WILSON, T., PAPAHADJOPOULOS, D. and TABER, R. (1977). Biological properties of poliovirus encapsulated in lipid vesicles: antibody resistance and infectivity in virus-resistant cells. Proc. Natl. Acad. Sci. USA, 74, 3471.

19) WILSON, T., PAPAHADJOPOULOS, D. and TABER, R. (1979). The introduction of poliovirus RNA into cells via lipid vesicles (liposomes). Cell, 17, 77.

20) OLSON, F., HUNT, C.A., SZOKA, F.C., VAIL, W.J. and PAPAHADJOPOULOS, D. (1979). Preparation of liposomes of defined size distribution by extrusion through polycarbonate membranes.

Biochem. Biophys. Acta, in press.

21) POSTE, G. and PAPAHADJOPOULOS, D. (1978). The influence of vesicle membrane properties on the interaction of lipid vesicles with cultured cells. Ann. N.Y. Acad. Sci., 308, 164.

22) PAPAHADJOPOULOS, D., MAYHEW, E., POSTE, G., SMITH, S. and VAIL, W.J. (1974). Incorporation of lipid vesicles by mammalian cells provides a potential method for modifying cell behavior. Nature, 252, 163.

23) PAGANO, R.E. and HUANG, L. (1975). Interactions of phospholipid vesicles with mammalian cells. II. Studies of Mechanism. J. Cell Biol., 67, 49.

24) POSTE, G. and PAPAHADJOPOULOS, D. (1976). Lipid vesicles as carriers for introducing materials into cultured cells: Influence of vesicle lipid composition on the mechanism of vesicle incorporation into cells. Proc. Natl. Acad. Sci., 73, 1603.

25) MARTIN, F.J. and MACDONALD, R.C. (1976). Lipid vesicle-cell interactions. II. Introduction of cell fusion. J. Cell. Biol., 70, 506.

26) MARTIN, F.J. and MACDONALD, R.C. (1976). Lipid vesicle-cell interactions. III. Introduction of a new antigenic determinant into erythrocyte membranes. J. Cell Biol., 70, 515.

27) WEISSMANN, G., COHEN, C. and HOFFSTEIN, S. (1977). Introduction of enzymes, by means of liposomes, into non-phagocytic human cells *in vitro*. Biochim. Biophys. Acta, 498, 375.

28) SCHROIT, A.J. and PAGANO, R.E. (1978). Introduction of antigenic phospholipids into the plasma membrane of mammalian cells: Organization and antibody-induced lipid redistribution. Proc. Natl. Acad. Sci., 75, 5529.

29) BATZRI, S. and KORN, E.D. (1975). Interaction of phospholipid vesicles with cells. Endocytosis and fusion as alternate mechanisms for the uptake of lipid-soluble and water-soluble molecules. J. Cell Biol., 66, 621.

30) COHEN, C.M., WEISSMANN, G., HOFFSTEIN, S., AWASTHI, U.C. and

SRIVASTAVA, S.K. (1976). Introduction of purified hexosaminidase A into Tay-Sachs leukocytes by means of immunoglobulin-coated liposomes. Biochem., 15, 452.

31) PAGANO, R.E. and TAKEICHI, M. (1977). Adhesion of phospholipid vesicles to Chinese hamster fibroblasts: role of serum proteins. J. Cell Biol., 74, 531.

32) SZOKA, F., JACOBSON, K. and DERZKO, Z. (1978). Phospholipid vesicle-cell interactions studied by fluorescence techniques. Ann. N.Y. Acad. Sci., 308, 437.

33) PAGANO, R.E., SANDRA, A. and TAKEICHI, M. (1978). Interactions of phospholipid vesicles with mammalian cells. Ann. N.Y. Acad., 308, 185.

34) KOCH, G. and BISHOP, J.N. (1968). The effect of polycation on the interaction of viral RNA with mammalian cells: studies on the infectivity of single- and double-stranded poliovirus RNA. Virology, 35, 9.

35) SZOKA, F., JACOBSON, K. and PAPAHADJOPOULOS, D. (1979). On the use of aqueous space markers to determine the mechanism of interaction between phospholipid vesicles (liposomes) and cells. Biochim. Biophys. Acta, 551, 295.

36) PAPAHADJOPOULOS, D. and VAIL, W.J. (1978). Incorporation of macromolecules within large unilamellar vesicles (LUV). Ann. N.Y. Acad. Sci., 308, 252.

37) LONBORG-HOLM, K. and PHILLIPSON, L. (1974). Early interactions between animal viruses and cells. Monographs in Virol., 9, 1.

38) DIMITRIADIS, G.J. (1978). Translation of rabbit globin mRNA introduced by liposomes into mouse lymphocytes. Nature, 274. 923.

39) OSTRO, M., GIACOMONI, D., LAVELLE, D., PAXTON, W. and DRAY, S. (1978). Evidence for the translation of rabbit globin mRNA after liposome-mediated insertion into a human cell line. Nature, 274, 921.

LIPOSOMES IN DRUG TARGETING

G. Gregoriadis

Clinical Research Centre
Watford Road, Harrow
Middlesex HA1 3UJ, England

1. INTRODUCTION

Transport of drugs to target tissues, cells or subcellular organelles by the use of carrier systems is now a recognized useful method of improving drug selectivity. The types of carrier that have been proposed to date include macromolecules, cells, viruses and synthetic systems (1). However, it is already apparent that most of these are limited in range and quantity of drugs they can accommodate and in their ability to prevent contact of the drug moiety with the normal biological milieu or to promote its access to areas in need of drug action. Further limitations relate to the toxicity of the carrier's components, their availability and to technical problems such as, for instance, the preparation of the drug-carrier unit. Therefore, extensive efforts have been made towards the development of the ideal drug-carrier (1, 2). As discussed elsewhere (2) such a carrier should be capable of delivering a wide variety of agents into the precise site of action within the biological entity and at the same time provoke no adverse effects. It has become evident during the last decade that liposomes possess many of the qualities expected from a multifunctional carrier and success in applying these to membrane research has now been extended to biology and pharmacology (3, 4).

Liposomes are a family of artificial phospholipid vesicles made of one or more lipid bilayers which alternate with aqueous spaces (5) and can be charged by the incorporation of a negative or positive amphiphile. Using appropriate methods, water soluble drugs are passively entrapped within the aqueous phase of liposomes and lipid soluble drugs accommodated within the lipid structure. The latter's permeability to ions or stability, can be adjusted accordingly by the incorporation of sterols or other lipid molecules (for a comprehensive list of agents that have been associated with liposomes see Ref. 1). Preparation of liposomes with or without entrapped solutes is carried out by a variety of methods which will give the classical multilamellar structures as well as small or large unilamellar or oligolamellar vesicles. Each of these types of liposomes is intended to suit particular needs in biology or pharmacology.

Initial reports (6-8) on the fate of protein-containing liposomes injected intravenously into rats, established some of the principles governingliposomal behaviour *in vivo*. Latency of liposomal enzymes, for instance, was found to be largely retained in the blood implying maintenance of the structural integrity of liposomes during their circulation in the blood. Further, examination of a number of tissues established that liposomes and their contents were taken up mostly by the liver and spleen through the process of endocytosis to end up in the lysosomal apparatus. These findings made apparent that the system was particularly attractive as a means of delivering agents into the intracellular environment, especially the lysosomes, from where agents could subsequently gain entry to other cell compartments (9). In addition to being localized into specific areas in the cell, liposomal agents were also found capable of action, following their liberation from the carrier. Thus, by 1973 it had already been demonstrated in cell culture that liposomes carrying invertase could deliver the enzyme in its active form into the sucrose-laden lysosomes of invertase-deficient cells (10). Subsequent work from this laboratory and from numerous others has now uncovered an intriguing variety of aspects related to the transport potential of liposomes and there are others which will, no doubt, be revealed as more and more disciplines in need of a drug carrier adopt the system (11). Attempts will be made here to summarize some of the basic facets of the interaction of the liposomal carrier with living systems and discuss possibilities and problems relevant to selective drug action and its applications in biology and medicine.

2. *IN VIVO* BEHAVIOUR OF LIPOSOMES

The considerable amount of information amassed regarding the interaction of liposomes with biological entities *in vivo* has been reviewed by a number of workers (3, 4, 12-14). One of the first observations was that after the intravenous injection of unilamellar or multilamellar liposomes containing radiolabels in both their lipid (e.g. cholesterol) and aqueous phase (e.g. drug) the ratio of the two labels in the blood often remained similar to that in the injected preparation. From this it was inferred that the carrier retains its structural integrity in the circulation. This is an essential prerequisite for effective drug delivery since it not only will warrant quantitative transport of drugs to target sites it will also protect these (e.g. enzymes in replacement therapy, certain drugs in cancer chemotherapy, nucleic acids in genetic engineering) from inactivation in the blood and prevent their wastage through premature excretion. However, the possibility exists that a labelled drug can form a complex with the labelled lipid marker and circulate in the blood as such, even after disruption of liposomes. On the other hand, because of the variety of paired markers used (e.g.

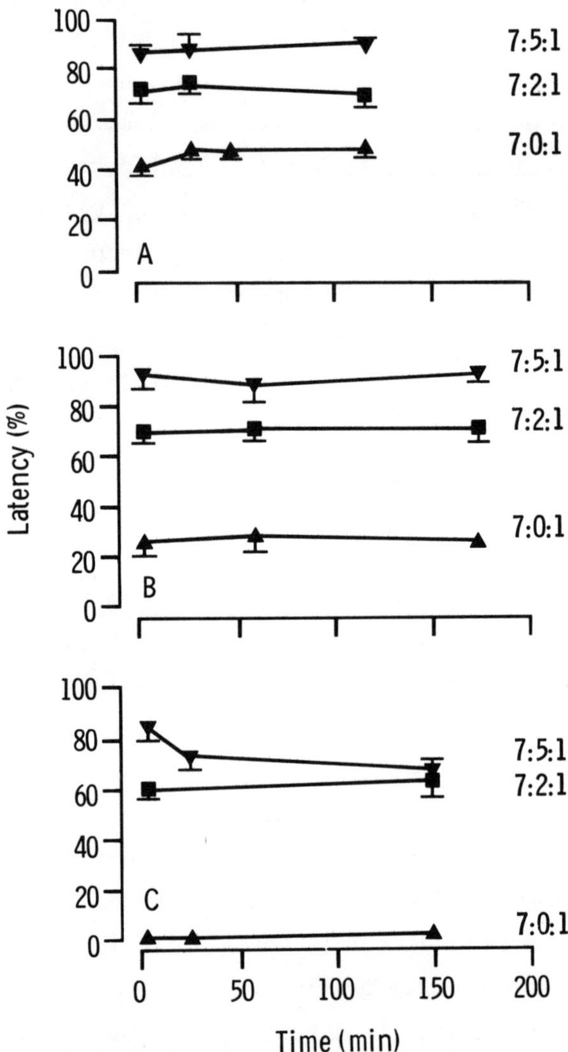

Fig. 1. *The effect of cholesterol content of liposomes on the latency of entrapped β-fructofuranosidase.* Liposomes containing β-fructofuranosidase and composed of PC and PA or PC, CHOL and PA at the molar ratios shown were injected intravenously into rats (A) or incubated with rat whole blood (B) or rat serum (C). Latent β-fructofuranosidase in blood or serum is expressed as % ± SD of the latent enzyme in the injected preparation.

cholesterol and albumin (7), dipalmitoyl phosphatidylcholine and albumin (15), cholesterol and bleomycin (16), cholesterol and methotrexate (17), such a possibility seems unlikely. It is, nevertheless, true that liposomes of certain lipid compositions become, in the presence of plasma (or even *in vivo* in the circulating blood) (18, 19) permeable to entrapped solutes of small molecular weight (20).

Our recent work (21-23) suggests that liposomal stability *in vivo* (blood circulation) and *in vitro* (in the presence of serum, plasma or whole blood) is related to the proportion of cholesterol relative to the phospholipid present in the lamellae. To avoid possible complex formation between lipid and aqueous markers we have used systems which reflect liposomal integrity *per se*. This is achieved by measuring the extent to which the latency of a given agent entrapped in the aqueous phase of liposomes changes within a biological milieu. Latency is defined here as the portion of the agent (% of the total) which cannot be measured unless liposomes are disrupted with a detergent (e.g. Triton X-100). When, for instance, the latency of a liposomal enzyme after coming into contact with, say, blood is equal to that observed in the preparation before use, one can then assume that the integrity of the preparation has not been altered by blood, at least in terms of substrate penetration through the lipid bilayers. Fig. 1A shows that in rats injected intravenously with invertase-containing small multilamellar liposomes, stability of liposomes in the blood (measured by the extent to which sucrose permeates the bilayers and reaches the enzyme) is dependent on the amount of cholesterol incorporated into the liposomal structure relative to that of phospholipid. With cholesterol-rich liposomes (7:5 phospholipid to cholesterol molar ratio) stability is nearly equal to that observed in the preparation before injection. However, with the proportion of cholesterol decreasing, liposomal stability is reduced accordingly (as soon as 2 min after injection) to reach low values with cholesterol-free liposomes. Similar results are ob-

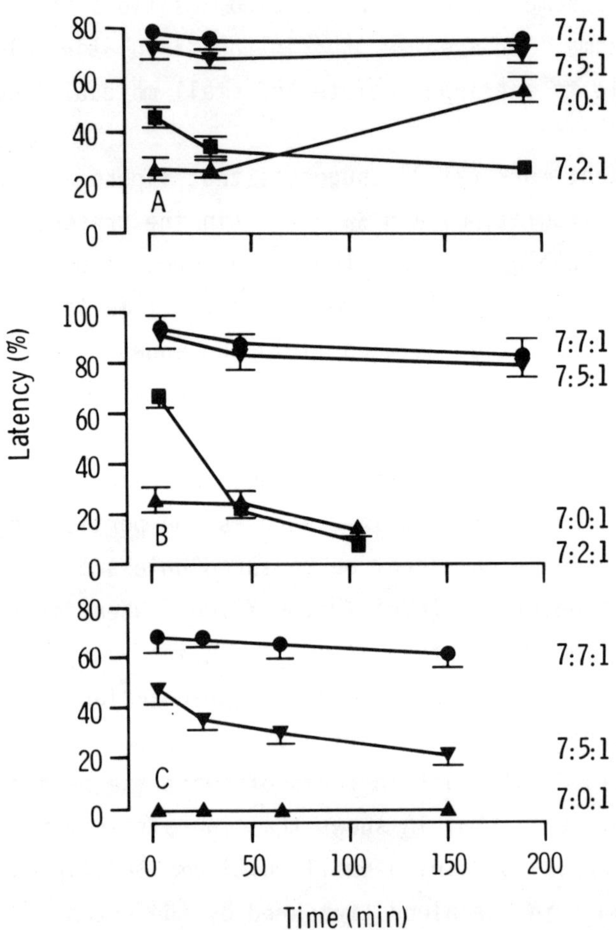

Fig. 2. *The effect of cholesterol content of liposomes on the latency of entrapped 6-CF.* Liposomes containing 6-CF and composed as in Fig. 1 were injected intravenously into rats (A) or incubated with rat whole blood (B) or rat serum (C). Latent 6-CF in blood or serum is expressed as % ± SD of the latent dye in the injected preparation (21).

tained with such liposomes exposed to whole blood *in vitro* (Fig. 1B) but in the presence of serum, loss of stability is more pronounced to become total with cholesterol-free liposomes (Fig. 1C). Dependence of liposomal stability of cholesterol content was also shown in rats injected with small multilamellar liposomes containing 0.25M 6-carboxyfluorescein (Fig. 2). At this concentration the dye is quenched but when, for any reason, the dye escapes into the medium, ensuing dilution enables it to fluoresce (24). It again appeared that the presence of a sufficient amount of cholesterol (e.g. 7:7 or 7:5 phospholipid to cholesterol molar ratio) is a prerequisite for the maintenance of their stability (in terms of dye leakage) after liposomes come into contact with blood *in vivo* (Fig. 2A) and also *in vitro* in the presence of whole blood (Fig. 2B) or serum (Fig. 2C). Work with unilamellar liposomes containing 0.25M 6-carboxyfluorescein indicates that a 7:7 phospholipid to cholesterol ratio results in total (100%) retention of liposomal stability in the blood of injected mice (Fig. 3) or in the presence of whole blood or plasma (23). Even when exposed to serum, stability loss in such liposomes is only minor (23). Additional evidence for full stability retention in cholesterol-rich unilamellar liposomes is obtained from monitoring the ratio of ^{14}C-cholesteryl oleate incorporated into the liposomal structure and 6-carboxyfluorescein entrapped in the aqueous phase (Table 1). For up to 150 min after intravenous injection of mice, the ratio retains almost at its initial value of unity the implication being that the two labels (i.e. aqueous and lipid phase of the carrier) are cleared from the circulation of nearly identical rates.

The mechanism by which cholesterol preserves liposomal stability is probably related to the fact that its presence in phospholipid bilayers leads to the packing of phospholipid molecules and to the reduction in the permeability to entrapped small molecules (25). Our experiments (21-23) show that in the absence of serum, loss of 6-CF from cholesterol-free liposomes is relatively slow but it becomes almost instantaneous in its presence. Other workers (20)

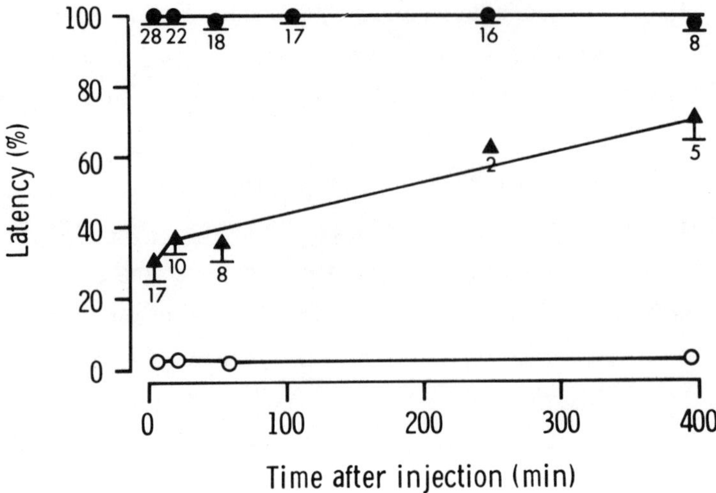

Fig. 3. *Latency of liposomal 6-CF in the blood of injected mice.* Mice were injected intravenously with 6-CF, free or entrapped in unilamellar liposomes. 6-CF latency values in blood at time intervals are % ± SD of latencies in the respective injected preparations. O, free 6-CF; ▲, cholesterol-free liposomes; ●, cholesterol-rich liposomes (23).

have found that such loss of solutes results from the destruction of liposomes because of liposomal phospholipid transfer to high density lipoproteins. On the basis of the present findings (Figs. 1-4 and Table 1) it is tempting to speculate that, in the presence of blood or serum, cholesterol, by virtue of the molecular packing it imposes, not only retards ion diffusion, it also prevents phospholipid molecules from being transferred to lipoproteins. Since the action of cholesterol in promoting liposomal stability in whole blood (Figs. 1A, B; 2A, B; 3) is more efficient than in serum alone (Figs. 1C; 2C) it is clear that blood cells *in vitro* and *in vivo* play a significant role in minimizing the detrimental effect of serum. Blood cells are known to interact with high density lipoproteins in terms of phospholipid movement (26) and it may be that when both liposomes and erythrocytes are present, such movement be-

Table 1. ^{14}*C:6-carboxyfluorescein ratios in the blood of mice injected with 6-carboxyfluorescein entrapped in* ^{14}*C-labelled liposomes.*

Treatment		^{14}C:6-carboxyfluorescein ratio ± SD				
		2 min	20 min	110 min	150 min	450 min
Intravenous	A	1.09±0.08(6)	1.09±0.09(6)	1.05±0.0(3)	1.02±0.0(4)	N.D.
	B	2.1, 2.3	5.5 ±0.8 (3)		9.2 ±3.1(3)	
	C	3.4, 6.0	11.5,4.8 (3)		14.3, 18,3	
Intra-peritoneal	A	N.D.	1.01±0.0 (4)	1.05±0.1(4)	1.06±0.0(4)	0.97±0.0(4)

Mice were injected intravenously or intraperitoneally with 6-carboxyfluorescein entrapped in cholesterol-rich (A), cholesterol-poor (B) and cholesterol-free (C) small unilamelar liposomes labelled with ^{14}C-cholesteryl oleate ($3.9 \times 10^4 - 4.1 \times 10^5$ d.p.m.). The ratio of ^{14}C:6-carboxyfluorescein in the injected preparations was taken as unity.
Numbers in parentheses denote animals used. N.D., not used. From Kirby *et al.* (23).

tween liposomes and lipoproteins diminishes or becomes non-existent. Regardless of the way by which cholesterol and blood cells protect liposomal stability, it is encouraging that liposomes are now available which, depending on their cholesterol content, can release entrapped agents *in vivo* at specific rates. Indeed, our recent work has shown that this applies to a number of drugs related to cancer (e.g. vincristine, melphalan, bleomycin) and antimicrobial (chloroquine, primaquine) therapy (C. Kirby, J. Clarke and G. Gregoriadis, unpublished data).

In vivo leakage of liposomal contents may also be prevented by accommodating these into the lipid framework of the carrier, by the use of agents which can interact electrostatically with liposomal lipid components or by linking agents on to already entrapped macromolecules or appropriate acceptors. For instance, when the lipid soluble actinomycin D is incorporated into the lipid phase of liposomes, its rate of clearance from the blood of injected rats is very similar to that of the carrier (18). The same applies to the lipid soluble colchicine (15) and daunomycin or vinblastine (27). In the "second carrier" approach (28) polyglutamic acid is incorporated into liposomes which are then allowed to interact with melphalan or methotrexate in the presence of carbodiimide. This results in the formation of a polyglutamic acid-drug complex and escape of the drug from liposomes in the circulation following their injection into rats is then prevented. Similar results are obtained when entrapped DNA serves as a second carrier for daunomycin or actinomycin D. (28).

Liposomal size and charge, among other factors, control the rate of elimination of liposomes from the blood. Thus, large liposomes are removed more rapidly than those of small size and this is reflected in the biphasic rate or clearance of liposomes of mixed sizes (7). Regarding surface charge, it appears that negatively charged liposomes are removed more rapidly than neutral or positively charged liposomes (23, 29, 30). This is probably related to the fact that liposomes, regardless of their initial charge, become negatively charged upon contact with blood plasma (31). However, the way by which such charge modulates rates of elimination is not known. It is possible that the surface charge originally present in liposomes controls the extent to, or even the fashion by, which plasma components associate with liposomes to cause their uptake by cells *in vivo*.

The cells responsible for liposome uptake are those of the reticuloendothelial system namely hepatic Kupffer cells and spleen macrophages (32, 33) and per unit weight participation of the two tissues is roughly similar (7, 16). It has been observed that even with liposomal preparations made under identical conditions and which are expected to transport entrapped agents to tissues at comparable rates, apparent total uptake of the agents by tissues can differ. This is because agents, depending on their nature, will behave differently once intracellularly. For instance, some agents will leak out while others will be degraded or metabolized with products being released extracellularly. The participation of hepatic parenchymal cells in the uptake of liposomes is still unclear in spite of extensive investigations (32-34); although it is conceivable that liposomes smaller than 100 nm in diameter can reach parenchymal cells and be subsequently interiorized by them. It is also unknown whether liposomes, even at their smallest size (about 15 nm) succeed in diffusing through capillary walls to reach extravascular areas. Liposomes are known, however, to cross membranes lining the peritoneal cavity. For instance, when small or large liposomes containing ^{125}I-labelled polyvinylpyrrolidone are given intraperitoneally, radioactivity is recovered in the blood and liver to an extent which is far above that expected to occur with the free polymer (35). It can thus be assumed that most of the radioactivity recover-

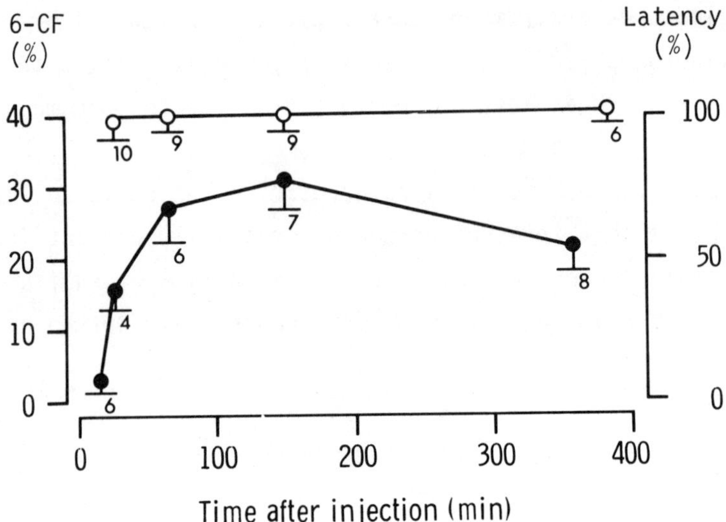

Fig. 4. *Latency and levels of liposomal 6-CF in the blood of injected mice.* Mice were injected intraperitoneally with 6-CF entrapped in unilamellar cholesterol-rich liposomes. 6-CF latency (O) and concentration (●) in total blood are expressed as % ± SD of the latency and the amount of the dye, respectively, in the injected preparation (23).

ed in these tissues is transported there by means of liposomes. Crossing of the peritoneum membranes has been shown beyond reasonable doubt in recent experiments in which mice were injected intraperitoneally with small unilamellar liposomes containing 0.25M 6-carboxyfluorescein (23). Fig. 4 shows that the dye penetrates the blood circulation in a fully quenched form supporting passage of intact liposomes. Further evidence for liposome transport through membranes comes from studies in which the rat testicle was injected with radiolabelled albumin or actinomycin D (36). When large liposomes were given, they remained quantitatively at the site of injection and disintegrated with released agents diffusing into the blood circulation. The fate of small liposomes was different in that entrapped agents were transported either to the lymph nodes draining the injected tissue or into the blood and tissues. Whether entrance in the blood occurred after direct crossing of the capillaries, via the lymphatic circulation or both is not known.

Further support for membrane crossing comes from experiments with tumour-bearing mice designed to investigate parameters related to the effect of size of the liposomal carrier (as well as that of entrapped agents) on its localization in malignant tissues. It was found (16, 35) that when small liposomes were used (about 80 nm average diameter) uptake of the liposomal ^{111}In-labelled bleomycin by Meth 'A', 6C3HED and Lewis lung carcinoma cells implanted in a variety of mouse strains and by Novikoff hepatoma in Wistar rats, was several-fold greater (up to about 7% of the dose per gram mouse tumour tissue) than that obtained with large liposomes. Because there was a parallel reduction in the uptake of the marker by the liver and spleen, it was reasoned that extended circulation of such liposomes in the blood enabled them to undergo transcapillary passage and reach tumour cells. Other workers (37) have recently confirmed these results in rats implanted with Walker 256 carcinoma. There are, however, at least three alternative explanations for such findings: as small liposomes circulate in the blood for longer periods of time, drug may be released slowly to reach the extravascular space more effectively. In addition, liposomes may interact in some way with the capillary walls, without actually crossing them. Again, by virtue of their longer survival in the circulation, small liposomes would be more efficient in doing so. The possibility also exists that liposomes are transported by macrophages which are known to infiltrate tumours.

Regarding the crossing of membranes at the subcellular level, there is now considerable evidence to support the notion that, *in vivo*, liposomes and their contents are endocytosed by cells to end up in the lysosomes (7-9, 33, 34, 39). Indeed, lysosomal localization of liposomes is far from being an unusual finding. Fixed macrophages of the liver and spleen are known to endocytose avidly macromolecules and particulate matter in the circulating blood and there is no reason to expect that liposomes would be an exception. Even stronger, although indirect, evidence for lysosomal localization of liposomes is the finding that in rats injected with liposomal radiolabelled albumin, the radioactivity content of the liver (which initially increases to high levels almost immediately after injection) declines rapidly, presumably as a result of albumin degradation and release of iodinated fragments into the circulation (8, 29). Such behaviour, also seen with liposomes containing enzymes (7, 8, 29, 39) is not exhibited by liposomal polyvinylpyrrolidone or ^{111}In which cannot be degraded or otherwise metabolized (16, 35).

In vivo interaction of cells with liposomes through fusion of the respective membranes, an event which would allow the introduction of agents directly into the cell's cytoplasm, is unlikely to occur to any significant extent: (a) although various morphological studies *in vivo* have provided ample evidence for endocytosis, they have failed to reveal liposome-entrapped material in the cytoplasm, unequivocally not surrounded by membranes; (b) erythrocytes and other blood cells which come into close contact for several hours with intravenously injected liposomes, do not incorporate any measurable proportion of liposomal agents.

3. INTERACTION OF LIPOSOMES WITH CELLS *IN VITRO*

The ability of liposomes to direct enzymes and other agents into the lysosomes of cells (7, 8) raised the question as to whether agents transported into these organelles could free themselves from the liposomal envelope and survive in an active form in their intralysosomal environment. In work carried out to show that liposomes could control cell metabolism (10) we found that cultured cells were capable of taking up liposomes the contents of which (in this case a hydrolytic enzyme) were delivered into the lysosomes where after the disintegration of the carrier, they were set free to act. Uptake of liposomes by cells, localization in lysosomes and their subsequent disruption were expected to occur not only because a similar fate of liposomes had been observed *in vivo*, but also because most cells are expected to endocytose soluble or particulate matter when exposed to it. Obviously, with "professional" endocytosers uptake will be more rapid than with other cells (e.g. fibroblasts). The fate and effect of agents entering lysosomes by endocytosis of the liposomal carrier depends on the physical characteristics of such agents. Thus, those which are stable in the lysosomal milieu can act within it (e.g. hydrolytic enzymes, metal chelating agents, certain antimicrobial drugs) or cross lysosomal membranes to reach, and act in, other cellular sites.

An alternative mechanism of cell-liposome interaction, namely fusion of the respective membranes, has been suggested (40-42). This has opened the possibility for a method of introducing agents entrapped in the aqueous space of liposomes directly into extralysosomal areas. On the other hand agents incorporated into the lipid phase of liposomes could, according to this mechanism, incorporate themselves into the cellular membrane. Although there has been a considerable amount of indirect experimental data to support fusion (12) doubts still exist as to its actual occurrence. Indeed, there is at least one mechanism which could provide an alternative explanation for such results: interaction of liposomes with cells may lead to the destabilization of the membranes of both entities with entrapped agents escaping from leaky liposomes to enter equally leaky cells at the points of contact.

4. DIRECTION OF LIPOSOMES TO TARGET SITES

As already mentioned, unmodified liposomes present in blood

circulation are taken up mostly by the cells of the reticuloendothelial system and also the hepatic parenchymal and endothelial cells. Obviously, in situations where biologically active agents are to be introduced into these cells, such localization can find good use. There are several instances, however, in which uptake of liposomes by alternative targets is desirable and therefore some versatility of the carrier's tissue distribution is required. This would not necessarily imply complete avoidance of non-target areas, especially in cases where drugs can be tolerated by such areas. In the treatment of enzyme deficiencies, for instance, with exogenous enzymes or of microbial diseases with certain antibiotics, participation of non-diseased cells is unlikely to be detrimental to their well-being. However, selective uptake by cytotoxic drugs would be essential for successful targeting, unless such drugs can be tolerated or inactivated by normal tissues.

In addition to variables pertaining to the carrier itself (e.g. size, surface charge, fluidity, etc.) other parameters also are known to influence liposome-target interaction. These have been tentatively classified (43) into two categories, namely those related to the biological space travelled by the carrier (e.g. blood, various membranes) or to the target itself (e.g. cell membrane composition, endocytic capacity, receptors). Consideration of such factors may help in rationalizing targeting and also in designing the overall carrier unit. Thus, there are a number of cases in which simple modifications of the liposomal carrier have been sufficient for its effective association with target areas. It was found, for instance, that by imposing a positive or negative charge on the surface of 99Tc-containing liposomes, there was a greater degree of radioactivity localization in infarcted myocardial regions of injected dogs (44). Furthermore, in the treatment of diabetic rats by the intragastric route with liposomal insulin, the choice of dipalmitoyl-phosphatidylcholine (which is less likely to be attacked by pancreatic phospholipases at 37°C or disrupted efficiently by bile salts), as the basic ingredient of liposomes helped us (45) to improve the glucose-lowering effect of the hormone. An example of modifying the non-target environment so as to improve localization of liposomal agents in specific areas is the administration of excess "empty" (buffer-loaded) liposomes of large average size together with smaller drug-carrying liposomes. Since large vesicles can compete successfully for the liver (29) with those of smaller size, these will circulate in the blood for longer periods of time and thus reach less accessible areas in the body. In experiments with tumour-bearing mice, for instance, large liposomes given at about the same time with small ones allowed the latter to localize their drug content in tumour tissues (16). Although such modifications of the liposomal carrier or the biological environment may, in certain cases, optimize drug action, there will be instances where a more sophisticated approach is needed. Towards selective association of cells with liposomes we have proposed (46) coating of the latter's surface with molecules possessing a specific affinity for the target. It is anticipated that these molecules will, by attaching themselves onto the relevant receptors of, say, cells mediate association of the liposomal moiety and its drug contents with the target. This idea was originally tested in my laboratory (46, 47) using antitumour cell antibodies or desialylated fetuins which along with other desialylated glycoproteins (48) binds specifically to the hepatic parenchymal cells. Proteins were associated with liposomes in a way that the Fab regions of antibodies (responsible for the recognition of the relevant antigens) and the terminal galactose molecules of desialylated fetuin (responsible for the specific receptors on the hepatocytes) (48) become available on the liposomal surface. We found that both types of macromolecules were capable of mediating uptake of liposomal agents by the respective receptor-carrying targets (i.e. tumour cells *in vitro* and hepatic parenchymal cells *in vivo*). However, application of the antibody-coated liposome system *in vivo* in tumour-bearing mice was not as successful (16). It appeared that antibodies raised against a variety of tumour cell surface antigens (whole cells were used for the immunization of rabbits) also shared by liver and spleen cells, were targeting liposomes to these cells as well.

Other proposed approaches for targeting include (a) coating of liposomes with isologous aggregated immunoglobulins which were found to mediate (through their Fc regions) association of liposome-entrapped horseradish peroxidase and hexosaminidase A with phagocytes from *Mustelus canis* and from a Tay-Sachs disease patient, respectively (49, 50); (b) incorporation into the liposome structure of a sialoglycoprotein extracted from the membrane of erythrocytes could, in the presence of lectins, facilitate binding of such liposomes to the cells *in vitro* (51); (c) ganglioside GM_1 incorporated in liposomes was shown to mediate selective uptake of the liposome moiety by receptors on the surface of hepatic parenchymal cells (52). Cell selectivity of liposomes coated with antibodies has recently found application in the specific stimulation or killing of cells (53). It was shown that, *in vitro*, liposomes containing anti-line 10 hepatocarcinoma cells immune RNA and coated with antilymphocyte antibodies were capable of stimulating lymphocytes to become specifically cytotoxic to line 10 tumour cells. In addition, actinomycin D-containing liposomes coated with anti-line 10 hepatocarcinoma cell antibodies were highly cytotoxic to such cells. It has been recently suggested (54) that selective uptake of liposomal agents by cells may not always be followed by the interiorization of the carrier. Obviously, interiorization will depend on the endocytic capacity of individual cell types.

5. APPLICATIONS IN BIOLOGY AND MEDICINE

The use of pharmacologically active agents in the elucidation or the control of cell behaviour and metabolic processes is often handicapped by problems related to the inability of such agents to enter cells or to reach specific intracellular organelles. Liposomes with their ability to associate with, or penetrate, cells in a variety of ways, is a unique system for the transport of agents into otherwise inaccessible cellular regions both *in vivo* and *in vitro*. Some of the applications in biology include studies of the role of the fluid state of the cell membrane in cellular regulatory mechanisms (55), the introduction of a new antigenic determinant into the surface of human erythrocytes (56), investigations on the nature of restrictions imposed by the cell membrane to certain drugs (57, 58), induction of interferon *in vivo* (59, 60) and *in vitro* (61), production of rabbit globin by cells exposed to liposome-entrapped rabbit mRNA coding for the globin (62, 63) and gene transfer by using liposomes containing metaphase chromosomes (64).

The increasing use of liposomes in medical research is the outcome of efforts to harness drug action by means of appropriate drug carriers (2). There is now a wide range of conditions in therapeutic and preventive medicine where liposomes hold promise. These include diseases in which the lysosomal apparatus is involved. For instance, liposomes can be employed for the delivery of missing enzymes in lysosomal storage diseases (65), of chelators for the removal of intralysosomally deposited metals (66) or of antimicrobial agents for the killing of intralysosomal parasites (67-69). In cancer chemotherapy (2) it is hoped that liposomes will prevent cytotoxic drugs from reaching normal rapidly dividing cells while at the same time directing drugs to tumour tissues. Liposomes may also find use in cases where administration of drugs by the oral route is preferable both for convenience, and also because it is often important that drugs enter the periphery via the portal circulation (e.g. administration of insulin in diabetes) (45). Finally, in preventive medicine liposomes could serve as immunological adjuvants for the potentiation of antibody response to bacterial (70) and viral (71) antigens.

6. CONCLUSIONS

During the last few years, the use of liposomes as membrane models has been extended to that of a drug carrier. The popularity of liposomes in research is based on two attractive features of the system, namely similarity to natural membranes and versatility. Owing to their semi-synthetic nature, liposomes can vary widely in size, surface characteristics and composition and can be made to accommodate a wide range of pharmacologically active substances including antitumour and antimicrobial drugs, enzymes, hormones, vaccines and informational molecules (12). However, in spite of the multitude of potential applications, knowledge on how liposomes interact with the biological milieu remains relatively poor. It is also correct to say that up to very recently the use of the liposomal carrier in terms of lipid composition, size, etc. was almost random. This is now being rapidly replaced by more rationalized and, in some instances, sophisticated fashions. Undoubtedly, there are difficulties to face. It should, nevertheless, be remembered that with many diseases affecting very large numbers of individuals, drugs have not fulfilled original hopes that followed their discovery. Similarly, many problems encountered in biological research remain, for reasons discussed earlier, unsolved. It follows that until there is considerable progress in achieving drug specificity, liposomes are likely to play important roles in optimizing drug action.

7. ACKNOWLEDGEMENT

I thank Mrs. Dorothy Seale for excellent secretarial work.

8. REFERENCES

1) Drug Carriers in Biology and Medicine (ed., G. Gregoriadis).

(1979). Academic Press, London, New York, San Francisco.
2) GREGORIADIS, G. (1977). Targeting of drugs. Nature, 265, 407.
3) GREGORIADIS, G. (1976). The drug-carrier potential of liposomes in Biology and Medicine. New Eng. J. Med., 295, 704.
4) GREGORIADIS, G. (1976). The drug-carrier potential of liposomes in Biology and Medicine. New Eng. J. Med., 295, 765.
5) BANGHAM, A.D., STANDISH, M.M. and WATKINS, J.C. (1965). Diffusion of univalent ions across the lamellae of swollen phospholipids. J. Mol. Biol., 13, 238.
6) GREGORIADIS, G., LEATHWOOD, P.D. and RYMAN, B.E. (1971). Enzyme entrapment in liposomes. FEBS Lett., 14, 95.
7) GREGORIADIS, G. and RYMAN, B.E. (1972). Fate of protein containing liposomes injected into rats. An approach to the treatment of storage diseases. Eur. J. Biochem., 24, 485.
8) GREGORIADIS, G. and RYMAN, B.E. (1972). Lysosomal localization of β-fructofuranosidase-containing liposomes injected into rats. Some implications in the treatment of genetic disorders. Biochem. J., 129, 123.
9) BLACK, C.D.V. and GREGORIADIS, G. (1974). Intracellular fate and effect of liposome-entrapped actinomycin D injected into rats. Biochem. Soc. Trans., 2, 869.
10) GREGORIADIS, G. and BUCKLAND, R.A. (1973). Enzyme-containing liposomes alleviate a model for storage diseases. Nature, 244, 170.
11) Liposomes in Biological Systems (eds., G. Gregoriadis and A.C. Allison) (1980). John Wiley and Sons, Chichester, New York, Brisbane, Toronto.
12) GREGORIADIS, G. (1980). The liposome drug-carrier concept: Its development and future. In: "Liposomes in Biological Systems", (eds., G. Gregoriadis and A.C. Allison), p. 25, John Wiley and Sons, Chichester, New York, Brisbane, Toronto.
13) TYRRELL, D.A., HEATH, T.D., COLLEY, C.M. and RYMAN, B.E. (1976). New aspects of liposomes. Biochim. Biophys. Acta, 457, 259.

14) KIMELBERG, H.K. and MAYHEW, E. (1978). Properties and biological effects of liposomes and their uses in pharmacology and toxicology. In: "CRC Critical Reviews in Toxicology". (ed., L Goldberg), p. 25, CRC Press Inc., West Palm Beach, Florida.

15) JULIANO, R.L. and STAMP, D. (1975). The effect of particle size and charge on the clearance rates of liposomes and liposome-encapsulated drugs. Biochem. Biophys. Res. Comm, 63, 651.

16) GREGORIADIS, G., NEERUNJUN, E.D. and HUNT, R. (1977). Fate of a liposome-associated agent injected into normal and tumour-bearing rodents. Attempts to improve localization in tumour tissues. Life Sci., 21, 357.

17) KIMELBERG, H.K. (1976). Differential distribution of liposome-entrapped [^{3}H] methotrexate and labelled lipids after intravenous injection in a primate. Biochim. Biophys. Acta, 448, 531.

18) GREGORIADIS, G. (1973). Drug entrapment in liposomes. FEBS Lett., 36, 292.

19) KIMELBERG, H.K., MAYHEW, E. and PAPAHADJOPOULOS, D. (1975). Distribution of liposome-entrapped cations in tumour-bearing mice. Life Sci., 17, 715.

20) ZBOROWSKI, J., ROERDINK, F. and SCHERPHOF, G. (1977). Leakage of sucrose from phosphatidylcholine liposomes induced by interaction with serum albumin. Biochim. Biophys. Acta, 497, 183.

21) GREGORIADIS, G. and DAVIS, C. (1979). Stability of liposomes *in vivo* and *in vitro* is promoted by their cholesterol content and the presence of blood cells. Biochem. Biophys. Res. Comm., 89, 1287.

22) DAVIS, C. and GREGORIADIS, G. (1979). The effect of lipid composition of liposomes on their stability *in vivo*. Biochem. Soc. Trans., 7, 680.

23) KIRBY, C., CLARKE, J. and GREGORIADIS, G. (1979). The effect of the cholesterol content of small unilamellar liposomes on their stability *in vivo* and *in vitro*. Biochem. J., in press.

24) WEINSTEIN, J.N., YOSHIKANI, S., HENKART, P., BLUMENTAL, R. and

HAGINS, W.A. (1977). Liposome-cell interaction: transfer and intracellular release of a trapped fluorescent marker. Science, 195, 489.

25) LADBROOKE, B.D., WILLIAMS, R.M. and CHAPMAN, D. (1968). Studies on lecithin-cholesterol-water interactions by differential scanning calorimetry and X-ray diffraction. Biochem. Biophys. Acta, 150, 333.

26) JAMES, A.T., LOVELOCK, J.E. and WEBB, P.W. (1959). The lipids of whole blood. 1. Lipid biosynthesis in human blood *in vitro*. Biochem. J., 73, 106.

27) JULIANO, R.L. and STAMP, D. (1978). Pharmacokinetics of liposome-encapsulated anti-tumour drugs. Biochem. Pharmacol., 27, 21.

28) GREGORIADIS, G., DAVISSON, P.J. and SCOTT, S. (1977). Binding of drugs onto liposome-entrapped macromolecules prevents diffusion of drugs from liposomes *in vitro* and *in vivo*. Biochem. Soc. Trans., 5, 1323.

29) GREGORIADIS, G. and NEERUNJUN, E.D. (1974). Control of the rate of hepatic uptake and catabolism of liposome-entrapped proteins injected into rats. Possible therapeutic applications. Eur. J. Biochem., 47, 179.

30) TAGESSON, C., STENDAHL, O. and MAGNUSSON, K.-E. (1977). The clearance of liposomes after intravenous injection into mice in relation to their physico-chemical properties as assessed by partitioning in an aqueous biphasic system. Studia Biophysica, 64, 151.

31) BLACK, C.D.V. and GREGORIADIS, G. (1976). Interaction of liposomes with blood plasma proteins. Biochem. Soc. Trans., 4, 256.

32) SEGAL, A.W., WILLS, E.J., RICHMOND, J.E., SLAVIN, G., BLACK, C.D.V. and GREGORIADIS, G. (1974). Morphological observations on the cellular and subcellular destination of intravenously administered liposomes. Br. J. Exp. Pathol., 55, 320.

33) WISSE, E., GREGORIADIS, G. and DAEMS, W.Th. (1976). The uptake of liposomes by the rat liver. In: "The Reticuloendothelial

System in Health and Disease: Functions and Characteristics". (eds., S.M. Reichard, M.R. Escobar and H. Friedman), p. 237, Plenum Publishing Co., New York.

34) RAHMAN, Y.-E. and WRIGHT, B.J. (1975). Liposomes containing chelating agents. Cellular penetration and a possible mechanism of metal removal. J. Cell Biol., 65, 112.

35) DAPERGOLAS, G., NEERUNJUN, E.D. and GREGORIADIS, G. (1976). Penetration of target areas in the rat by liposome-associated bleomycin, glucose oxidase and insulin. FEBS Lett., 63, 235.

36) SEGAL, A.W., GREGORIADIS, G. and BLACK, C.D.V. (1975). Liposomes as vehicles for the local release of drugs. Clin. Sci. Mol. Med., 49, 99.

37) RICHARDSON, V.J., JEYASINGH, K., JEWKES, R.F., RYMAN, B.E. and TATTERSALL, M.H. (1977). Properties of [^{99m}Tc] Technetium-labelled liposomes in normal and tumour-bearing mice. Biochem. Soc. Trans, 5, 290.

38) GREGORIADIS, G., PUTMAN, D., LOUIS, L. and NEERUNJUN, E.D. (1974). Comparative fate and effect of non-entrapped and liposome-entrapped neuraminidase injected into rats. Biochem. J., 140, 323.

39) STEGER, L.D. and DESNICK, R.J. (1977). Enzyme therapy. VI. Comparative *in vivo* fates and effects on lysosomal entegrity of enzyme entrapped in negatively and positively charged liposomes. Biochim. Biophys. Acta, 464, 530.

40) GRANT, C.W.M. and McCONNELL, H.M. (1973). Fusion of phospholipid vesicles with viable Acholeplasma laidlawii. Proc. Nat. Acad. Sci. USA, 70, 1238.

41) PAPAHADJOPOULOS, D., POSTE, G. and MAYHEW, E. (1974). Cellular uptake of cyclic AMP captured within phospholipid vesicles and effect on cell growth behaviour. Biochim. Biophys. Acta, 363, 404.

42) PAGANO, R.E. and HUANG, L. (1975). Interaction of phospholipid vesicles with cultured mammalian cells. J. Cell Biol., 67, 49.

43) GREGORIADIS, G. (1978). Liposomes in Therapeutic and Preventive Medicine. The development of the drug carrier concept. Ann. N.Y. Acad. Sci., 308, 343.

44) CARIDE, V.J. and ZARET, B.L. (1977). Liposome accumulation in regions of experimental myocardial infarction. Science, 198, 735.

45) DAPERGOLAS, G. and GREGORIADIS, G. (1976). Hypoglycaemic effect of liposome-entrapped insulin administered intragastrically into rats. Lancet, 2, 824.

46) GREGORIADIS, G. (1974). Structural requirements for the specific uptake of macromolecules and liposomes by target tissues. In: "Enzyme therapy in Lysosomal Storage Diseases" (eds., J.M. Tager, G.J.M. Hooghwinkel and W.Th. Daems), p. 131, North Holland Publishing Co.

47) GREGORIADIS, G., NEERUNJUN, E.D. (1975). Homing of liposomes to target cells. Biochem. Biophys. Res. Comm., 65, 537.

48) GREGORIADIS, G. (1975). Catabolism of glycoproteins. In: "Lysosomes in Biology and Pathology". (eds., J.T. Dingle and R.T. Dean), p. 265, North Holland Publishing Co.

49) WEISSMANN, G., BLOOMGARDEN, D., KAPLAN, R., COHEN, C., HOFFSTEIN, S., COLLINS, T., GOTTLIEB, A. and NAGLE, D. (1975). A general method for the introduction of enzymes, by means of immunoglobulin-coated liposomes, into lysosomes of deficient cells *in vitro*. Proc. Natl. Acad. Sci. USA, 72, 88.

50) COHEN, C.M., WEISSMANN, G., HOFFSTEIN, S., AWASTHI, Y.C. and SRIVASTAVE, S.K. (1976). Introduction of purified hexosaminidase A into Tay-Sachs leucocytes by means of immunoglobulin-coated liposomes. Biochemistry, 15, 452.

51) JULIANO, R.L. and STAMP, D. (1976). Lectin-mediated attachment of glycoprotein bearing liposomes to cells. Nature, 261, 235.

52) SUROLIA, A. and BACHHAWAT, B.K. (1977). Monosialyganglioside liposome-entrapped enzyme uptake by hepatic cells. Biochim. Biophys. Acta, 497, 760.

53) MAGEE, W.E., GRONENBERGER, J.H. and THOR, D.E. (1979). Marked stimulation of lymphocyte-mediated attack on tumour cells by target-directed liposomes containing immune RNA, Cancer Res., 38, 1173.

54) WEINSTEIN, J.N., BLUMENTHAL, R., SPARROW, S.O. and HENKART, P.A. (1978). Antibody-mediated targeting of liposomes. Binding to lymphocytes does not ensure incorporation of vesicle contents into the cells. Biochim. Biophys. Acta, 509, 272.

55) INBAR, M. and SHINITZKY, M. (1974). Increase of cholesterol level in the surface membrane of lymphoma cells and its inhibitory effect on ascites tumour development. Proc. Nat. Acad. Sci. USA, 71, 2128.

56) MARTIN, F.J. and McDONALD, R.C. (1976). Lipid vesicle-cell interactions. III. Introduction of a new antigenic determinant into erythrocyte membranes. J. Cell Biol., 70, 515.

57) PAPAHADJOPOULOS, D., POSTE, G., WAIL, W.J. and BIEDLER, J.L. (1976). Use of lipid vesicles as carriers to introduce actinomycin D into resistant tumour cells. Cancer Res., 36, 2988.

58) SCHIFFMAN, F.I. and KLEIN, I. (1977). Rapid induction of amphotericin B sensitivity in L1210 leukemia cells by liposomes containing ergosterol. Nature, 269, 65.

59) STRAUB, S.X., GARRY, R.F. and MAGEE, W.E. (1974). Interferon induction by poly(I):poly(C) enclosed in phospholipid particles. Infect. Immun., 10, 783.

60) MAGEE, W.E., TALCOTT, M.L., STRAUB, S.X. and VRIEND, C.Y. (1976). A comparison of negatively and positively charged liposomes containing entrapped polyinosinic polycytidylic acid for interferon induction in mice. Biochim. Biophys. Acta, 451, 610.

61) MAYHEW, E., PAPAHADJOPOULOS, D., O'MALLEY, J., CARTER, W.A. and VAIL, W.J. (1977). Cellular uptake and protection against virus infection by polyinosinic-polycytidylic acid entrapped within phospholipid vesicles. Molec. Pharmacol., 13, 488.

62) DIMITRIADIS, G.J. (1978). Translation of rabbit globin mRNA in-

troduced by liposomes into mouse lymphocytes. Nature, 274, 423.

63) OSTRO, M.J., GIACOMONI, D., LAVELLE, D., PAXTON, W. and DRAY, S. (1978). Evidence for translation of rabbit globin mRNA after liposome-mediated insertion into a human cell line. Nature, 274, 921.

64) MUKHERJEE, A.B., ORLOFF, S., BUTLER, J.D., TRICHE, T., LALLEY, P. and SCHULMAN, J.D. (1978). Entrapment of metaphase chromosomes into phospholipid vesicles (lipochromosomes): Carrier potential in gene transfer. Proc. Nat. Acad. Sci. USA, 75, 1361.

65) BELCHETZ, P.E., BRAIDMAN, I.P., CRAWLEY, J.C.W. and GREGORIADIS, G. (1977). Treatment of Gaucher's disease with liposome-entrapped glucocerebroside:β-glucosidase. Lancet, 2, 116.

66) RAHMAN, Y.-E., ROSENTHAL, M.W. and CERNY, E.A. (1973). Intracellular plutonium: removal by liposome-encapsulated chelating agents. Science, 180, 300.

67) BLACK, C.D.V., WATSON, G.J. and WARD, R.J. (1977). The use of Pentostam liposomes in the chemotherapy of experimental leishmaniasis. Transp. Roy. Soc. Trop. Med. Hyg., 71, 550.

68) NEW, R.R.C., CHANCE, M.L., THOMAS, S.C. and PETERS, W. (1978). Antileishmanial activity of antimonials entrapped in liposomes. Nature, 274, 55.

69) BONVENTRE, P. and GREGORIADIS, G. (1978). Killing of intraphagocytic *Staph. Aureus* by dehydrostreptomycin entrapped in liposomes. Antimicrobial Agents and Chemotherapy, 13, 1049.

70) ALLISON, A.C. and GREGORIADIS, G. (1974). Liposomes as immunological adjuvants. Nature, 252, 252.

71) MANESIS, E.K., CAMERON, C. and GREGORIADIS, G. (1979). Hepatitis B surface antigen-containing liposomes enhance humoral and cell-mediated immunity to the antigen. FEBS Lett., 102, 107.

FUSION OF CELL FRAGMENTS AS A METHOD IN CELL GENETICS

T. Ege

Department of Medical Cell Genetics
Medical Nobel Institute
Karolinska Institutet
S-104 01 Stockholm 60, Sweden

1. INTRODUCTION

Prior to the early sixties mammalian genetics had been concerned almost exclusively with the mechanisms by which genetic information was transmitted through the germ cells. Although this is still a central area recent technical developments now make it possible to analyze the organization and function of genes in somatic cells. Somatic cell genetics is a new subfield of genetics which aims to define genetic mechanisms involved in differentiation, neoplasia, inborn errors of metabolism, cell-virus interactions and other hereditary phenomena in somatic cells. The methodology of this new field includes generation and selection of mutant cell lines, phenotypic analysis of cultured cells, cell hybridization and gene transfer methods to mention but a few of the methods currently used.

The technique of somatic cell hybridization is based on the observation that several viruses will cause an increase in the percentage of multinucleated cells during infection. Their appearance is due to fusion of infected cells (1) caused by agents in the virus envelope (2). From a technical point of view it is of interest that cell fusion can also be induced by inactivated virus or virus envelopes in the absence of an infection (3).

In conventional cell hybridization, the immediate fusion product of two different cells is a binucleated cell (heterokaryon) with a mixed cytoplasm consisting of components from both the parental cells. By comparing the pattern of gene expression seen in the heterokaryon with that of the parental cells it is possible to obtain information about the factors controlling gene expression (for a review, see 4).

The analysis of the nuclear-cytoplasmic interaction in heterokaryons is complicated to some extent by the presence of two nuclei in a *mixed* cytoplasm, and also by the limited amount of material and short lifespan of such cells. When heterokaryons go into mitosis, occasionally daughter cells appear which contain the full genetic complement of the two parental cells. The analysis of such growing hybrid cells has given important information about factors controlling gene expression in somatic cells (for a review, see 4), although the interpretation of these experiments is complicated by the frequent loss of chromosomes from one or both of the parental complements (5). To avoid some of the problems associated with the analysis of heterokaryons, formed by fusion of two intact cells, and growing hybrid cells, cell fragments can be used as one or both fusion partners.

2. REACTIVATION OF CHICK ERYTHROCYTE NUCLEI

(i) Reactivation in intact cells

Mature chick erythrocytes are inactive with respect to DNA,

RNA, and protein synthesis (for review, see 6). The inactive erythrocyte nuclei can be reactivated by virus induced fusion of chick erythrocytes to growing mammalian cells (7, 8). Most of the cytoplasm of the erythrocyte is lost to the surrounding medium due to the hemolytic activity of the virus (9, 10). Therefore, practically all the cytoplasm in the resulting heterokaryon will be of mammalian origin. This type of experiment, therefore, comes very close to being a transplantation of an inactive avian genome into the cytoplasm of a mammalian "host" cell. In the heterokaryon, the chick nucleus undergoes a series of morphological and chemical changes starting with physiochemical changes in the chromatin followed by a rapid swelling and increase in dry mass, and activation of chick RNA and DNA synthesis. After som days chick genes are reexpressed in the heterokaryons. This system has been used to gather information about events that take place during the activation of a large number of inactive genes in the hope that this may give an insight into the mechanisms that operate when specific genes are activated during embryonic development and in response to specific stimuli (for a review, see 6 and 8).

The increase in dry mass of the chick erythrocyte nucleus takes place also when chick macromolecule-synthesis is blocked (8, 11) indicating that host materials accumulate in the chick nucleus during the reactivation process. It therefore seemed reasonable to assume that among these macromolecules there were factors which activated chick genes. In order to examine further the types of macromolecules that accumulate in the reactivating chick nuclei, heterokaryons were examined by immunological methods.

After fusion of chick erythrocytes with human cells (12) the reactivation and migration of host macromolecules into the chick nucleus can be followed using antibodies directed against human macromolecules and indirect immune fluorescence. As a source of antibodies we used immune sera from patients suffering from *Lupus Erythematosus*; these sera contain autoantibodies to various antigens (for a review, see 13). By analyzing a large number of sera from different patients, we were able to select three showing a high titer of antibodies directed against a nucleolar, a nucleoplasmic and a cytoplasmic component, respectively. In addition these sera were also species-specific as they showed no cross-reactivity with several types of chick cells.

In HeLa-chick erythrocyte heterokaryons the chick nuclei became positive for human nuclear antigens. The percentage of chick nuclei showing uptake of the two human nuclear antigens increased continuously with time and there was also an increase in the intensity of the immune fluorescence of the individual chick nuclei. No uptake of antigens characteristic of human cytoplasm was ever observed. The location of the antigens characteristic for human nucleoli changed during the reactivation of the chick erythrocyte nucleus. At an early stage the staining was weak and localized to a few regions in the erythrocyte nucleus, but this changed with time to show strong staining of 2-3 distinct spots which corresponded with the location of the nucleoli seen in phase contrast microscopy.

These results offered direct evidence that human macromolecules move into the chick erythrocyte nucleus during their reactivation in human-chick heterokaryons. They also showed that this uptake is selective for nucleus-specific material, as demonstrated by the lack of uptake of cytoplasmic antigens. Several pieces of evidence seem to exclude nucleic acids and point towards the proteinaceous nature of the nuclear antigens. In mitotic cells, the antigenic material is present in the cytoplasm but absent from the chromosomes. Furthermore, the antibody binding is resistant to pretreatment with DNase, suggesting that the antigenic material is not DNA or a DNA-protein complex. In experiments where chick erythrocytes have been fused to cells prelabelled with ^{3}H-uridine, we have been unable to detect accumulation of radioactivity in the chick nucleus. This, together with the fact that antibody binding is uninfluenced by RNase digestion, suggests that the antigen is not RNA or a RNA-protein complex.

Several reports have appeared that confirm and extend the results on the accumulation of host specific material in the chick nucleus during reactivitation. Using cytochemical methods Appels *et al.* (14) showed that the overall protein content of the chick erythrocyte nucleus increased 2-3-fold during reactivation largely due to an early accumulation of non-histone proteins. These results were confirmed using chemical analysis of the proteins from isolated, reactivated erythrocytes (15). During the early stages, the erythrocyte nucleus preferentially accumulated host non-histone proteins relative to histones. Furthermore, the accumulation of proteins of molecular weights below 60,000 daltons was more rapid than that of larger proteins and was independent of whether the proteins had been synthesized before or after fusion thus indicating that the deposition of nuclear proteins was not linked to their synthesis.

Specific proteins accumulating during the reactivation process include RNA polymerase A and B (16), DNA repair enzymes (17), and the T-antigen of SV40 transformed cells (18), all of which show a nuclear location in the host cell. Specific host cell proteins that do not accumulate include the cytoplasmic enzymes lactate dehydrogenase, isocitrate dehydrogenase and malate dehydrogenase (14). These proteins are also absent from the host nucleus. However, it is not possible to draw conclusions about cause and effect relationships from the above data and the exact role that the accumulated proteins play in the reactivation process is still unknown. It seems likely, however, that, among the mammalian nucleospecific proteins that do accumulate, there are some which should be considered as signals of direct regulatory importance.

The rate of reactivation of the chick nucleus has been shown to be reduced when the ratio of chick/host nuclei in heterokaryons is high (19). This indicates that the erythrocyte nuclei compete for some factor(s) present in the heterokaryons and that these are rate limiting for the reactivation process. Experiments by Carlsson *et al.* (16) indicated that the rate limiting factors were macromolecular since competition was also observed in an *in vitro* assay for endogenous RNA polymerase activity where the ionic environment was controlled and nucleotides were present in excess.

(ii) Reactivation in enucleated cells

As the nuclei in heterokaryons are quite often seen to be in close contact, the possibility exists that the accumulation of host macromolecules and factors rate limiting for the reactivation might take place through a direct internuclear transfer. To examine this possibility, reconstituted cells were produced (20) by fusing chick erythrocytes with cells that had been enucleated (see below) prior to fusion. Similar experiments had already been performed by two other groups (21, 22) but their results were conflicting and difficult to interpret. In the experiments reported by Poste and Reeve (21) no sign of reactivation was found when erythrocytes were fused with enucleated cells. Ladda and Estensen (22), however, reported nuclear swelling and initiation of RNA synthesis when chick erythrocytes were fused with intact cells that were later enucleated under conditions that preferentially removed the host nucleus.

In our experiments, the kinetics of reactivation of the chick nucleus was similar in both heterokaryons and enucleated cells during the first 12 h after fusion. Uptake of host specific nuclear antigen, nuclear swelling and RNA synthesis was evident in most erythrocyte nuclei. In addition, the percentage of chick nuclei synthesizing DNA was found to be the same in both heterokaryons and enucleated cells.

Fortyeight hours post fusion, a small fraction of chick nuclei in reconstituted cells showed the presence of a chick specific nucleolar antigen. This antigen normally appears at late stages of chick erythrocyte reactivation in heterokaryons, but is absent in mature chick erythrocytes and in erythrocyte nuclei reactivated in heterokaryons in which chick RNA synthesis is blocked. We therefore interpret the presence of this antigen as evidence for *de novo* chick protein synthesis in some of the reconstituted cells.

A decreased rate of RNA synthesis and nuclear swelling was observed during later stages of reactivation, and at 48 h after fusion RNA synthesis was negligible. This might explain the failure of Poste and Reeve to detect erythrocyte reactivation in enucleated cytoplasms, as their enucleation procedure required several hours to elapse between the enucleation process and the introduction of a new nucleus into the cytoplasm.

Although the reconstituted cells remained attached to the substratum longer than did enucleated cells, they eventually disappeared. The survival of reconstituted cells could be prolonged by using enucleated chick cells and immature chick erythrocytes in which RNA synthesis had not been completely inactivated. However, no cells capable of long term survival and multiplication have been found. This could be due to the relatively slow reactivation of the chick nucleus, which may result in a delayed supply of vital components to the cytoplasm.

The fact that chick erythrocyte nuclei reactivate in both heterokaryons and reconstituted cells does not exclude the possibility that inter-nuclear transfer of macromolecules might occur in the former, but does show that this is not the only method of transfer. A more likely explanation is probably that the cytoplasm contains a pool of the macromolecules, and/or the machinery to synthesize them, and that these are taken up directly by the chick nucleus. The presence of such a pool is indicated by the fact that protein synthesis is not required after fusion for this uptake to take place (23, 24).

3. RECONSTITUTION OF CELLS

Fusion products of chick erythrocyte nuclei and enucleated cytoplasms are only produced in low yield and fail to give rise to growing cells. For this reason they have a limited applicability as a system for studying the influence of the cytoplasm on nuclear gene activity. A more favourable system would be one where an active nucleus from a cell with one pattern of gene expression is transplanted into the cytoplasm of a cell with a different pattern of gene expression. Such experiments involving artificial transfer of cytoplasm and nucleus, have been accomplished with unicellular organisms. Cybrids and hybrids can be formed in *Acetabularia* by grafting enucleated or intact cells, showing one cap-type with intact cells of another cap-type. Analysis of the cap-types of the fusion-products showed that the caps formed were of an intermediate type in the hybrids and of the type characteristic for the nuclear donor in the cybrids (25, 26), indicating that the form of the cap is under nuclear control.

In amoebae, nuclei of one species can be transferred to enucleated cells of another species of amoebae. Such reconstituted amoebae survive and multiply for years. Some properties of these clones (division rate and nuclear diameter) are determined by the cytoplasmic donor, others (shape when migrating) are intermediate, while other still are under nuclear control (27, 28).

Similar experiments with mammalian cells had met with little success until the early seventies. Attempts had been made to transfer isolated nuclei into other cells, but although these were taken up by the cells, the experiments failed due to degradation of the nuclei (29). A different approach became possible, however, with the introduction of a technique that allowed the preparation of nucleated and enucleated cell fractions which still retained the potential for fusion with *Sendai* virus.

(i) Preparation of cell fragments

In 1967, Carter (30) observed that one of the effects of the fungal metabolite *cytochalasin B*, was to cause a partial extrusion of the nuclei of exposed cells. With some cell types this extrusion became complete in a low percentage of the cells. This allowed the separation of the enucleated cell fragments from intact cells and nucleated fragments by density gradient centrifugation. However, it was not until Prescott *et al.* (31) discovered that the enucleation frequency could be dramatically increased by applying centrifugal force to *cytochalasin B* treated cells, that it became possible to perform large scale enucleation experiments.

The method involves centrifugation of cells, adhering to glass or plastic slides, in medium containing *cytochalasin B*. During centrifugation, the nucelus is drawn out from the main cell body until only a thin cytoplasmic strand connects the nucleated part with the rest of the cell. This eventually breaks, so giving rise to nucleated and enucleated fragments.

The enucleated cells (cytoplasms) remain attached to the slide, while the nucleated fragments can be recovered from the pellet in the bottom of the tube. We have used L6 cells, a rat myoblast cell line, for our model experiments (32) which were designed to characterize the cell fragments obtained after enucleation. These cells have several characteristics which make them suitable for enucleation experiments, the most important being the homogeneity of the cell population, the high plating efficiency and the strong adherence of the cells to the substratum. The general conclusions obtained from these experiments, however, have been confirmed for other cell types by ourselves and other groups.

Cytoplasms. Immediately after enucleation of L6 cells, the enucleated fragment has a drawn out morphology, but it will recover and show the normal, flattened out appearance of intact cells within one hour. Dry mass measurements have shown that the mass is approximately 50-60% that of intact cells. The anucleate cells retain several characteristics of the intact cells such as membrane ruffling, active cell movement and endocytosis (unpublished results, 33, 34). In addition, electron microscopical examination show cytoplasmic organelles in a ground substance which is surrounded by an intact cell membrane similar to that found in untreated cells (see also 34, 35, 36). While no RNA or DNA synthesis can be detected, the rate of protein synthesis soon after enucleation is similar to that of intact cells if the smaller size is taken into account (31, 34). However, there is a gradual decrease in the rate of protein synthesis (31, 34) so that after 12-18 h many anucleate cells fail to show amino acid incorporation. Most anucleate cells die between 15 and 30 h after enucleation.

From the above results, it seems that the enucleation process does not result in irreversible damage to cultured cells. Shortly after enucleation they behave like intact cells in several respects, for instance the information for cell-morphology and locomotion is present in enucleated cells and is preserved through trypsinization and replating. It is also of interest to note that when normal and transformed cells are enucleated, the resulting enucleated cells retain their typical parental responses upon contact with other cells (34).

Minicells. After enucleation, the extruded nuclei are found as a pellet on the bottom of the centrifuge tube. Chemical analysis of the protein content of this fraction indicated that at least 75% of the original cytoplasm had been lost. This agrees well with the observation that the enzyme activity of cytoplasmic enzymes were reduced to a level of 25-35% that of intact cells. However, in addition to nucleated fragments, the pellet also contained a high percentage of very small cytoplasmic fragments and so the true value for the cytoplasmic content of individual nucleated fragments was lower than that indicated by chemical measurements made on the whole pellet. The cytoplasmic fragments can be separated from nucleated fragments on the basis of their lower density and smaller size using a Ficoll-gradient at unit gravity (37). Dry mass measurement and cytochemical analysis of the protein content of individual nucelated fragments showed that they contained a maximum of 10% of the original cytoplasm. This figure agrees well with estimations from electron microscopical pictures of serially sectioned pellet material and with results obtained by other methods. One such method of determining cytoplasmic contamination is based on feeding cells polystyrene particles. When cells are grown in the presence of polystyrene beads (0.5-1.0 μm) in diameter, the beads are taken up by the cells (36) and accumulate in the cytoplasm. When such labelled cells are enucleated, about 2% of the beads present in intact cells can be found associated with the cytoplasmic rim of the nucleated fragments, so providing a rough estimate of the cytoplasmic contamination of these fragments. However, such an analysis assumes, firstly, that there is an even distribution of beads in the cytoplasm of the intact cells, and secondly that the bead distribution is uninfluenced by the enucleation conditions, neither of which might be true. Lucas *et al.* (37), determined the cytoplasmic contamination of nucleated fragments of mouse L929 cells to be 4% using the above mentioned bead-method and about 8% using the amount of cytoplasmic ribosomal RNA associated with the nuclei after enucleation. These figures agree well with our own results both for L6 cells and other cell types (unpublished observations).

Most of the nucleated fragments exclude trypan blue indicating that they are surrounded by an intact cell membrane. Electron microscopy confirms this observation, showing that the nucleated fragments consist of a nucleus, with a normal morphology, surrounded by a thin rim of cytoplasm and a cell membrane.

Such structures have been given the name minicells. Serial sectioning of the minicells shows that they are lacking a Golgi-apparatus, and only rarely can mitochondria be found. Vesicular and cisternal elements of the cytoplasmic reticulum are usually absent, and free ribosomes and matrix substance dominate. Similar observations have been made by Prescott and Kirkpatrick (36, 39) who also showed that the centriole remained in the anucleate fragment.

About 80-90% of the minicells are viable immediately after preparation as determined by trypan blue exclusion and the ability to synthesize RNA. During incubation under normal tissue culture conditions, where intact cells survive and multiply, the percentage of trypan blue positive minicells increases with time after preparation. Two days after preparation only a small percentage of the original population are intact as judged by the trypan blue exclusion test. These are probably intact cells, present as contamination in the minicell fraction, rather than minicells which are capable of surviving since continuous observation of a large number of minicells and intact cells demonstrated that all minicells followed (>300) were found to lyse while intact cells in the same culture survived and multiplied during the observation period. Further evidence supporting this conclusion comes from experiments with minicells prepared from bead labelled cells. When such minicells are incubated under normal tissue culture conditions for one week, a low percentage of the incubated cells have formed colonies. If these colonies originated from minicells that have regenerated a new cytoplasm and divided, one would expect each of the colonies to contain a low number of beads, comparable to that found in minicells immediately after preparation. However, all such clones contain a bead number similar to that found in the intact cells used for minicell preparation, indicating that all colonies arise from intact cells contaminating the minicells pellet. Similar results have been obtained with other cell types (unpublished results).

In contrast to these results Lucas *et al.* (37) found that 30% of the minicells prepared from L929 cells attache to the surface of the culture vessel and that 10% proceed to divide.

(ii) Fusion of minicells and cytoplasms

Fusion of cells with *Sendai* virus requires that the virus can bind to the cells through specific virus receptors present on the cell membrane. As both minicells and cytoplasms are surrounded by a cell membrane containing *Sendai* virus receptors, it should be possible to fuse these two cell fragments together. The development of such a technique would permit the construction of reconstituted cells in which the nucleus is derived from one parental cell type and most of the cytoplasm from another cell type.

The identification of growing reconstituted cells is hampered by a low fusion frequency and the presence of a small percentage of intact cells in both preparations of cell fragments. For these reasons it is important to use parental cells which differ with respect to genetic markers and/or to use artificial markers. Genetic markers can be either nuclear (absence of enzymes due to mutations, chromosome markers, chromocenters, sex chromatin, etc.), cytoplasmic (mitochondrial drug resistance mutants) or artificial markers such as phagocytosed particles (polystyrene beads, carbon and tantalum particles). Another type of artificially induced marker is the use of isotope labelling, e.g. thymidine labelling of DNA and amino acid labelling of proteins. The drawback of all forms of induced markers is that they are transient and so are only useful for a short period of time following fusion.

In the first attempts (40) to generate reconstituted cells by fusion of minicells and cytoplasms from a rat myoblast cell line, we used isotopic labels. The cytoplasmic donor cells were labelled with ^{3}H-leucine and the nuclear donors with ^{3}H-thymidine. Autoradiography performed on the parental cells showed a weak labelling all over the cytoplasmic donor, and a strong nuclear labelling over the minicell donor. Reconstituted cells would be expected to show a heavy nuclear and a weak cytoplasmic labelling. Cells fulfilling these criteria could be identified at an early stage after fusion and the number of such cells was dependent on the addition of virus.

(iii) Viability of reconstituted cells

Although it had been shown that reconstituted cells could be formed using the same cell type as both nuclear and cytoplasmic donor, it was uncertain whether interspecific combinations were possible, nor was it known whether reconstituted cells were capable of giving rise to viable daughter cells. Both these properties would greatly improve the usefulness of reconstituted cells as a system in which several aspects of cell biology could be studied. However, it was evident that our previous method for identifying reconstituted cells would be unable to demonstrate these properties and so a different method was adopted. This utilized minicell and cytoplasmic donors, each labelled with latex beads of different sizes, as described by Veomett *et al.* (38). In addition, the cytoplasmic donor was deficient in an enzyme which rendered it incapable on incorporating exogenously added hypoxanthine, and so we could use the following criteria for differentiating reconstituted cells from parental cells and other fusion products:

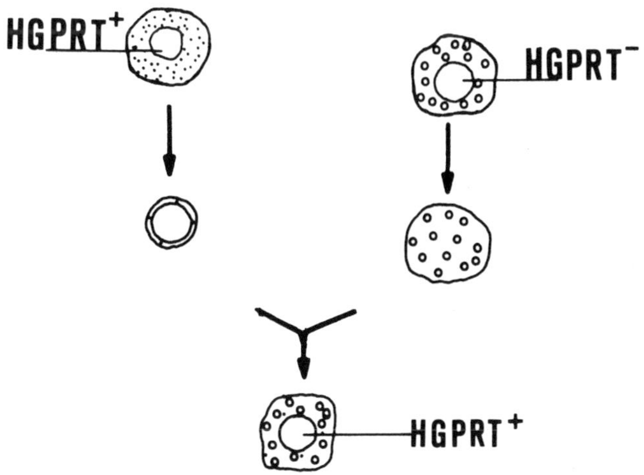

Fig. 1. *Labelling pattern of parental and reconstituted cells.*

Nuclear donor cells would have a high number of small latex spheres and would show incorporation of radioactive hypoxanthine. Cytoplasmic donors would have a large number of large latex spheres, and would be unable to incorporate hypoxanthine. Reconstituted cells will carry a high number of large latex spheres, and will be distinguished from intact cytoplasmic donors on the basis of the ability of the added nucleus to incorporate hypoxanthine. Furthermore, reconstituted cells will only contain a fraction of the small beads present in the cytoplasm of the nuclear donor cells since the majority of the cytoplasm will be removed during the preparation of the minicells. Although other combinations of beads and hypoxanthine labelling are also possible as the result of other cell/fragment fusions, these can be easily differentiated from reconstituted cells.

Using rat cells as cytoplasmic donors and both rat and mouse cells as nuclear donors, minicells and cytoplasms were prepared as outlined above and then mixed in the presence or absence of virus (41). At different times after fusion the cells were given a short pulse of radioactive hypoxanthine and immediately processed for autoradiography.

Preparations that did not receive virus only showed cells with those labelling patterns expected of contaminating parental cells, while preparations receiving virus contained cells with a variety of labelling patterns. All cells that were unlabelled in autoradiograms had a high number of large beads and were probably contaminating intact cytoplasmic donors. Among those cells incorporating hypoxanthine, three types of bead labelling pattern were found: firstly, cells with many small beads only, secondly, cells with a high number of both small and large beads and finally cells with a few small and many large beads. Only the last category satisfied the criteria set for reconstituted cells, the two former labelling pattern representing intact minicell donors and fusion products between intact minicell donors and enucleated cytoplasms, respectively.

Preparations fixed soon after fusion contained only a few well separated cells satisfying the criteria set for reconstituted cells. Those preparations fixed later, however, showed several pairs of cells identifiable as reconstituted cells, as well as reconstituted cells in different stages of mitosis, indicating that reconstituted cells were able to enter mitosis and form viable daughter cells. The results of experiments using rat and mouse cells as nuclear donors did not differ significantly, showing that a species differences between the two fused fragments was of little importance.

(iv) Isolation of growing reconstituted cells

As mentioned above, experiments involving nuclear transplantation in unicellular organisms have convincingly demonstrated that cytoplasmic substances control nuclear gene activity. The procedures discussed above show that nuclear transplantation experiments can also be performed with cultured mammalian cells and that such reconstituted cells are at least capable of limited proliferation. The advantage of the latter technique is that cytoplasms and nuclei may be obtained from various differentiated cell types and therefore the technology allows the recombination of a wide spectrum of nuclei and cytoplasms. If growing cell lines of reconstituted cells could be isolated, they would provide excellent material for the analysis of the effects of cytoplasmic substances on nuclear gene activity and cell differentiation.

Prolonged survival and growth of reconstituted cells were first reported by Lucas and Kates (42) in an intraspecific cell combination. However, the effect of the cytoplasm of these parameters was unclear since a significant proportion of the minicells used in these experiments were capable of regenerating a new cytoplasm. It was therefore necessary to find out if an interspecific combination of minicells and cytoplasms from cells of different phenotypes could be used for rescuing the minicells. Resulting fusion products could then be examined to see whether cell lines of reconstituted cells could be isolated free of contaminating parental cells.

As the previous identification scheme involved fixation and

close microscopical examination of the cells in the fusion mixture to reveal their identity, this was unsuitable for the purpose of isolating growing cell lines. Therefore, a new selective system was

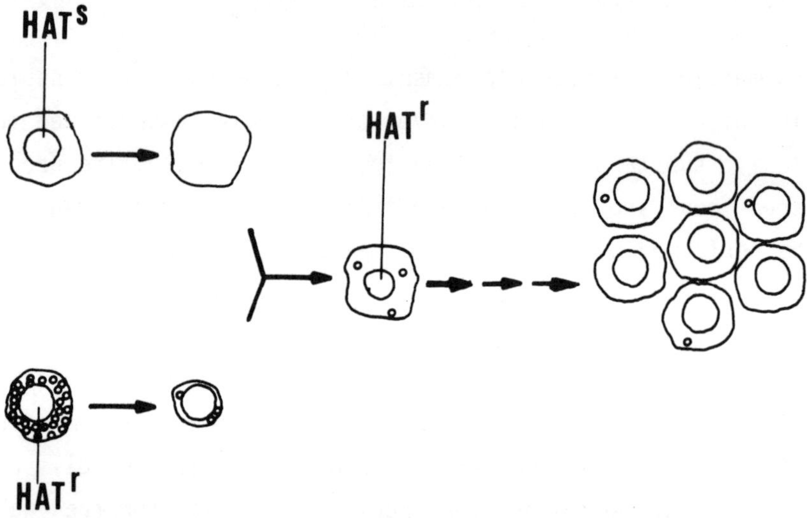

Fig. 2. *Labelling pattern of parental and reconstituted cells.*

devised based upon observations (unpublished results, (43)) of the properties of bead labelled cells. The presence of beads in the cytoplasm does not seriously interfere with the growth and division of the labelled cells as the plating efficiency and size of colonies arising from such cells is equal to that of unlabelled cells. In addition, colonies arising from bead labelled cells contain the same number of beads as the cells from which they originated, indicating that loss of phagocytosed beads only occurs by dilution through cell division. Furthermore, it was found that minicells prepared from extensively labelled cells only carry a few percent of the beads originally present in the intact cell. Therefore, by using minicells prepared from extensively labelled cells, and a cytoplasmic donor that is unable to grow in HAT-selective medium (44, 45), reconstituted cells can be selected on HAT-medium. Colonies originating from intact minicell donors can be distinguished from those originating from reconstituted cells as the latter will contain a much lower bead number than the former.

Using the markers and selection system described above, we fused minicells prepared from rat myoblasts with cytoplasts from mouse fibroblastic cells (46). Those preparations which contained complete fusion mixtures formed 2-3 times as many colonies as controls in which *Sendai* virus has been omitted. In order to identify the types of cells present in the resulting colonies, the number of beads per colony was counted. The number of beads in colonies arising from control cultures was comparable to that of the intact minicell donor. These colonies, therefore, must all be derived from intact cells contaminating the minicell preparations.

In the presence of virus, two types of colonies were observed. One type contained as many beads as did colonies in control preparations while the other contained very few beads. The cells in this latter type of colony were interpreted to be the progeny of reconstituted cells. Using conventional cloning techniques, such colonies were isolated and expanded in separate culture vessels. Chromosome analysis of these cells confirmed that their karyotype was indistinguishable from that of the nuclear donor. This excludes the possibility that the isolated cells originated from surviving cytoplasmic donor cells.

Using the same selection system and the same myoblast-fibroblast cell combination described above, Ringertz *et al.* (47) analyzed the phenotype of reconstituted cells. When myoblast nuclei were introduced into enucleated fibroblast cytoplasms, it was found that the resulting reconstituted cells retained the capacity to undergo the same myogenic differentiation as the minicell donors, resulting in myosin producing, cross striated myotubes. This indicates that the fibroblast cytoplasm had no long-lasting, irreversible effect on the genes expressed in the myoblast nucleus. Short term effects could not be investigated due to the heterogenous cell population present soon after fusion. Whether the lack of a long lasting influence from the cytoplasmic donor is a general phenomenon could not be concluded from these limited data, but must await further experiments with other cell combinations.

Muggelton-Harris and Hayflick (48) have reconstituted cells by fusing minicells and cytoplasms from young and old fibroblasts, in order to study nuclear and cytoplasmic factors which influence cell aging. The reconstituted cells showed stable growth characteristics similar to those of the minicell donor, indicating that the cytoplasm had no lasting irreversible influence.

In experiments where intact cells have been fused with enucleated cells to form cybrids, similar and conflicting results have been obtained. Cybrids formed between multipotent teratocarcinoma cells and enucleated cytoplasms with dissimilar properties have been reported to retain their protein synthesis pattern (49) and developmental potency (50). However, some cellular properties of the intact cells such as the tumorigenicity (51) and hemoglobin inducibility in Friend cells (52) have been reported to be effected in cybrids.

From these limited data, no firm conclusions can yet be drawn about the effect of cytoplasmic components on the gene expression pattern. Some properties seem to be changed, while others do not, but confirmation of the generality of the effects has to wait until further experiments have been performed with other cell combinations.

A new selection method has recently been introduced for the selection of reconstituted cells and cybrids. The method is based on the development of mitochondrial chloramphenical-resistant (CAP^r) mutants (53, 54) and the observation that this resistance is cytoplasmically inherited (55, 56). By fusing normal minicells or intact cells (CAP^s) with enucleated cytoplasms from cells carrying CAP^r-mitochondria, reconstituted cells (57) and cybrids (50, 52, 55, 56) could be selected on media containing chloramphenicol.

There are a number of antibiotics other than CAP which interfere specifically with mitochondrial function in mammalian cells (58-60). The possibility therefore exists that cells carrying mitochondrial mutants which are resistant to the lethal effects of these drugs could be selected. If this is the case, reconstituted cells will provide an invaluable means of studying both cytoplasmic effects on the gene expression pattern and mitochondrial genetics in higher cells.

4. MICROCELL HETEROKARYONS

It is a well-known characteristic of interspecies somatic cell hybrids that they lose chormosomes (for review, see 61). This chromosome segregation is progressive and apparently more or less random, except that the loss may selectively affect the chromosomes of one of the parental cells. For instance mouse-human hybrids usually show a preferential loss of human chromosomes. In extreme cases, hybrid clones may lose all but one or two human chromosomes and yet retain all of the mouse chromosomes. By analyzing a variety of hybrid clones it has been possible to demonstrate that some genetic markers always appear and disappear together, i.e. to establish linkage relationships. In some cases the presence or absence of a specific human chromosome has been correlated with the presence or absence of specific gene products, i.e. synteny relationships have been established. With the aid of this technique genes have been assigned to all human chromosomes except the Y-chromosome and chromosome 22 and 23 (for review, see 62).

One major problem in using hybrid cells in the mapping of human chromosomes is that in several cell hybrid systems, chromosome segregation may be slow and unpredictable. In order to overcome this problem we have tried to devise a rapid method for obtaining cell hybrids with a severely reduced chromosome complement from one of the parental cells. This technique used cell fragments containing micronuclei as vehicles for the transfer of partial genomes from one cell to another.

(i) Preparation of microcells

The presence of cells with many small nuclei (micronucleated cells) in pathological material and in cells grown *in vitro* has been observed for many years. Agents that will induce micronucleation have also been found. Observations by Levan (63) and others (64, 65, 66) suggested that the micronucleated cells arise during abnormal mitosis when chromosome fragments, single chromosomes or small groups of chromosomes were surrounded by a nuclear membrane, so giving rise to subdiploid micronuclei.

Large numbers of micronucleated cells can be obtained by exposing cultured animal cells to inhibitors which affect the formation of the mitotic spindle. These cells become arrested in metaphase but, after a lag period, the arrested cells proceed into interphase and give rise ot extensively micronucleated cells. Under optimal conditions the number of micronuclei per cell was found to equal but never exceed the number of chromosomes of that cell (64). This indicates that individual micronuclei often contain a quantity of DNA equivalent to that of a single chromosome.

When micronucleated cells were exposed to cytochalasin B in combination with strong centrifugal force under similar conditions to those used during enucleation of mononucleated cells, enucleated cytoplasms and nucleated fragments, smaller than the size of minicells were produced (67).

Electron microscopical analysis showed the fragments to consist of a small nucleus with normal interphase chromatin, surrounded by a thin rim of cytoplasm and a cell membrane. The plasma membrane appeared to be intact since 80-90% of the small subcellular fragments exclude trypan blue. The term microcells was used to describe these fragments.

Cytochemical analysis by Feulgen microspectrophotometry showed that most microcells prepared from L6 cells contained a subdiploid nucleus, the smallest having a DNA content equivalent to 1/30 of the G1 level of intact nuclei. This would be equivalent to one or two chromosomes as these cells have a chromosome number of 40. This conclusion is also supported by DNA measurements on micronuclei from rat kangaroo cells (68). In this case the comparison of DNA content and chromosome number is facilitated by the fact that this species has only 6 pairs of chromosomes.

Because the smallest microcells contain the lowest amount of genetic material, these are the most useful in chromosome transfer experiments. To separate small microcells from larger ones, a linear 1-3% bovine serum albumin gradient can be used (69) where cell fragments are allowed to sediment at unit gravity. Analysis of gradient fractions after sedimentation show that the smallest microcells remain near the top of the gradient, while larger microcells and contaminating intact cells are found nearer the bottom.

(ii) Fusion of microcells

If microcells fuse with intact cells, the resulting heterokaryons should be binucleated cells with one small and one normal sized nucleus. Such cells can readily be observed when *Sendai* virus is added to mixtures of microcells and intact cells. The formation of microcell heterokaryons was verified by fusing ^{3}H-thymidine labelled microcells to unlabelled recipient cells. The cells used for microcell preparation were allowed to incorporate radioactive thymidine for 24 h before and during the period of micronucleation which resulted in almost 100% labelling of the micronuclei. Fusion of microcells, prepared from labelled donors, with intact cells gave rise to microcell heterokaryons with one labelled and one unlabelled nucleus.

The fact that both nuclei of the microcell heterokaryons incorporate radioactive uridine suggest that micronuclei are at least able to synthesize RNA, and might also be able to supply gene products to the microcell heterokaryon.

When microcell heterokaryons divide, each pair of daughter cells formed contains only a small fraction of the chromosomes present in the normal microcell donor, thereby creating a heterogenous population of microcell hybrids. By using mutant cells as microcell recipients and selective medium, Fournier and Ruddle (70, 71) have selected microcell hybrids where the mutant defect is complemented. All such hybrids were found to contain the microcell donor chromosome carrying the gene complementing the defect of the mutant, in addition to a few other chromosomes. Microcells may therefore be of use in obtaining hybrids suitable for gene assignment and chromosome mapping.

A completely different method for the production of subdiploid cell fragments has been reported by R.T. Johnson and coworkers (72, 73). Exposure of cells arrested in mitosis to low temperatures overnight resulted in the aberrant formation of cleavage furrows when the cells were brought back to normal temperatures, thereby separating individual mitotic chromosomes or groups of chromosomes into different cell compartments. These chromosomes were found to be enclosed by nuclear membranes and formed micronuclei with a dispersed interphase chromatin. By exposing the micronucleated cells to a mechanical shearing force, the partly cleaved cells were broken up into a number of subdiploid fragments referred to as mini-segregants. Each such mini-segregant was found to consist of a micronucleus surrounded by a cytoplasm and an intact cell membrane and therefore corresponded very closely to microcells. The mini-segregants, too, can be fused with recipient cells (74), thus serving as vehicles for the transfer of genetic information from one cell to another.

Microcell mediated gene transfer is only one of the methods available for transferring subdiploid amounts of genetic material. However, microcells and mini-segregants appear to be the only methods in which the transferred material can be reproducibly identified as intact chromosomes. Isolated DNA (75, 76, 77) and metaphase chromosomes (78) are also taken up by tissue culture cells, but gene products characteristic of the donor cell can only be identified in a very low fraction of the treated cells. Furthermore, in the latter example, donor chromosomes have been identified in only a few cases. The different methods offer different possibilities of transferring genetic material from one cell to another, since it seems that the recipient cell retains the foreign DNA in different froms dependent of the method used. Hence, the choice of method will depend on the purpose of the transfer.

5. REFERENCES

1) OKADA, Y. (1958). The fusion of Ehrlich's tumor cells caused by HVJ virus *in vitro*. Bikens J., 1, 103.

2) OKADA, Y & MURAYAME, F. (1968). Fusion of cells by HVJ: Requirement of concentration of virus particles at the site of contact of two cells for fusion. Exptl. Cell Res., 52, 34.

3) OKADA, Y. and TADOKORO, J. (1962). Analysis of giant polynuclear cell formation caused by HVJ virus from Ehrlich's tumor cells. II. Quantitative analysis of giant polynuclear cell formation. Exptl. Cell Res., 26, 108.

4) RINGERTZ, N.R. and SAVAGE, R.E. (1976). Cell hybrids, Academic Press, New York, 1976.

5) WEISS, M.C. and GREEN, H. (1967). Human-mouse hybrid cell lines containing partial complements of human chromosomes and functioning human genes. Proc. Natl. Acad. Sci. USA, 58, 1104.

6) RINGERTZ, N.R. and BOLUND, L. (1974). Reactivation of chick erythrocyte nuclei by somatic cell hybridization. In, Int. Rev. Exptl. Pathol., Vol. XIII, p. 83 (ed., G.W. Richter and M.A. Epstein). Academic Press, New York.

7) HARRIS, H. (1967). The reactivation of the red cell nucleus. J. Cell Sci., 2, 23.

8) HARRIS, H. (1970). Cell fusion. The Dunham Lectures, Oxford University Press, London and New York.

9) DUPUY-COIN, A.-M., BOUTEILLE, M., EGE. T. and RINGERTZ, N.R. (1976). Ultrastructure of chick erythrocyte nuclei undergoing reactivation in heterokaryons and enucleated cells. Exptl. Cell Res., 101, 355.

10) SCHNEEBERGER, E.E. and HARRIS, H. (1966). An ultrastructural study of interspecific cell fusion induced by inactivated *Sendai* virus. J. Cell Sci., 1, 401.

11) BOLUND, L., DARZYNKIEWICZ, Z. and RINGERTZ, N.R. (1969). Growth of hen erythrocyte nuclei undergoing reactivation in heterokaryons, Exptl. Cell Res. 56, 406.

12) RINGERTZ, N.R., CARLSSON, S.-A., EGE, T. and BOLUND, L. (1971). Detection of human and chick nuclear antigens in nuclei of chick erythrocytes during reactivation in heterokaryons with HeLa cells. Proc. Natl. Acad. Sci. USA, 68, 3228.

13) KOFFLER, D., CARR, R. AGNELLO, V., THOBURN, R. and KUNKEL, G.H. (1971). J. Exptl. Med., 134, 294.

14) APPELS, R., TALLROTH, E., APPELS, D.M. and RINGERTZ, N.R. (1975). Differential uptake of protein into the chick nuclei of HeLa x chick erythrocyte heterokaryons. Exptl. Cell Res., 92, 70.

15) APPELS, R., BOLUND, L. and RINGERTZ, N.R. (1974). Biochemical analysis of reactivated chick erythrocyte nuclei isolated from chick x HeLa heterokaryons. J. Mol. Biol., 87, 339.

16) CARLSSON, S.-A., MOORE, G.P.M. and RINGERTZ, N.R. (1973). Nucleocytoplasmic protein migration during the activation of chick erythrocyte nuclei in heterokaryons. Exptl. Cell Res., 76, 234.

17) DARZYNKIEWICZ, Z. and CHELMICKA-SZORE, E. (1972). Unscheduled DNA synthesis in hen erythrocyte nuclei reactivated in heterokaryons. Exptl. Cell Res., 74, 131.

18) ROSENQVIST, M., STENMAN, S. and RINGERTZ, N.R. (1975). Uptake of SV40 T-antigen into chick erythrocyte nuclei in heterokaryons. Exptl. Cell Res., 92, 515.

19) EGE, T., CARLSSON, S.-A. and RINGERTZ, N.R. (1971). Immune microfluorimetric analysis of the distribution of species specific nuclear antigens in HeLa-chick erythrocyte heterokaryons. Exptl. Cell Res., 69, 472.

20) EGE, T., ZEUTHEN, J. and RINGERTZ, N.R. (1975). Reactivation of chick erythrocyte nuclei after fusion with enucleated cells. Somatic Cell Gen., 1, 65.

21) POSTE, G. and REEVE, P. (1972). Enucleation of mammalian cells by cytochalasin B. II. Formation of hybrid cells and heterokaryons by fusion of anucleate and nucleated cells. Exptl. Cell Res., 73, 287.

22) LADDA, R.L. and ESTENSEN, R.D. (1970). Introduction of a heterologous nucleus into enucleated cytoplasms of cultured mouse L cells, Proc. Natl. Acad. Sci. USA, 67, 1528.

23) GOTO, S. and RINGERTZ, N.R. (1974). Preparation and characterization of chick erythrocyte nuclei from heterokaryons. Exptl. Cell Res., 85, 182.

24) APPELS, R. BOLUND, L., GOTO, S. and RINGERTZ, N.R. (1974). The kinetics of protein uptake by chick erythrocyte nuclei during reactivation in chick-mammalian heterokaryons. Exptl. Cell Res, 85, 182.

25) HÄMMERLING, J. (1943). Über Genomwirkungen und Formbildingsfähigkeit bei *Acetabularia*. Arch. Entwick-Mech. Org., 132, 424.

26) HÄMMERLING, J. (1953). Nucleo-cytoplasmic relationships in the development of *Acetabularia*. In, Intern. Rev. Cytol., 2, 475.

27) LORCH, I.J. and DANIELLI, J.F. (1950). Transplantation of nucleic from cell to cell. Nature, 166, 329.

28) DANIELLI, J.F., LORCH, I.J., ORD, M.J. and WILSON, E.C. (1955). Nucleus and cytoplasm in cellular inheritance. Nature, 176, 1114.

29) POSTE, G. (1973). Anucleate mammalian cells: Applications in cell biology and virology, In:Methods in Cell Biol., Vol. VIII, p. 123, (ed., D.M. Prescott), Academic Press, New York.

30) CARTER, S.B. (1967). Effects of cytochalasins on mammalian cells. Nature, 213, 261.

31) PRESCOTT, D.M., MYERSON, D. and WALLACE, J. (1972). Enucleation of mammalian cells with cytochalasin B. Exptl. Cell Res., 71, 480.

32) EGE, T., HAMBERG, H., KRONDAHL, U., ERICSSON, J. and RINGERTZ, N.R. (1974). Characterization of minicells (nuclei) obtained by cytochalasin enucleation. Exptl. Cell Res., 87, 365.

33) GOLDMAN, R.D., POLLACK, R. and HOPKINS, N. (1973) Preservation of normal behaviour by enucleated cells in culture. Proc. Natl. Acad. Sci. USA, 70, 750.

34) GOLDMAN, R.D. and POLLACK, R. (1974). Uses of enucleated cells. In:Methods of Cell Biol., Vol. VIII, p. 123 (ed., D.M. Prescott), Academic Press, New York.

35) WISE, G.E. and PRESCOTT, D.M. (1973). Ultrastructure of enucleated mammalian cells in culture. Exptl. Cell Res., 81, 63.

36) SHAY, J.W., PORTER, K.R. and PRESCOTT, D.M. (1974). The surface morphology and fine structure of CHO (Chinese hamster ovary) cells following enucleation. Proc. Natl. Acad. Sci. USA,71,3059.

37) LUCAS, J.J., SZEKELY, E. and KATES, J.R. (1976). The regeneration and division of mouse L-cell karyoplasts. Cell, 7, 115.

38) VEOMETT, G., PRESCOTT, D.M., SHAY, J. and PORTER, K.R. (1974). Reconstruction of mammalian cells from nuclear and cytoplasmic components separated by treatment with cytochalasin B. Proc. Natl. Acad. Sci. USA, 71, 1999.

39) PRESCOTT, D.M. and KIRKPATRICK, J.B. (1973). Mass enucleation of cultured animal cells, In: Methods in Cell Biol., Vol. VII, p. 189, (ed., D.M. Prescott), Academic Press, New York.

40) EGE, T., KRONDAHL, U. and RINGERTZ, N.R. (1971). Introduction of nuclei and micronuclei into cells and enucleated cytoplasms by *Sendai* virus induced fusion. Exptl. Cell Res., 88, 428.

41) EGE, T. and RINGERTZ, N.R. (1975). Viability of cells reconstituted by virus-induced fusion of minicells with anucleate cells. Exptl. Cell Res., 94, 469.

42) LUCAS, J.J. and KATES, J.R. (1976). The construction of viable nuclear-cytoplasmic hybrid cells by nuclear transplantation. Cell, 7, 397.

43) LEVINE, M.R. and COX, R.P. (1978). Use of latex particles for analysis of heterokaryon formation and cell fusion. Somatic Cell Gen., 4, 507.

44) LITTLEFIELD, J.W. (1964). Three degrees of guarylic acid-inosinic acid pyrophosphorylase deficiency in mouse fibroblasts. Nature, 203, 1142.

45) SZYBALSKI, W., SZYBALSKI, E.H. and RAGNI, G. (1962). Genetic studies with human cell lines. Natl. Ca. Inst. Monogr., 7, 75.

46) KRONDAHL, U., BOLS, N., EGE, T., LINDER, S. and RINGERTZ, N.R. (1977). Cells reconstituted from cell fragments of two different species multiply and form colonies. Proc. Natl. Acad. Sci. USA, 74, 606.

47) RINGERTZ, N.R., KRONDAHL, U. and COLEMAN, J.R. (1978). Reconstitution of cells by fusion of cell fragments. I. Myogenic expression after fusion of minicells from rat myoblasts (L6)

with mouse fibroblast (A9) cytoplasm. Exptl. Cell Res., 113, 233.

48) MUGGLETON-HARRIS, A.L. and HAYFLICK, L. (1976). Cellular aging studied by the reconstruction of replicating cells from nuclei and cytoplasms isolated from normal human diploid cells. Exptl. Cell Res., 103, 321.

49) LINDER, S. BRZEŞKI, H. and RINGERTZ, N.R. (1979). Phenotypic expression in cybrids derived from teratocarcinoma cells fused with myoblast cytoplasms. Exptl. Cell Res., 120, 1.

50) WATANABL, T., DEWEY, M.J. and MINTZ, B. (1978). Teratocarcinoma cells as vehicles for introducing specific mutant mitochondrial genes into mice. Proc. Natl. Acad. Sci. USA, 75, 5113.

51) HOWELL, A.N. and SAGER, R. (1978). Tumorigenicity and its suppression in cybrids of mouse and Chinese hamster cell lines. Proc. Natl. Acad. Sci. USA., 75, 2358.

52) GOPALAKRISHNAN, T.V., THOMPSON, E.B. and ANDERSON, W.F. (1977). Extinction of hemoglobin inducibility in Friend erythroleukemia cells by fusion with cytoplasm of enucleated mouse neuroblastoma or fibroblast cells. Proc. Natl. Acad. Sci. USA, 74, 2461.

53) SPOLSKY, C.M. and EISENSTADT, J.M. (1972). Chloramphenicol-resistant mutants of human HeLa cells. FEBS Lett., 25, 319.

54) KISLEV, N, SPOLSKY, C.M. and EISENSTADT, J.M. (1973). Effect of chloramphenicol on the ultrastructure of mitochondria in sensitive and resistant strains of HeLa cells. J. Cell Biol., 57, 571.

55) BUNN, C.L., WALLACE, D.C. and EISENSTADT, J.M. (1974). Cytoplasmic transfer of chloramphenical resistance in mouse tissue culture cells. Proc. Natl. Acad. Sci. USA, 71, 1681.

56) WALLACE, D.C., BUNN, C.L. and EISENSTADT, J.M. (1975). Cytoplasmic transfer of chloramphenical resistance in human tissue culture cells. J. Cell Biol., 67, 174.

57) SHAY, J.W. (1977). Selection of reconstituted cells from karyoplasts fused to chloramphenical-resistant cytoplasts. Proc. Natl. Acad. Sci. USA, 74, 2461.

58) KROON, A. (1970). Nuclear and chloroplast control of chloroplast structure and function in Chlamydomonas Reinhardi. In: Control of Organelle Development, p. 13 (ed. P.L. Miller) University Printing House, Cambridge.

59) TOWERS, N.R., DIXON, H., KELLERMAN, G.M. and LINNANE, A.W. (1972). Biogenesis of Mitochondria. 22. The sensitivity of rat liver mitochondria to antibiotics; a phylogenetic difference between a mammalian system and yeast. Arch. Biochem. Biophys., 151, 361.

60) DENSLOW, N.D. and O'BRIEN, T.W. (1974). Susceptibility of 55 S mitochondrial ribosomes to antibiotics inhibitory to prokaryotic ribosomes, Lincomycin, Chloramphenical and PA 114 A. Biochem. Biophys. Res. Comm., 57, 9.

61) RUDDLE, F.H. (1974). Human genetic linkage and gene mapping by somatic cell genetics. In: Somatic Cell Hybridization, p. 1 (ed., R.L. Davidson) Raven Press, New York.

62) Human Gene Mapping 3. Baltimore Conference 1975. Third Intern. Workshop of Human Gene Mapping. Birth Defects: Original Article Series, Vol. XII, No. 7 (The National Found., New York, 1976).

63) LEVAN, A. (1954). Colchicine-induced C-mitosis in two mouse ascites tumours. Hereditas, 40, 1.

64) PHILLIPS, S.G. and PHILLIPS, D.M. (1969). Sites of nucleolus production in cultured Chinese hamster cells. J. Cell Biol., 40, 248.

65) STUBBLEFIELD, E. (1964). DNA synthesis and chromosomal morphology of Chinese hamster cells cultured in media containing N-deacetyl-N-methylcolchisine (colcemid). In: Cytogenetics of Cells in Culture, Vol. III, p. 223.

66) HERNANDEZ-VERDUN, D., BOUTEILLE, M., EGE, T. and RINGERTZ, N.R. (in press). Fine structure of nucleoli in micronucleated cells. Exptl. Cell.

67) EGE, T. and RINGERTZ, N.R. (1974). Preparation of microcells by enucleation of micronucleate cells. Exptl. Cell Res. 87, 378.

68) SEKIGUCHI, T., SHELTON, K. and RINGERTZ, N.R. (1978). DNA-content of microcells prepared from rat, kangaroo and mouse cells. Exptl. Cell Res., 113, 247.

69) HECHT, T.T., RUDDLE, N.H. and RUDDLE, F.H. (1975). Analysis of differentiating B lymphocytes from mouse spleens. Fed. Proc., 34, 995.

70) FOURNIER, R.E.K. and RUDDLE, F.H. (1977). Microcell-mediated transfer of murine chromosomes into mouse, Chinese hamster, and human somatic cells. Proc. Natl. Acad. Sci. USA, 74, 319.

71) FOURNIER, R.E.K. and RUDDLE, F.H. (1977). Stable association of the human transgenome and host murine chromosomes demonstrated with trispecific microcell hybrids. Proc. Natl. Acad. Sci. USA, 74, 3937.

72) JOHNSON, R.T., MULLINGER, A.M. and SKAER, R.J. (1975). Pertubation of mammalian cell division. I. Human mini segregants derived from mitotic cells. Proc. R. Soc. B., 189, 591.

73) SCHOR, S.L., JOHNSON, R.T., MULLINGER, A.M. (1975). Pertubation of mammalian cell division. II. Studies of the isolation and charecterization of human mini segregant cells. J. Cell Sci. 19,281.

74) TOURIAN, A., JOHNSON, R.T., BURG, K., NICOLSON, S.W. and SPERLING, K. (1978). Transfer of human chromosomes via human mini segregant cells into mouse cells and the quantitation of the expression of hypoxanthine phosphoribosyltransferase in the hybrids. J. of Cell Sci., 30, 193.

75) BAECHETTI, S. and GRAHAM, F.L. (1977). Transfer of the gene for thymidine kinase to thymidine-kinase deficient human cells by purified Herpes Simplex Viral DNA, Proc. Natl. Acad. Sci. USA, 74, 1590.

76) MAITLAND, N.J. and MCDOUGALL, J.K. (1977). Biochemical transformation of mouse cells by fragments of Herpes Simplex Virus DNA, Cell, 11, 233.

77) WIGLER, M., SILVERSTEIN, S., Lee, L.-S., PELLICER, A. CHENG, Y.-C. and AXEL, R. (1977). Transfer of purified Herpes virus

thymidine kinase gene to cultured mouse cells. Cell, 11, 223.

78) MCBRIDE, O.W. and OZER, H.L. (1973). Transfer of genetic information by purified metaphase chromosomes. Proc. Natl. Acad. Sci. USA, 70, 1257.

B-CELL AND EPSTEIN-BARR VIRUS (EBV) ASSOCIATED FUNCTIONS IN HUMAN CELLS AND HYBRIDS

J. Zeuthen* and G. Klein#

**Institute of Human Genetics*
The Bartholin Building
University of Aarhus
8000 Aarhus C, Denmark

#*Department of Tumor Biology*
Karolinske Institutet
104 01 Stockholm, Sweden

1. INTRODUCTION

In this review, we will discuss some aspects of current work related to the control mechanisms involved in the selective expression of B-cell differentiated markers, as well as the control mechanisms involved in the expression and function of Epstein-Barr virus (EBV) associated markers in human cells.

EBV is a lymphotropic herpesvirus in man (1). Its main target is the human B-lymphocyte (2), though other cell types might be infectible by EBV, provided that the membrane barrier is surpassed. EBV is known to be the causative agent of infectuous mononucleosis (3), and is associated with two completely different human malignant tumors: African Burkitt's lymphoma (BL) - malignant proliferation of B-cells (4) -, and nasopharyngeal carcinoma (NPC) - malignant proliferation of epithelial carcinoma cells (5). In both cases the presence of the EBV genome has been demonstrated by the presence of EBV-DNA as well as by the presence of EBV-specific antigens. From BL tumor cells a large number of established B-cell lines have been obtained while it has not yet been possible to obtain epithelial carcinoma lines from NPC tumors.

Infection of B-lymphocytes with EBV regularly leads to transformation (more commonly referred to as "immortalization" (6)) into so-called lymphoblastoid cell lines (LCL). Normally, B-lymphocytes are transitory cells, located within a chain of differentiation, proceeding from primitive stem cells towards mature, immunoglobin secreting end cells (plasma cells). EBV cannot infect stem cells or plasma cells. Infection of B-lymphocytes is sharply restricted to surface immunoglobulin and complement (C3) receptor positive B-cells (7). IgM producer cells represent the most usual target. Recently, studies in progress (8), have found IgM+IgD-cells to be "switched" to IgM+IgD+ following immortalization into LCL lines. This finding might suggest that minor changes in the differentiated phenotype of B-cells can occur after EBV-induced transformation. The cell lines of BL origin appear to represent a clonal proliferation of neoplastic cells with phenotypic characteristics of the corresponding normal target cells, i.e. surface immunoglobulin and C3 receptor positive B-cells. In addition to cell lines of BL or LCL origin cell lines from other neoplastic cells of hematopoietic origin have been established which present similar clonal proliferation of cells with a developmental arrest at a given stage in their differentiation pathway. An example of the normal B-cell lineage with the corresponding lymphoproliferative disorders is given in Table 1 (adapted from 9).

Table 1. *Human lymphoproliferative disorders. Functional differentiation and relationship to the normal B-cell lineage.* 1)

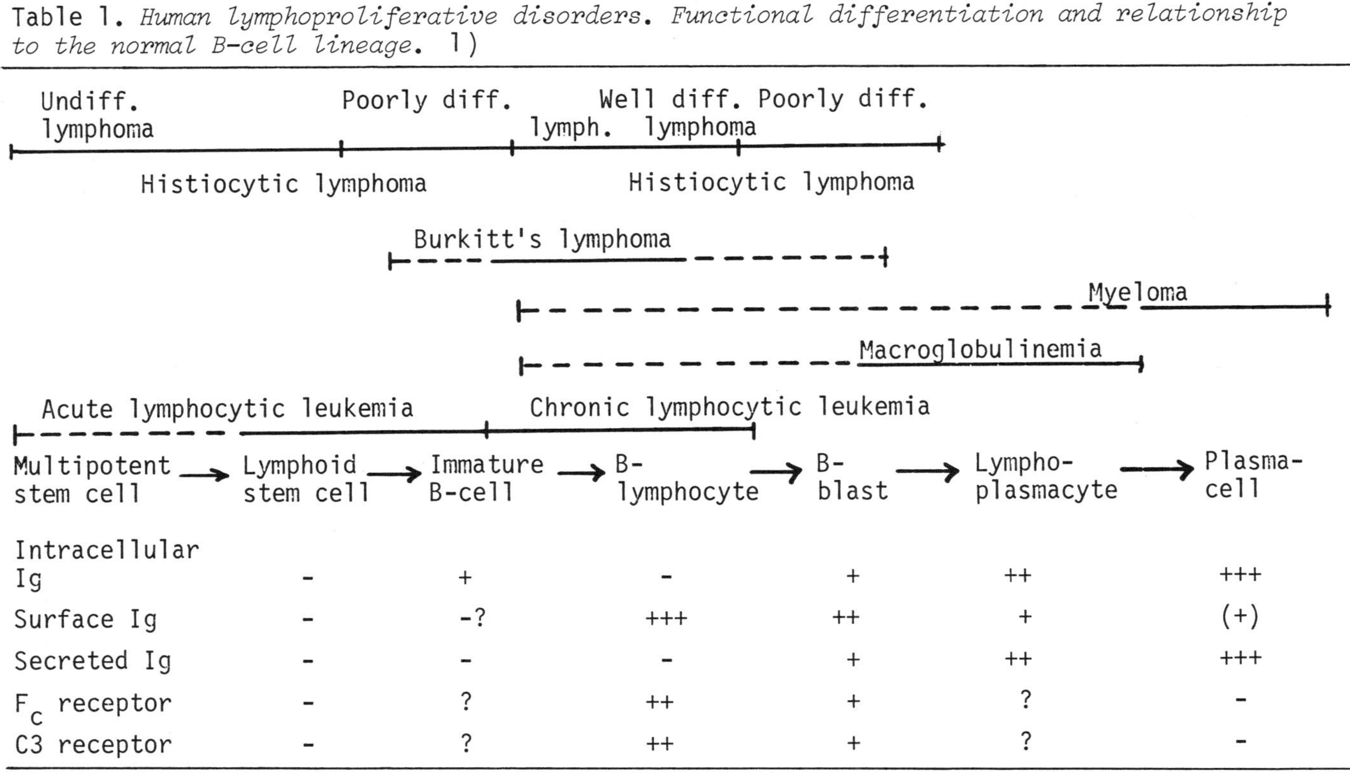

	Multipotent stem cell →	Lymphoid stem cell →	Immature B-cell →	B-lymphocyte →	B-blast →	Lympho-plasmacyte →	Plasma-cell
Intracellular Ig		-	+	-	+	++	+++
Surface Ig		-	-?	+++	++	+	(+)
Secreted Ig		-	-	-	+	++	+++
F_c receptor		-	?	++	+	?	-
C3 receptor		-	?	++	+	?	-

1) From Ref. 9.

2. IMMUNOGLOBULIN AND SURFACE MARKER EXPRESSION

(i) Lymphoid cell lines

Membrane bound immunoglobulin synthesized by neoplastic B-cells represents an important marker for the monoclonality of B-cell proliferation (10). In chronic lymphocytic leukemia and Waldenström macroglobulinemia, the cells of the proliferating clone usually bear both surface IgD and IgM, whereas in B-cell derived lymphomas and acute leukemias, the cells usually have high density surface IgM with little or no surface IgD (11). EBV-transformation of EBV-negative lymphoma cells have recently been observed to "switch" IgM+IgD- cells to IgM+IgD+ (8). Myeloma cells produce monoclonal and secretory immunoglobulin at a high rate, but little if any surface immunoglobulin is expressed (12). B-lymphoma lines express almost invariably surface IgM, though rare IgG (13) and nonproducing lines have been described. Immunoglobulins in lymphoma lines are almost exclusively destined for plasma membrane integration (14,15). In contrast to B-lymphoma lines, LCL lines appear to synthesize higher amounts of immunoglobulin, some of which is secreted (16). It is now possible to obtain specific antibody producing LCL lines by antigen preselection and EBV transformation (17), which might represent a useful alternative in order to obtain human monoclonal antibodies.

In addition to immunoglobulin, a number of other markers are of interest in order to define the state of differentiation of lymphoid cell lines. An important group of markers are the B-cell or Ia-like antigens which are defined by means of antisera that react with B-cell glycoprotein (18,19). Primitive non-B, non-T cell lines are Ia-like antigen positive, while myeloma lines only express a small amount of Ia-like antigen (20). Other markers are F_c receptors that are scored by adsorption of aggregated IgG (21) or by rosette formation with IgG sensitized sheep erythrocytes

(EA rosettes, 22), and complement receptors (C3b and C3d) detected by rosette formation with sheep erythrocytes sensitized with IgM and human and mouse complement, respectively (EAC rosettes, 22). The relationship of these markers to normal B-cell differentiation is represented in Table I. While BL cells usually express high amounts of all of these three markers, LCL cells show a similar profile except for a significantly lower density of F_c receptors. Standard sheep erythrocyte rosettes (E rosettes) serve as a standard T-cell marker (23), and is absent on all B-cell derived lines.

In spite of the fact that human lymphoma cells represent a rather narrow range of differentiation, their B-cell phenotype show a rather wide range with respect to the presence of these markers. The profiles of a few representative lines are given below (Table II).

Table II. *B-cell phenotypes of different BL cell lines.*

	Ia-antigens	Surface Ig	F_c receptor	C3 receptor
Raji	+	± (IgM kappa)	±	++(C3b+C3d+)
Daudi	+	+++ (IgM kappa)	+++	++(C3b-C3d+)
BJAB	+	+++ (IgM kappa)	±	±(C3b-C3d+)
HRIK-BJAB	+	+++ (IgM kappa)	±	++(C3b-C3d+)

±designates weak reaction. Data from Ref. 24 and 25.
All lines except Daudi are HLA+Beta-2 microglobulin+.
BJAB is an EBV-negative BL line, HRIK-BJAB and EBV-positive EBV-converted derivative of BJAB.

In the data above, it is of interest ot note that Daudi representing an unique HLA-,Beta-2 microglobulin-cell line (24,26) is Ia-like antigen positive suggesting a lack of association of Ia-like antigens with HLA. A further point of interest is the comparison between the EBV-negative BL-lymphoma line BJAB and its EBV-converted derivative HRIK-BJAB (25). A significant increase in the density of complement receptors is observed after EBV-conversion and also a parallel decrease in the density of EBV receptors was observed in this and other EBV-converted EBV-negative lymphoma lines (25). It appears therefore likely that EBV-conversion brings about a steric change in the membrane affecting increased complement receptor activity and decreased EBV receptor activity. This finding fits with more direct tests of a steric relationship between complement and EBV receptors on human B-cells.(27,28).

(ii) Hybrid Cells

The fate of immunoglobulin expression in somatic cell hybrids has been studied in several laboratories. Most work has been done with established mouse cell lines, but results are also available from hybridization of human BL, LCL, and myeloma lines. The results appear to fall into two main categories: 1) fusion of immunoglobulin producing cells with other cells of lymphoid origin, and 2) fusion of immunoglobulin producing cells with unrelated cell types. In the first group, cells continue to synthesize the immunoglobulins made by their parental cells, i.e. coexpression in the case both parents were producers. In the second group of experiments, the most common observation has been total loss of immunoglobulin synthesis, i.e. extinction, though a few experiments have shown the retention of immunoglobulin synthesis, in most cases at a reduced level. Some of the results obtained on human B-cell derived lines are summarized in Table III.

Table III. *Expression of immunoglobulin synthesis in hybrids with human B-cell derived cell lines.*

Retention of immunoglobulin synthesis in hybrids between lymphoid cells.	
BL x BL (H x H)	Ref. 29
LCL x LCL (H x H)	Ref. 30
Leukemia x myeloma (H x M)	Ref. 31
Retention of immunoglobulin synthesis in hybrids between lymphoid and non-lymphoid cells.	
LCL x 3T3 fibroblast (H x M)	Ref. 32
Loss of immunoglobulin synthesis in hybrids between lymphoid and non-lymphoid cells.	
Myeloma x L fibroblast (H x M)	Ref. 33
BL x Leukemia (H x H)	Ref. 34

(H = human, M = mouse)

In hybrids between the two BL lines Raji and Namalwa (29) which express either small amounts of IgM kappa (Raji) or large amounts of IgM lambda (Namalwa) it was possible to quantitate the amounts of the two different types of light chains on the cell surface by means of radioimmunoassay. In this experiment, coexpression of the two types of light chains was observed in analogy with some of the other results recorded in Table III, and with other results not mentioned from hybrids between mouse lymphoid cells. An interesting aspect of these quantitative measurements was that in several clones investigated, the quantitative determinations of the amounts of kappa and lambda light chains expressed were similar to those of the parental cells individually. Typical results were as follows (29): Raji: $18.6 \pm 10.2 \times 10^3$ kappa chains/cell; Namalwa: $159 \pm 147 \times 10^3$ lambda chains/cell; Raji/Namalwa hybrid (1-1): $14.5 \pm 4.0 \times 10^3$ kappa chains/cell, $212.5 \pm 147.8 \times 10^3$ lambda chains/cell. This type of result argues for a relatively fixed level of expression of immunoglobulin molecules in hybrids between BL cells, even when as here studied at the level of membrane expression. In other cases we do, however, find evidence for more complex control mechanisms. In one hybrid combination Raji/BJAB (24), where both parents produce relatively high amounts of IgM kappa, surface immunoglobulin showed an intermediate or suppressive pattern, whereas intracellular kappa chain content showed an amplification in the hybrid.

The more general observation by these and other experiments - that immunoglobulin producing hybrid cells made from two producers allow both parental phenotypes to be expressed - is the basis for the remarkable success of using hybrids between myeloma cells and antigen-stimulated lymphocytes for the production of antigen-specific antobody. When hybrids of this combination (socalled hybridoma cells) are cloned, monoclonal antibodies are produced from the cloned hybridomas (35). Until now this approach has been used in the mouse system, but the selection of appropriately marked human myeloma cells should make it possible to adapt this system for the production of desired human monoclonal antibodies.

The finding of extinction of antibody production is the most common observation in studies of hybrids made by fusing immunoglobulin producing cells with non-lymphoid cells. In the hybrid between human myeloma cells (266B1) producing IgE with mouse L cells (33), early passages of the hybrid population were studied in order to eliminate as much as possible the preferential loss of human chromosomes, and the majority of human chromosomes found present by chromosome analyses and isozyme electrophoresis. In spite of this, IgE as detected by sensitive radioimmunoassay was lost completely (i.e. the myeloma parent produced IgE at a rate of 8.3×10^3 ng/10^6 cells/48 h; the hybrid population less than 0.1 ng/10^6 cells/48 h). This finding suggests that regulatory factors are involved in the loss of immunoglobulin production. In an additional study (36), the primary fusion products, binucleate heterokaryons, were analyzed for cytoplasmic content of immunoglobulin (lambda chains) by immunofluorescence, and a similar loss of immunoglobulin found early after cell fusion. This result again suggests the possible involvement of regulatory factors in the control of immunoglobulin expression in the fusion products of myeloma cells with unrelated cell types.

In subsequent studies we have characterized immunoglobulin expression in hybrids with more closely related cells. For these studies we used a cell line derived from chronic myeloid leukemia (CML) (37). CML derived cells can show a variety of paths of differentiation, which may be differentiated from each other using appropriate markers. Either the CML phase or the acute blast crisis (seen as Philadelphia (Ph^1) chromosome positive acute leukemia) may be present first. Different clones representing different differentiation lineages (lymphoid, myeloid, and granulocytic) may be present simultaneously, and all of these are Ph^1-positive.

The particular CML derived line (K562) (37) contained a Ph^1-derived marker (38,39) and lacked B- and T-cell markers (39). Subsequent studies have found the K562 line to lack expression of myeloid antigens, and to express glycophorin (gp42) (40), a property of erythroid cells, as well as to be inducible for hemoglobin synthesis by either Na-butyrate (41) or haemin (42). This particular phenotype (shared by or stock of K562 cells) strongly argues, that at least some K562 sublines are erythroleukemic cells, i.e. a human analogue of mouse Friend cells. Recent controversy among different laboratories observing different phenotypes in K562 sublines might suggest the exciting possibility that the original isolate could represent a Ph^1-positive pluripotential stem cell that has shown diverse differentiation in different sublines. Recent evidence suggests a common stem cell origin for CML cells and B-cells (43). Therefore, K562 in spite of its apparent erythroid differentiation would be expected to be relatively closely related to B-cells. Hybrids were obtained by fusing K562 with two BL lines Daudi and P3HR-1 (34,44). The hybrid between K562 and Daudi was shown to be an almost complete hybrid with a modal chromosome number close to the sum of the two parental cell lines (69(K562) + 46(Daudi)). Daudi expresses membrane associated IgM strongly, whereas K562 being a non-lymphoid cell, does not express immunoglobulin. The K562/Daudi hybrid likewise did not express membrane associated IgM (Table IV) .

Since the K562 line is erythroid one could expect a dominance of erythroid phenotype in the K562/Daudi hybrid. This possibility was tested by measuring haeme levels in the three different cell types below (Table IV) .

Table IV. *Phenotype of K562/Daudi hybrid.*

Quantitative immunofluorescence (microfluorimetry), IgM	
Daudi	12.74 ± 4.16 (arbitrary units)
K562	0.67 ± 0.49 - -
K562/Daudi	0.82 ± 0.76 - -
Haeme levels (^{59}Fe incorporation)	
Daudi	0.0185 picomoles/10^6 cells
K562	0.2700 - - -
K562/Daudi	5.3334 - - -

These results suggest a dominance of the erythroid phenotype that even seems to be amplified in the K562/Daudi hybrid. Similar results were obtained for the K562/P3HR-1 hybrid. Further studies are in progress to determine more precisely the apparent dominance of the erythroid phenotype of the K562/BL hybrids, which was unexpected in view of the relatively close relatedness of the two lineages (43).

In contrast to differentiated functions, other "household" functions are usually coexpressed. This pertains to isoenzyme markers used for hybrid characterization, and also to HLA antigens which likewise have been useful in identifying intraspecific hybrids between human cells as those already discussed. In a few cases we have observed abnormalities with respect to HLA expression in our collection of human cell lines. These cases are the Daudi cell line, already mentioned as being HLA-, Beta-2 microglobulin - (24,26), and the K562 line that in contrast to Daudi shows normal intracellular amounts of Beta-2 microglobulin, but contains extremely low if any membrane associated Beta-2 microglobulin and also is HLA negative (24,26,34). The correlation between lack of membrane associated Beta-2 microglobulin and HLA is understandable in view of the current view that HLA antigens are present in the cell membrane in the form of Beta-2 microglobulin-HLA dimers. Since Daudi cells type as Ia+ (24) it is likely that this is not the case for Ia-like antigens, although Ia-like antigens have been suggested to be HLA (probably D locus) - controlled (45,46). Daudi cells carry an interstitial deletion of one of its chromosomes 15 (26), carrying the structural gene for Beta-2 microglobulin (47). The extent of this deletion (q14-q21) is in good agreement with recent results from regional mapping of the gene for Beta-2 microglobulin on chromosome 15 (48,49). If this association is not a mere coincidence, it would present a rather unique case of lack of one gene on an autosome leading to total loss of activity. A Raji/Daudi hybrid (24, 50) showed expression of additional HLA specificities (A10,B38,B17) not present on Raji (or Daudi). These new specificities are interpreted to arise by genetic complementation of the Beta-2 microglobulin deficiency of Daudi cells, bringing out hidden HLA specificities in the hybrid in the form of membrane associated Beta-2 microglobulin-HLA dimers, constituting a genetic argument in favor of this hypothesis. With special interest in relation to B-cell differentiation, anchorage sites for cellular differentiation antigens have been proposed to be the Beta-2 microglobulin-HLA dimer (51). In accordance with this hypothesis, the male H-Y antigen has been found to be shedded into culture supernatants of Daudi cells from which it has been isolated and purified (52,53). A possibility which should be tested is if similar B-cell specific differentiation antigens could be characterized similarly. In the K562/P3HR-1 hybrid (34), membrane expressed Beta-2 microglobulin was strongly suppressed as compared to the P3HR-1 parental line. Interestingly, there was a low degree of HLA expression (specificity A3, P3HR-1 derived), whereas another P3HR-1 derived specificity (A3) was undetectable. An explanation for this finding would be that A3 more efficiently competes for limited amounts of Beta-2 microglobulin than B17. In the K562/Daudi hybrid (44), Beta-2 microglobulin was expressed in similar low amounts as in K562, but a small subcytotoxic quantity of HLA-B17 specified by Daudi was reexpressed, indicating weak complementation between the two defects leading to lack of HLA expression in K562 and Daudi. In contrast to Daudi cells, the K562/Daudi hybrid did not express Ia-like antigens, in accordance with the behavior of Ia-like antigens as B-cell specific differentiated markers similarly to what has already been discussed for membrane IgM in this particular hybrid combination.

In hybrids between different B-cell BL cell lines, differentiated B-cell markers (Ia-like antigens, F_c receptors, C3 receptors, EBV receptors) generally are expressed but do show examples of more complex interactions. In Raji/Daudi and Raji/BJAB hybrids (24) surface markers behaved as represented in Table V.

Table V. *Schematic summary of surface marker tests in Raji/Daudi and Raji/BJAB hybrid cells.*

	Raji	Daudi	Raji/Daudi	BJAB	Raji/BJAB
Surface Ig (IgM kappa)	-	+++	±	+++	++++
F_c receptors	-	++	++	++	++
Complement:					
C_3b (EAC rosettes)	+++	-	+++	-	+++
Complement staining	+++	+++	+++	±	±
Complement consumption	high	medium	medium	low	medium
EBV receptor staining	+++	++	+++	+	+++
EBV absorption test	high	medium	high	low	high

(From Ref. 24)

Points of interest is a suppressive pattern of surface immunoglobulin in one hybrid combination (Raji/Daudi) while surface immunoglobulin appears to be amplified in another (Raji/BJAB). F_c receptors in this and other cases appear to be controlled in a dominant fashion. The three types of complement tests give different results: dominant expression in the rosette test, suppression in staining, and intermediate levels in complement consumption. This is hardly surprising, since the three tests measure different complement dependent phenomena. Quantitative measurements of the EBV receptor by absorption show that the high concentration of Raji dominates in both hybrid combinations. In another hybrid combination (Daudi/P3HR-1) surface immunoglobulin was dominant, while complement and EBV receptors were suppressed (54). These data (represented in Table VI) show that widely different results are obtained depending upon the hybrid combination studied. Further generalizations involving the dominance of the pattern of a given parents expression pattern will require the study of further hybrid combinations.

Table VI. *Surface markers on Daudi, P3HR-1 and Daudi/P3HR-1 hybrid.*

	Daudi	P3HR-1	Daudi/P3HR-1
IgM (MF)	>90%	0	>90%
kappa (MF)	>90%	0	>90%
Beta-2 microglobulin (MF)	0	>90%	>90%
C3 receptor (EAC rosettes)	76±15%	13±3%	23±5%
C3 receptor (CMF)	87±13%	5±2%	42±8%

MF = Membrane fluorescence (living cells)
CMF = Complement membrane fluorescence
Data from Ref. 54.

3. CELLS INFECTED BY EBV.

As already discussed, infection of B-lymphocytes is sharply restricted to human surface immunoglobulin and complement (C3) positive B-cells (7). This explains the rather narrow range of differentiated B-cell lineage phenotypes seen with EBV transformed or immortalized B-cell lines. This narrow range of cells infectible with EBV is explained by considering the expression of EBV receptors related to the complement receptor on human B-cells (27,28). The apparent specificity can therefore in most cases be explained by the presence of EBV receptors restricted to human B-lymphocytes at a specific stage in their differentiation (see Table I). The possibility therefore remains that other cell types could be infected and transformed by EBV, provided that a means of penetrating the membrane barrier is provided. This problem is of particular relevance for the understanding of how EBV containing malignant epithelial carcinoma cells arise in NPC. One of the means of achieving this goal is to use direct microinjection of the viral particles into cells by means of glass microcapillaries (55). In preliminary experiments we have microinjected a concentrated preparation of EBV (100 x concentrated B95-8 supernatant) into human epithelial amnion cells, and between 50 and 100% of the microinjected cells became positive for the Epstein-Barr virus nuclear antigen (EBNA) within 4 days after microinjection (56). These results demonstrate that the early events of EBV transformation can be achieved in a system unrelated to human B-cells. This process and the phenotype of EBV microinjected epithelial cells is now the subject of further studies.

4. EXPRESSION OF EBV, THE EBNA ANTIGEN AND CELLULAR TRANSFORMATION

Multiple copies of EBV viral genomes are present in EBV-carrying B-cells, both of BL and LCL origin (57). These cells invariably contain the EBV-determined nuclear antigen EBNA (58). The EBNA antigen is detected by a three-layer anticomplementary immunofluorescence (58) or by two-layer indirect immunoperoxidase staining(59) since it is present in extremely low amounts, in the order of 10^4 molecules per cell. The amount of EBNA antigen in different EBV-carrying lines is proportional to the number of EBV genomes present (60), suggesting autonomous expression of this part of the viral genome. While EBNA is present in all EBV-transformed cell lines, two additional viral antigens,early antigen (EA) (61), and viral capsid antigen (VCA) (62) are only expressed when the virus enters the lytic cycle. These two antigens are detected by direct or indirect immunofluorescence or immunoperoxidase staining. To detect the antigens mentioned selected patient (usually BL) sera are used; it is therefore possible that the simple designations like EA or VCA could cover a range of antigenic specificities. Recent immunochemical studies on EBV associated early and late antigens (63) have found 15 polypeptides to be associated with the EBV lytic cycle, two of which could be classified as late viral products. These are probably minimal estimates of the numbers of viral polypeptides involved.

The expression of EBV antigens during the productive viral cycle is associated with the appearance of two additional membrane antigens, early membrane antigen (EMA) and late membrane antigen (LMA), and the productive cycle is further associated with the appearance of an EBV associated thymidine kinase (TK) (64). The sequence may be represented as follows:

(Infection ⟶ EBNA) ⟶ EMA, EA ⟶ viral DNA synthesis, TK ⟶ VCA, LMA (⟶ virus release)

A similar sequence to the above is seen after induction of latent virus in EBV-carrying cell lines, which can be brought about by inducers like IUdR (65), Na-butyrate (66), anti-IgM (67) and tumor promoting phorbol ester (TPA) (68) as well as superinfection with exogenous EBV. Different cell lines show a wide range in capacity to produce early and late functions spontaneously (and after induction). Lines might therefore be classified as being non-producer, abortive producer, or producer cell lines (Table VII). Release of infectuous virus even from producer lines is a relatively rare event, restricted to a few human and a larger number of non-human primate cell lines.

Table VII. *Main types of EBV-carrying cell lines.*

	Antigens expressed			
	EBNA	EA	VCA	Typical BL lines
Non-producer	+	-	-	Namalwa
Abortive producer	+	+	+/-	Raji
Producer	+	+	+	Daudi, P3HR-1

The early events after EBV infection of B-cells have been characterized to some extent. Virus adsorption and penetration is followed by the induction of EBNA, RNA synthesis, activation of polyclonal immunoglobulin production, DNA synthesis (S-phase), and mitosis (69-73). The first detectable change is the appearance of EBNA in nuclei after a lag of 12 - 25 h. This is followed by

DNA synthesis in EBNA positive nuclei after 40 h and mitosis after 48 h. The sequence may therefore be represented as:

B-lymphocyte + EBV	→	RNA synthesis	→	EBNA	→	RNA+DNA synthesis	→	mitosis
Hours after infection:		5		12-25		40		48

The accumulation of EBNA in nuclei is slower than that observed for T antigens of the small DNA viruses, polyoma and SV40 (74,75). The accumulation of EBNA into nuclei preceding the first S-phase suggests however that in analogy to these systems, EBNA could be directly involved in the control of this DNA synthesis.

The phenotypic changes induced by EBV have been largely studied by comparing clonal, EBV-negative but EBV-susceptible B-lymphoma lines (BJAB and Ramos) with their *in vitro* converted, EBV- and EBNA-positive sublines. Such comparisons are probably more meaningful than comparisons with uninfected, resting B-cells, since they dissociate the virally induced phenotypic changes from the pleiotropic consequences of polyclonal B-cell activation that accompany the transformation of lymphocytes by EBV. When such cell lines are compared, the karyotypes were maintained and no major changes in surface immunoglobulin and F_c receptors, but changes in complement and EBV receptor densities were found (25). Interestingly, EBV-conversion is observed to induce increased resistance to saturation conditions, decreased serum dependence, independence of dialyzable serum factor(s), decreased capping of surface markers, increased lectin agglutinability and an increased ability to activate the alternative complement pathway (76-82). Most of these effects are surprisingly similar to those induced by the classical transforming small DNA viruses (polyoma and SV40) in monolayer cultures. This is surprising since the systems are so different: EBV is a large DNA virus (100 x 10^6 daltons DNA), its target is a lymphoid cell that grows in suspension, and these effects were found on comparing EBV-converted cells with EBV-negative cells already of malignant origin. The common denominator between these systems could be sought in the ability of all transforming viruses (EBV included) to emancipate their targets from the need for exogenous stimulation *in vitro*, i.e. the basic change implied by the term "immortalization". In particular this is suggested by the decrease in serum requirement that may result from reorganization of the cell membrane and improved utilization of serum-carried growth factors (83).

The EBNA antigen is the only known viral function regularly expressed in all EBV-DNA carrying cells (58). So far, there is no known exceptions to this rule, even for as diverse biological material as EBV-carrying cell lines of human and simian origin, BL and NPC biopsies, somatic cell hybrids between EBV-carrying cells and EBV-negative cells of human or rodent origin, as well as simian tumors induced by EBV (84-95). In hybrids between EBV-carrying BL or NPC tumor cells with mouse cells no correlation has been possible associating EBV with any particular human chromosomes (92-95). The question if the presence of EBV and EBNA is directly related to tumorigenicity has been addressed in two studies on hybrids between NPC biopsy or BL biopsy cells and a mouse cell line (IT-22), which is non-tumorigenic when injected subcutaneously in nude mice (94,95). In these experiments tumorigenicity was observed for EBV-DNA- and EBNA-negative hybrid cells, suggesting that the presence of EBV-DNA and EBNA might not be directly involved in tumorigenicity, though it is possible that the presence of EBV could be somehow related to the initiation of a tumorigenic state. A further observation of relevance to the relationship of EBV to tumorigenicity is the finding that EBV-carrying LCL cells (in contrast to BL cells) are non-tumorigenic when implanted subcutaneously in nude mice (96), showing that further changes are necessary to produce tumorigenicity. LCL lines are usually normal diploid, whereas BL derived lines show secondary chromosomal changes: most BL lines carry a specific translocation (8q-/14q+ translocation (97)) which could be directly involved in malignancy. This relationship is the subject of further studies.

The EBV-carrying cell lines as mentioned can be classified into three categories: non-producers, abortive producers, and producers. Producer cell lines spontaneously contain a small proportion of EA+ cells, and a smaller proportion of VCA+ cells. The number of positive cells can be increased by means of inducers whose only common denominator is a known effect on differentiated cell markers in other cell systems. Abortive producers switch on production of EA in a very small proportion of cells, but these do not proceed to viral DNA synthesis and VCA production (98). The inducing agents amplify this process of EA production, but cannot push the cells beyond the block to viral DNA replication. This block could be due to either viral defectiveness or to some negative cellular control. The latter is more likely, since we have recently found that hybridization of the typical, abortively inducible line Raji with the EBV-negative BL line BJAB lifts the block to viral DNA replication and VCA production.

Somatic cell hybridization experiments between EBV-carrying cell lines have also given us some information on the controls involved. With certain minor variations, the picture is consistent: When EBV-carrying B-lymphoma lines are fused, producer status tends to dominate over non-producer status and inducibility over non-inducibility (54,99-102). This suggests positive controls, either viral or cellular. The fact that the inducers used (e.g. IUdR, Na-butyrate, TPA) are substances that interfere with cell differentiation, while standard mutagenic or carcinogenic agents as a rule are non-inducers (68), speaks for cellular control mechanisms. EBV-carrying B-cell lines have been fused with cells of different lineages, such as human or murine fibroblasts (87,91) or mouse or human carcinoma cells (92,102-105). In the cases where B-cells were hybridized with fibroblasts, virus production and inducibility were switched off in spite of the continued presence of EBV-DNA in multiple genome copies per cell, while EBNA expression was uninfluenced. In our recent studies on hybrids between the two producer lines Daudi and P3HR-1 with the K562 leukemic line (34,44), EBV production and inducibility was suppressed in spite of the fact that the lymphoid cells and the leukemic line must be assumed to be much closer related in differentiation than lymphoid cells and fibroblasts. The K562/P3HR-1 hybrid carried 26 EBV-DNA copies per cell and was 100% EBNA positive. The parental P3HR-1 subline was a low level producer, induced by IUdR, Na-butyrate and TPA to produce higher levels of EA and VCA. In contrast, the hybrid was completely non-permissive for both EA and VCA and non-inducible by any of the three inducers. The K562/Daudi hybrid in contrast was inducible, though at a much lower level than the parental Daudi cell line. The inducibility varied between the three inducers. The analogy of the expression of viral cycle antigens to differentiated B-cell markers has been mentioned (extinction in lymphoid x fibroblast hybrid cells, induction by inducers interfering with cell differentiation). It is therefore not surprising that the behavior of viral cycle antigens parallels the behavior of other B-cell markers in the hybrids with K562. An interesting exception to this observation is the behavior of the hybrids between EBV-carrying B-cells with human carcinoma cells (102-105). The human carcinoma cell partner, though EBV-negative, actually increases the permissiveness of the EBV-carrying cell, switching abortive producer lines (EA+VCA-) to full inducibility (EA+VCA+) in certain combinations. This observation might be of relevance to NPC, since epithelial carcinoma cells might be more compatible with EBV expression than other cells of non-B-cell origin. In contrast to the observations on human carcinoma/EBV-carrying B-cell hybrids (102-105), a mouse carcinoma/EBV-carrying B-cell hybrid was entirely non-permissive (92), suggesting some kind of species specificity.

Like the T antigens of the small DNA viruses, EBNA is a DNA-binding protein (106-111). In metaphase plates it is present on all chromosomes (58). This is the case both in hybrid cells where only one of the parental cells was EBV-carrying, as well as in an EBV-converted cell line carrying only one EBV genome copy per cell. The precise location of EBNA on chromosomes is not known,

Table VIII. *Presence of DNA-binding 53K and 48K components in different cell types.*

Cell	Derivation	53K	48K
Normal B-lymphocytes+	-	-	-
Protein A stimulated	-	-	-
B-lymphocytes+	-	-	-
Raji	EBV-carrying African BL	+	+
Namalwa	EBV-carrying African BL	+	+
Ramos	EBV-neg. American BL	+	-
AW-Ramos	In vitro EBV-conv. Ramos	+	+
BJAB	EBV-neg. BL-like lymphoma	+	-
DHL-4	B-cell lymphoma^{x}	+	-
DHL-7	B-cell lymphoma^{x}	+	-
Molt-4	T-cell ALL^{xx}	-	-
1301	T-cell ALL	-	-

Data from Ref.113.
$^{+}$from peripheral blood, ^{x}Diffuse histiocytic lymphoma, ^{xx}ALL, a-cute lymphatic leukemia.

but recent results suggest a preferential association with genetically inactive segments of mitotic chromosomes (R-bands)(112). Purified EBNA antigen (113) has a molecular weight of ∿ 180,000. On SDS gel electrophoresis, two major bands are obtained of 48,000 (48K) and 53,000 (53K) molecular weight, respectively. The 53K component is particularly interesting since a similar DNA-binding protein was found in EBV-negative lymphoma lines, but not in normal mitogen stimulated lymphocytes and not in T-cell lines as well as in histiocytic lymphoma lines of B-cell origin, that are derived from a different point in B-cell differentiation from lymphomas (Table VIII). It is therefore possible that the 53K protein is a normally occurring protein in certain types of B-cells.

It is of interest to note that similar host-cell specified 53K component has been found in SV40 T antigen (114), suggesting a further analogy between EBV and the small DNA viruses.

The question whether the DNA-binding EBNA protein is involved in the transforming action of EBV (changed growth control, immortalization) remains a subject to speculation. In the SV40 system, the number of DNA replication forks has been shown to be increased in SV40-transformed cells (115,116). Similarly, EBV-positive EBV-converted lymphoma cells show an increased number of DNA replication forks when compared to their EBV-negative counterparts (117). In recent preliminary experiments, we have microinjected purified EBNA into contact-inhibited 3T3 cells (113). EBNA was slowly accumulated into nuclei, and using erythrocyte-ghost-mediated microinjection (118), of contact-inhibited 3T3 cells, an apparent specific stimulation of DNA synthesis in EBNA-microinjected cultures as compared to control cultures microinjected with control protein (BSA, HMG protein) was observed (113). Further experiments have shown similar stimulation of EBNA-microinjected cultures of other cell types (BJAB EBV-neg. BL-like lymphoma, chinese hamster lung fibroblasts) under other conditions. This result would favor a direct role of EBNA in controlling host-cell DNA replication, which could be involved at least in some aspects of the transformed phenotype.

The choice between transformation and the lytic cycle during EBV-infection might be determined similarly as suggested for the SV40 system (55). If levels above a certain threshold of EBNA are produced during primary infection of B-cells, excess EBNA is available to induce viral DNA synthesis and late functions. If less than this amount is produced all available EBNA is bound to host-cell initiation sites for DNA synthesis, host-cell DNA synthesis is changed resulting in transformation and the few EBV-DNA copies are replicated under host-cell control. At the moment, quantitative measurements of EBNA in cells during the early steps of EBV transformation are not available, that could prove a test of this hypothesis. A further test would be to microinject EBNA into EBV-carrying cells and look for production of late functions.

5. CONCLUSIONS

The present review describes some aspects of current work concerning the phenotypes and control mechanisms involved in B-cell differentiation with special emphasis on EBV-transformed human cell lines (LCL and BL cells). B-cell differentiated markers include surface and secreted immunoglobulin, Ia-like antigens, F_c receptors, C3 receptors and EBV receptors. These properties behave like typical differentiated cell markers in hybrids with cells representing different pathways of differentiation. In hybrids with other B-cell derived lines, these markers are retained and coexpressed, but the quantitative levels of expression are changed in some hybrid combinations, suggesting cellular regulatory mechanisms that modify their expression. At the moment it is premature to generalize these results, since many different results are obtained depending on which hybrid combination is studied but it is hoped that a generalized picture will emerge by comparing the changes observed in several combinations of B-cell derived cell lines, derived from different steps of the differentiation lineage of B-cells as represented in Table I. Studies of hybrids of B-cells with the human erythroleukemic CML-derived line K562, showed that B-cell markers are suppressed in this combination. This observation was surprising, since the parental cells are not far from each other in their derivation.

The human intraspecific hybrids have been characterized by a number of methods: karyotypically, by isoenzyme patterns, and by their HLA profiles. The characterization of hybrid karyotypes has been very informative in all cases, since the parental cells have a number of specific markers which can be found in hybrid cells, for example Raji cells have 9 characteristic markers, while Namalwa have 7 characteristic markers, most of which can be positively in hybrid cells (29). In some cases, the isoenzyme profiles have been informative for a smaller number of chromosomes (e.g. 58), and in most cases the HLA profiles have been informative with respect to confirm the hybridity based on one chromosome (chromosome 6)(e.g. 24). The specific abnormality of Daudi lacking Beta-2 microglobulin and membrane-associated HLA (28,30) made it possible to look for genetic complementation resulting in the appearance of new HLA specificities, providing a genetic proof that Beta-2 microglobulin is a component of membrane-associated HLA.

Infection of B-lymphocytes is normally restricted to surface immunoglobulin and C3 receptor positive cells (7). EBV receptors have not been found on other types of cells. It is therefore a paradox that at least one other cell type - the epithelial carcinoma cell in NPC - carries the EBV genome. Recent studies aim at understanding this paradox, since they show that EBNA-positive cells do appear after microinjecting epithelial amnion cells with concentrated EBV. These results do suggest that if EBV somehow is able to penetrate the membrane barrier EBV-transformed cells might arise.

In EBV carrying cells (BL, LCL, NPC) multiple copies are present of EBV viral genomes. These cells all express the EBNA antigen, in amounts proportional to the number of genomes present. Other viral antigens (EA, VCA) are expressed in a variable fashion in different cell lines (non-producer (EA-VCA-), abortive producer (EA+VCA-), producer (EA+VCA+)). Viral cycle antigens like EA and VCA may be induced by inducers (IUdR, Na-butyrate, anti-IgM, TPA), or by superinfection with exogenous virus. In hybrids between different BL cell lines, producer status usually dominates over non-producer status, and inducibility over non-inducibility. In hybrids of BL cells with cells of other lineages (fibroblasts, K562 erythroleukemic cells) production of viral cycle antigens is suppressed. This finding suggests that the production of viral cycle antigens behave like differentiated B-cell functions. An interesting exception to the extinction of viral cycle antigen production is found in hybrids between BL cells and carcinoma cells: The carcinoma partner here did not suppress EA and VCA production, but in certain combinations EA+VCA- were actually switched to full inducibility (EA+VCA+). This observation might again be of relevance to NPC, since epithelial carcinoma cells might be more compatible with EBV expression than other non-B cells.

The EBNA antigen is associated with nuclei and mitotic chromosomes (58). Purified EBNA antigen (113) has a molecular weight of ∿180,000, and appears to consist of two subunits of 48K and 53K. The 48K component is probably EBV coded, since it is present only in EBV-transformed cells; the 53K component is interesting since it is present also in other types of B-lymphocyte derived tumro cells, and is probably host-coded (113). This observation is reminescent of similar results in the SV40-system (114). Recent results, (113) further show that microinjection of EBNA under some conditions stimulate DNA synthesis in quiescent cells. This result favors a direct role of EBNA that could be involved in controlling host-cell DNA replication. This is probably not a sufficient step in producing tumorigenic cells, since EBNA-positive LCL usually are non-tumorigenic in contrast to cells of BL origin. In hybrids between NPC and BL biopsy cells (94,95) EBNA-negative hybrid cells have been found to produce tumors in nude mice. This observation is puzzling, and suggests the possibility that while EBV and EBNA might be necessary to initiate tumorigenicity, secondary changes might occur that lead to tumorigenicity even in the absence of EBNA. EBNA could have a further function in promoting the decision between transformation and the lytic cycle. A possibility would be that this choice is made on the basis of the levels of EBNA produced during primary infection, similarly as has been suggested for the SV40-system (55).

6. ACKNOWLEDGEMENTS

We thank our colleagues for stimulating collaboration and exchange of information, without which many of the results reviewed in this article would have been absent. In addition we wish to thank our colleagues for permission to quote unpublished material.

Work in the authors' laboratories have been supported by the

Danish Natural Science Research Council, The Danish Cancer Society, Aarhus University; and by Contract No.N01 CP 33316 from the Division of Cancer Cause and Prevention, National Cancer Institute, Public Health Service Research Grant No. 5R01 CA 14054-05, and the Swedish Cancer Society.

7. REFERENCES

1) EPSTEIN, M.A. and ACHONG, B.G. (1977). Recent progress in Epstein-Barr virus research. Ann.Rev.Microbiol., 31, 421.

2) JONDAL, M. and KLEIN, G. (1973). Surface markers on human B and T lymphocytes. II. Presence of Epstein-Barr virus (EBV) receptors on B lymphocytes. J.Exp.Med., 138, 1365.

3) HENLE, G., HENLE, W., and DIEHL, V. (1968). Relation of Burkitt's tumor-associated herpes type virus to infectuous mononucleosis. Proc. Natl. Acad. Sci. USA, 59, 94.

4) FIALKOW, P.J., KLEIN, G., GARTLER, S.M., and CLIFFORD, P. (1970). Clonal origin for individual Burkitt tumours. Lancet, 1, 384.

5) KLEIN, G. (1979). The relationship of EB-virus to nasopharyngeal carcinoma. In "The Epstein-Barr virus" (eds. M.A. Epstein and B.G. Achong), in press.

6) MILLER, G. (1971). Human lymphoblastoid cell lines and Epstein-Barr virus. A review of their interrelationships and their relevance to the etiology of leukoproliferative states in man. Yale J. Biol. Med., 43, 358.

7) EINHORN, L., STEINITZ, M., YEFENOF, E., ERNBERG, I., BAKACS, T., and KLEIN, G. (1978). Epstein-Barr virus (EBV) receptors, complement receptors, and EBV infectability of different lymphocyte fractions of human peripheral blood. II. Epstein-Barr virus studies. Cell. Immunol., 35, 43.

8) ÅMAN, P. and SPIRA, G., unpublished.

9) NILSSON, K. (1978). Established human lymphoid cell lines as models for B-lymphocyte differentiation. In "Human lymphocyte differentiation: Its application to cancer" (eds. B. Serrou and C. Rosenfeld). p. 307. North-Holland Publishing Co., Amsterdam.

10) PREUD'HOMME, J.-L. and SELIGMANN, M. (1974). Surface immunoglobulins on human lymphoid cells. In "Progress in clinical immunology" (ed. R.S. Schwartz) vol. 2, p. 121. Grune and Stratton, New York.

11) PREUD'HOMME, J.-L., BROUET, J.-C., and SELIGMANN, M. (1977). Membrane bound IgD on human lymphoid cells, with special reference to immunoproliferative diseases. Immunol. Rev., 37, 127.

12) MATSUOKA, Y., TAKAHASHI, M., YAGI, Y., MOORE, G.E., and PRESSMAN, D. (1968). Synthesis and secretion of immunoglobulins by established cell lines of human hematopoietic origin. J.Immunol., 101, 1111.

13) KLEIN, E., NILSSON, K., and YEFENOF, E. (1975). An established Burkitt's lymphoma line with cell membrane IgG. Clin. Immunol. Immunopathol. 3, 575.

14) KLEIN, E., ESKELAND, T., INOUE, M., STROM, R., and JOHANSSON, B. (1970). Surface immunoglobulin-moieties on lymphoid cells. Exp. Cell Res., 62, 133.

15) ESKELAND, T. and KLEIN, E. (1971). Isolation of 7S IgM and Kappa chains from the surface membrane of tissue culture cells derived from a Burkitt lymphoma. J. Immunol., 107, 1367.

16) NILSSON, K. and PONTEN, J. (1975). Classification and biological nature of established human hematopietic cell lines. Int. J. Cancer, 15, 321.

17) STEINITZ, M., KOSKIMIES, S., KLEIN, G., and MÄKELÄ, O. (1978). Establishment of specific antibody producing human cell lines by antigen preselection and EBV transformation. In "Lympho-

cyte Hybridomas" (eds. F. Melchers, M. Potter, N. Warner), Curr. Topics in Microbiol. and Immunol., 81, 156, Springer-Verlag.

18) WELSH, K.I. and TURNER, M.J. (1976). Preparation of antisera specific for human B cells by immunization of rabbits with immune complexes. Tissue Antigens, 8, 1976.

19) TING, A., MICKEY, M.R., and TERASAKI, P. (1976). B-lymphocyte alloantigens in Caucasians. J. Exp. Med., 143, 981.

20) NILSSON, K., unpublished.

21) DICKLER, H.B. and KUNKEL, H. (1972). Interaction of aggregated IgG with human lymphocytes. J. Exp. Med., 136, 191.

22) JONDAL, M. (1974). Surface markers on human B- and T-lymphocytes. IV. Distribution of surface markers on resting and blast-transformed lymphocytes. Scand. J. Immunol., 3, 739.

23) BLOOM, B.R. and DAVID, J.R. (eds.)(1976). In "In vitro methods of cell-mediated and tumor immunity". Academic Press, New York.

24) KLEIN, G., TERASAKI, P., BILLING, R., HONIG, R., JONDAL, M., ROSEN, A., ZEUTHEN, J., and CLEMENTS, G. (1977). Somatic cell hybrids between human lymphoma lines. III. Surface markers. Int. J. Cancer, 19, 66.

25) KLEIN, G., ZEUTHEN, J., TERASAKI, P., BILLING, R., HONIG, R., JONDAL, M., WESTMAN, A., and CLEMENTS, G. (1976). Inducibility of the Epstein-Barr virus (EBV) cycle and surface marker properties of EBV-negative lymphoma lines and their in vitro EBV-converted sublines. Int. J. Cancer, 18, 639.

26) ZEUTHEN, J., FRIEDRICH, U., ROSEN, A., and KLEIN, E. (1977). Structural abnormalities in chromosome 15 in cell lines with reduced expression of Beta-2 microglobulin. Immunogenetics, 4, 567.

27) JONDAL, M., KLEIN, G., OLDSTONE, M., BOKISH, V., and YEFENOF, E. (1976). Surface markers on human B and T lymphocytes. VIII. Association between complement and Epstein-Barr virus (EBV)

receptors on human lymphoid cells. Scand. J. Immunol., 5, 401.

28) YEFENOF, E., KLEIN, G., JONDAL, M., and OLDSTONE, B. (1976). Surface markers on human B and T lymphocytes. IX. Two-color immunofluorescence studies on the association between EBV receptors and complement receptors on the surface of lymphoid cell lines. Int. J. Cancer, 17, 693.

29) ROSEN, A., CLEMENTS, G., KLEIN, G., and ZEUTHEN, J. (1977). Double immunoglobulin production in cloned somatic cell hybrids between two human lymphoid cell lines. Cell, 11, 139.

30) BLOOM, A.D. and NAKAMURA, F.T. (1974). Establishment of a tetraploid, immunoglobulin-producing cell line from the hybridization of two human lymphocyte lines. Proc. Natl. Acad. Sci. USA, 71, 2689.

31) LEVY, R. and DILLEY, J. (1978). Rescue of immunoglobulin secretion from human neoplastic lymphoid cells by somatic cell hybridization. Proc. Nat. Acad. Sci. USA, 75, 2411.

32) ORKIN, S.H., BUCHANAN, P.D., YOUNT, W.J., REISNER, H., and LITTLEFIELD, J.W. (1973). Lambda-chain production in human lymphoblast-mouse fibroblast hybrids. Proc. Natl. Acad. Sci. USA, 70, 2401.

33) ZEUTHEN, J. and NILSSON, K. (1976). Hybridization of a human myeloma permanent cell line with mouse cells. Cell Differentiation, 4, 355.

34) KLEIN, G., ZEUTHEN, J., ERIKSSON, I., TERASAKI, P., BERNOCO, M., ROSEN, A., MASUCCI, G., POVEY, S., and BER, R. (1979). Hybridization of a myeloid leukemia derived cell line (k562) with a Burkitt lymphoma line (P3HR-1): Surface marker and Epstein-Barr virus (EBV) studies. J. Natl. Cancer Inst., in press.

35) MELCHERS, F., POTTER, M., and WARNER, N.L. (eds.) (1978). "Lymphocyte hybridomas", Curr. Topics in Microbiol. and Immunol., 81, Springer-Verlag.

36) ZEUTHEN, J., STENMAN, S., FABRICIUS, H.-A., and NILSSON, K. (1976). Expression of immunoglobulin synthesis in hyman myeloma x non-lymphoid cell heterokaryons: Evidence for negative control. Cell Differentiation, 4, 369.

37) LOZZIO, C.B. and LOZZIO, B.B. (1973). Cytotoxicity of a factor isolated from human spleen. J. Natl. Cancer Inst., 50, 535.

38) LOZZIO, C.B. and LOZZIO, B.B. (1975). Human chronic myelogenous leukemia cell line with positive Philadelphia chromosome. Blood, 45, 321.

39) KLEIN, E., BEN-BASSAT, H., NEUMANN, H., RALPH, P., ZEUTHEN, J., POLLIACK, A., and VANKY, F. (1976). Properties of the K562 cell line derived from a patient with chronic myeloid leukemia. Int. J. Cancer, 18, 421.

40) ANDERSSON, L.C., NILSSON, K., and GAHMBERG, C.G. (1979). K562, a human erythroleukemic cell line. Int. J. Cancer, 23, 143.

41) ANDERSSON, L.C., JOKINEN, M., and GAHMBERG, C.G. (1979). Induction of erythroid differentiation in the human leukemia cell line K562. Nature, 278, 364.

42) RUTHERFORD, T.R., CLEGG, J.B., and WEATHERALL, D.J. (1979). K562 human leukaemic cells synthesize embryonic haemoglobin in response to haemin. Nature, 280, 164.

43) FIALKOW, P.J., DENMAN, A., JACOBSEN, R.J., LOWENTHAL, M.N. (1979). Chronic myelocytic leukemia: Origin of some lymphocytes from leukemic stem cells. J. Clin. Invest., in press.

44) KLEIN, G. et al., manuscript in preparation (1979).

45) MÖLLER, G. (ed.)(1976). Biochemistry and biology of Ia antigens. Transplant. Rev., 30.

46) SPRINGER, T.A., KAUFMAN, J.F., TERHORST, C., and STROMINGER, J.L. (1977). Purificant and structural characterization of human HLA-linked B cell antigens. Nature, 268, 213.

47) GOODFELLOW, P.N., JONES, E.A., VAN HEYNINGEN, V., SOLOMON, E., BOBROW, M., MIGGIANO, V., and BODMER, W.P. (1975). The B2 microglobulin gene is on chromosome 15 and not in the HLA region. Nature, 254, 267.

48) OLIVER, N., FRANCKE, U., and PELLEGRINO, M.A. (1978). Regional assignment of genes for mannose phosphate isomerase, pyruvate kinase 3, and B2-microglobulin expression on human chromosome 15 by hybridization of cells from a t(15;22) (q14;q13.3) translocation carrier. Cytogenet. Cell Genet., 22, 506.

49) PAJUNEN, L., SOLOMON, E., BURGESS, S., BOBROW, M., POVEY, S., and SWALLOW, D. (1978). Regional mapping of chromosome 15. Cytogenet. Cell Genet., 22, 511.

50) FELLOUS, M., KAMOUN, M., WIELS, J., DAUSSET, J., CLEMENTS, G., ZEUTHEN, J., and KLEIN, G. (1977). Induction of HLA expression in Daudi cells after cell fusion. Immunogenetics, 5, 423.

51) OHNO, S. (1977). The original function of MHC antigens as the general plasma membrane anchorage sites of organogenesis-directing proteins. Immunol. Rev., 33, 59.

52) BEUTLER, B., NAGAI, Y., OHNO, S., KLEIN, G., and SHAPIRO, I. (1978). The HLA dependent expression of testis-organizing H-Y antigen by human male cells. Cell, 13, 509.

53) NAGAI, Y., CICCARESE, S., and OHNO, S. (1979). The identification of human H-Y antigen and testicular transformation induced by its interaction with the receptor site of bovine fetal ovarian cells. Differentiation, 13, 155.

54) BER, R., KLEIN, G., MOAR, M., POVEY, S., ROSEN, A., WESTMAN, A., YEFENOF, E., and ZEUTHEN, J. (1978). Somatic cell hybrids between human lymphoma lines. IV. Establishment and characterization of a P3HR-1/Daudi hybrid. Int. J. Cancer, 21, 707.

55) GRAESSMANN, A., GRAESSMANN, M., and MUELLER, C. (1980). Biological activity of simian virus 40 DNA fragments and T-antigen tested by microinjection into tissue culture cells. This volume. (Further references to the technique of microcapillary microinjection are found in this article).

56) Jesper ZEUTHEN, Stella ROSENBAUM, and Edith TRØST SØRENSEN, unpublished.

57) ZUR HAUSEN, H. (1975). Oncogenic herpesviruses. Biochim. Biophys. Acta, 417, 25.

58) REEDMAN, B. and KLEIN, G. (1973). Cellular localization of an Epstein-Barr virus (EBV)-associated complement-fixing antigen in producer and non-producer lymphoblastoid cell lines. Int. J. Cancer, 11, 499.

59) KURSTAK, E., DE THE, G., VAN DEN HURK, J., CHARPENTIER, G., KURSTAK, C., TIJSSEN, P., and MORISSET, R. (1978). Detection of Epstein-Barr virus antigens by peroxidase-labeled specific immunoglobulins. J. Med. Virol., 2, 189.

60) ERNBERG, I., ANDERSSON-ANVRET, M., KLEIN, G., LUNDIN, L., and KILLANDER, D. (1977). Relationship between the amount of Epstein-Barr virus determined nuclear antigen per cell and the number of EBV-DNA copies per cell. Nature, 266, 269.

61) HENLE, W., HENLE, G., ZAJAC, B., PEARSSON, G., WAUBKE, R., and SCRIBA, M. (1970). Differential reactivity of human serums with early antigens induced by Epstein-Barr virus. Science, 169, 188.

62) HENLE, G. and HENLE, W. (1966). Immunofluorescence in cells derived from Burkitt's lymphoma. J. Bact., 91, 1248.

63) KALLIN, B., LUKA, J., and KLEIN, G. (1979). Immunochemical characterization of Epstein-Barr virus (EBV) associated early and late antigens in n-butyrate treated P3HR-1 cells. J. Virol., in press.

64) CHEN, S.-T., ESTES, J.E., HUANG, E.-S., and PAGANO, J.S. (1978). Epstein-Barr virus-associated thymidine kinase. J.

Virol., 26, 203.

65) KLEIN, G. and DOMBOS, L. (1973). Relationship between the sensitivity of EBV-carrying lymphoblastoid lines to superinfection and the inducibility of the resident viral genome. Int. J. Cancer, 11, 327.

66) LUKA, J., KALLIN, B., and KLEIN, G. (1979). Induction of the Epstein-Barr viral cycle in latently infected cells by n-butyrate. Virology, 94, 228.

67) TOVEY, M.C., LENOIR, G., and BERGNON-LOURS, J. (1978). Activation of latent Epstein-Barr virus by antibody to human IgM. Nature, 276, 270.

68) ZUR HAUSEN, H., BORNKAMM, G.W., SCHMIDT, R., and HECKER, E. (1979). Tumor initiators and promotors in the induction of Epstein-Barr virus. Proc. Natl. Acad. Sci. USA, 76, 782.

69) AYA, T. and OSATO, T. (1974). Early events in the transformation of human chord blood leukocytes by Epstein-Barr virus: Induction of DNA synthesis, mitosis and the virus associated nuclear antigen synthesis. Int. J. Cancer, 14, 341.

70) ROBINSON, J. and MILLER, G. (1975). Assay for Epstein-Barr virus based on stimulation of DNA synthesis in mixed leukocytes from human umbilical blood. J. Virol., 15, 1065.

71) EINHORN, L. and ERNBERG, I. (1978). Induction of EBNA precedes the first cellular S-phase after EBV-infection of human lymphocytes. Int. J. Cancer, 21, 157.

72) ERNBERG, I. (1979). Requirements for macromolecular synthesis during primary Epstein-Barr virus infection of lymphocytes. Submitted for publ.

73) ZERBINI, M. and ERNBERG, I. (1979). Epstein-Barr virus infection and growth stimulating effect in human B-lymphocytes. Submitted for publ.

74) HOGGAN, M.D., ROWE, W.P., BLACK, P.H., and HUEBNER, R.J. (1965). Production of tumor specific antigens by oncogenic viruses during acute cytolytic infection. Proc. Natl. Acad.

Sci. USA, 53, 12.

75) OXMAN, M.N., TAKEMOTO, K.K., and ECKHART, W. (1972). Polyoma T antigen synthesis by temperature-sensitive mutants of polyoma virus. Virology, 49, 675.

76) STEINITZ, M. and KLEIN, G. (1975). Comparison between growth characteristics of an Epstein-Barr virus (EBV)-genome negative lymphoma line and its EBV-converted subline in vitro. Proc. Natl. Acad. Sci. USA, 72, 3518.

77) STEINITZ, M. and KLEIN, G. (1976). Epstein-Barr virus (EBV)-induced change in saturation density and serum dependence of established, EBV-negative lymphoma lines in vitro. Virology, 70, 570.

78) STEINITZ, M. and KLEIN, G. (1977). Further studies on the differences in serum dependence in EBV negative lymphoma lines and their in vitro converted, virus-genome carrying sublines. Eur. J. Cancer, 13, 1269.

79) YEFENOF, E. and KLEIN, G. (1976). Difference in antibody induced redistribution of membrane IgM in EBV-genome free and EBV positive human lymphoid cells. Exp. Cell Res., 99, 175.

80) McCONNELL, I., KLEIN, G., LINT, T.F., and LACHMANN, P.J. (1978). Activation of the alternative complement pathway by human B cell lymphoma lines is associated with Epstein-Barr virus transformation of the cells. Eur. J. Immunol., 8, 453.

81) YEFENOF, E., KLEIN, G., BEN-BASSAT, H., and LUNDIN, L. (1977). Differences in the Con A - induced redistribution and agglutination patterns of EBV genome-free and EBV-carrying human lymphoma lines. Exp. Cell Res., 108, 185.

82) MONTAGNIER, L. and GRUEST, J. (1979). Cell-density-dependence for growth in agarose of two human lymphoma lines and its decrease after Epstein-Barr virus conversion. Int. J. Cancer, 23, 71.

83) HOLLEY, R.W., ARMOUR, R., BALDWIN, J.H., BROWN, K.D., and YEH, Y.-C. (1977). Density-dependent regulation of growth of

BSC-1 cells in cell culture: Control of growth by serum factors. Proc. Natl. Acad. Sci. USA, 74, 5046.

84) POVLSEN, C.O., FIALKOW, P.J., KLEIN, E., KLEIN, G., RYGAARD, J., and WIENER, F. (1973). Growth and antigenic properties of a biopsy-derived Burkitt's lymphoma in thymusless (nude) mice. Int. J. Cancer, 11, 30.

85) HUANG, D.P., HO, J.H.C., HENLE, W., and HENLE, G. (1974). Demonstration of Epstein-Barr virus-associated nuclear antigen in nasopharyngeal carcinoma cells from fresh biopsies. Int. J. Cancer, 14, 580.

86) KLEIN, G., GIOVANELLA, B.C., LINDAHL, T., FIALKOW, P.J., SINGH, S., and STEHLIN, J.S. (1974). Direct evidence for the presence of Epstein-Barr virus DNA and nuclear antigen in malignant epithelial cells from patients with poorly differentiated carcinoma of the nasopharynx. Proc. Natl. Acad. Sci. USA, 71, 4737.

87) KLEIN, G., WIENER, F., ZECH, L., ZUR HAUSEN, H., and REEDMAN, B. (1974). Segregation of the EBV-determined nuclear antigen (EBNA) in somatic cell hybrids derived from the fusion of a mouse fibroblast and a human Burkitt lymphoma line. Int. J. Cancer, 14, 54.

88) LINDAHL, T., KLEIN, G., REEDMAN, B.M., JOHANSSON, B., and SINGH, S. (1974). Relationship between Epstein-Barr virus (EBV) DNA and the EBV-determined nuclear antigen (EBNA) in Burkitt lymphoma biopsies and other lymphoproliferative malignancies. Int. J. Cancer, 13, 764.

89) KLEIN, G. (1975). Studies on the Epstein-Barr virus genome and the EBV-determined nuclear antigen in human malignant disease. Cold Spring Harbor Symp. Quant. Biol., 39, 783.

90) FRANK, A., ANDIMAN, W.A., and MILLER, G. (1976). Epstein-Barr virus and non-human primates: Natural and experimental infection. Adv. Cancer Res., 23, 171.

91) GLASER, R., ABLASHI, D.V., NONOYAMA, M., HENLE, W., and EASTON, J. (1977). Enhanced oncogenic behavior of human and mouse cells after cellular hybridization with Burkitt tumor cells. Proc. Natl. Acad. Sci. USA, 74, 2574.

92) SPIRA, J., POVEY, S., WIENER, F., KLEIN, G., and ANDERSSON-ANVRET, M. (1977). Chromosome banding, isoenzyme studies and determination of Epstein-Barr virus DNA content on human Burkitt lymphoma/mouse hybrids. Int. J. Cancer, 20, 849.

93) STEPLEWSKI, Z., KOPROWSKI, H., ANDERSSON-ANVRET, M., and KLEIN, G. (1978). Epstein-Barr virus in somatic cell hybrids between mouse cells and human nasopharyngeal carcinoma cells. J. Cell Physiol., 97, 1.

94) STACZEK, J., STEPLEWSKI, Z., WEINMANN, R., KLEIN, G., and KOPROWSKI, H. (1979). Manuscript in prep.

95) Jesper ZEUTHEN and George KLEIN, unpublished.

96) NILSSON, K., GIOVANELLA, B.C., STEHLIN, J.S., and KLEIN, G. (1977). Tumorigenicity of human hematopoietic cell lines in athymic nude mice. Int. J. Cancer, 19, 337.

97) MANOLOV, G. and MANOLOVA, Y. (1972). Marker band in one chromosome 14 from Burkitt lymphomas. Nature, 237, 33.

98) MOAR, M. and KLEIN, G. (1979). Abortive expression of the Epstein-Barr virus (EBV) cycle in a variety of EBV DNA containing cell lines, as reflected by nucelic acid hybridization in situ. Int. J. Cancer, in press.

99) NYORMOI, O., KLEIN, G., ADAMS, A., and DOMBOS, L. (1973). Sensitivity to EBV superinfection and TUdR inducibility of hybrid cells formed between a sensitive and a relatively resistant Burkitt lymphoma cell line. Int. J. Cancer, 12, 396.

100) KLEIN, G., CLEMENTS, G., ZEUTHEN, J., and WESTMAN, A. (1976). Somatic cell hybrids between human lymphoma lines. II. Spontaneous and induced patterns of the Epstein-Barr virus (EBV) cycle. Int. J. Cancer, 17, 715.

101) KLEIN, G., CLEMENTS, G., ZEUTHEN, J., and WESTMAN, A. (1977). Spontaneous and induced patterns of the Epstein-Barr virus (EBV) cycle in a new set of somatic cell hybrids. Cancer Letters, 3, 91.

102) MOAR, M.H., BER, R., KLEIN, G., WESTMAN, A., and ERIKSSON, I. (1978). Somatic cell hybrids between human lymphoma lines. V. IUdR inducibility and P3HR-1 superinfectability of Daudi/HeLa (DAD) and Daudi/P3HR-1 (DIP-1) cell lines. Int. J. Cancer, 22, 669.

103) GLASER, R. and RAPP, F. (1972). Rescue of Epstein-Barr virus from somatic cell hybrids of Burkitt lynphoblastoid cells. J. Virol., 10, 288.

104) GLASER, R. and NONOYAMA, M. (1973). Epstein-Barr virus: Detection of genome in somatic cell hybrids of Burkitt lymphoblastoid cells. Science, 179, 492.

105) TANAKA, A., NONOYAMA, M., and GLASER, R. (1977). Transcription of latent Epstein-Barr virus genomes in human epithelial/Burkitt hybrid cells. Virology, 82, 63.

106) LENOIR, G., BERTHELON, M.C., FAURE, M.C., and DE THE, G. (1976). Characterization of Epstein-Barr virus antigens. I. Biochemical analysis of the complement-fixing soluble antigen and its relationship with Epstein-Barr virus-associated nuclear antigen. J. Virol., 17, 672.

107) LUKA, J., SIEGERT, W., and KLEIN, G. (1977). Solubilization of the Epstein-Barr virus-determined nuclear antigen and its characterization as a DNA-binding protein. J. Virol., 22, 1.

108) LUKA, J., LINDAHL, T., and KLEIN, G. (1978). Purification of the Epstein-Barr virus-determined nuclear antigen from Epstein-Barr virus-transformed human lymphoid cell lines. J. Virol., 27, 604.

109) MATSUO, T.S., NISHI, H., HIRAM, H., and OSATO, T. (1977). Studies of Epstein-Barr virus related antigens. II. Bioche-

mical properties of soluble antigen in Raji Burkitt lymphoma cells. Int. J. Cancer, 19, 364.

110) OHNO, S., LUKA, J., LINDAHL, T., and KLEIN, G. (1977). Identification of a purified complement-fixing antigen as Epstein-Barr virus-determined nuclear antigen (EBNA) by its binding to metaphase chromosomes. Proc. Natl. Acad. Sci. USA, 74, 1605.

111) BARON, D. and STROMINGER, J.L. (1978). Partial purification and properties of Epstein-Barr virus-associated nuclear antigen. J. Biol. Chem., 253, 2875.

112) Edith TRØST SØRENSEN and Jesper ZEUTHEN, unpublished.

113) KLEIN, G., LUKA, J., and ZEUTHEN, J. (1979). Epstein-Barr virus (EBV)-induced transformation and the role of the nuclear antigen (EBNA). Cold Spring Harbor Symp. Quant. Biol., 44, in press.

114) LANE, D.P. and CRAWFORD, L.V. (1979). T antigen is bound to a host protein in SV40-transformed cells. Nature, 278, 261.

115) MARTIN, G. and OPPENHEIM, A. (1977). Initiation points for DNA replication in non-transformed and simian virus 40-transformed Chinese hamster lung cells. Cell, 11, 859.

116) OPPENHEIM, A. and MARTIN, A. (1978). Initiation points for DNA replication in non-transformed and simian virus 40-transformed BALB/c3T3 cells. J. Virol., 25, 450.

117) Ariella OPPENHEIM and Hannah BEN-BASSAT, unpublished.

118) KALTOFT, K. and CELIS, J.E. (1978). Ghost-mediated transfer of human hypoxanthine guanine phosphoribosyl transferase into deficient chinese hamster ovary cells by means of polyethylene glycol-induced fusion. Exp. Cell Res., 115, 423.

TUMORIGENICITY, ACTIN CABLES AND GENE EXPRESSION IN MOUSE CLID x CHO CELL HYBRIDS

R. Bravo, J.V. Small*, A. Celis, K. Kaltoft and J.E. Celis

Division of Biostructural Chemistry, Department of Chemistry, Aarhus University, 8000 Aarhus C, Denmark, and
**Institute of Molecular Biology of the Austrian Academy of Sciences, Salzburg, Austria*

1. INTRODUCTION

There is pressing need to search for assays of transformation that could be used to assess malignancy or tumorigenicity in cultured cells. A variety of reports have appeared correlating abnormal properties of transformed cells with the ability of these cells to produce tumors (1-10). Reported changes in cell cytoarchitecture, especially those of actin containing microfilament bundles following viral transformation (3, 6, 7, 10) promted us to look for similar changes in non-virally transformed cells (11). Quantitative analysis of the distribution and organization of microfilament bundles in several non-virally transformed cells as examined by indirect immunofluorescence using human actin antibodies (11, 12) and by electronmicroscopy of whole cells grown attached to support grids (13, 14) indicated that a loss or reduction of actin microfilament bundles was not essential for some of these cell lines to produce tumors in nude mice. From these studies, however, we could not exclude the possibility that the clearly different pattern of microfilament bundles ("crossed pattern") found in mouse CLID cells could be directly related to tumorigenicity. In this cell line the bundles radiated or crossed from a region close to the cell's center or near its projections and usually penetrated the projections.

To answer this question we have analysed the pattern of microfilament bundles and tumorigenicity in nude mice of cell hybrids produced by polyethylene glycol (PEG) fusion between tumorigenic mouse CLID cells and transformed, low tumorigenic chinese hamster ovary cells (CHO) having a normal pattern of microfilament bundles (15). The hybrid nature of the cell lines was confirmed by chromosome analysis as well as by high resolution two dimensional gel electrophoresis of [^{35}S]-methionine labelled polypeptides obtained from the parents as well as from the different hybrid cells.

Our studies on these hybrids clearly show that loss or alteration of the actin microfilament bundles cannot be used as a reliable assay to asses tumorigenicity at the cellular level in non-virally transformed cells. The possibility of using cell hybrids to map polypeptides to defined chromosomes will be discussed.

2. MORPHOLOGY OF THE PARENT AND HYBRID CELLS

The morphology of eight hybrids and of the parent cells is shown in Fig. 1. Hybrids 13, 14 and 41 resemble the shape of the CLID parent and are composed predominantly of spindle shape fibroblasts exhibiting numerous, frequently overlapping cytoplasmic processes. Hybrids 11 and 16 showed an intermediate morphology while hybrids 51 and 52 consisted of moderately large spread fibroblasts with cytoplasmic processes overlapping in dense cultures. Hybrid 12 is one of the most interest-

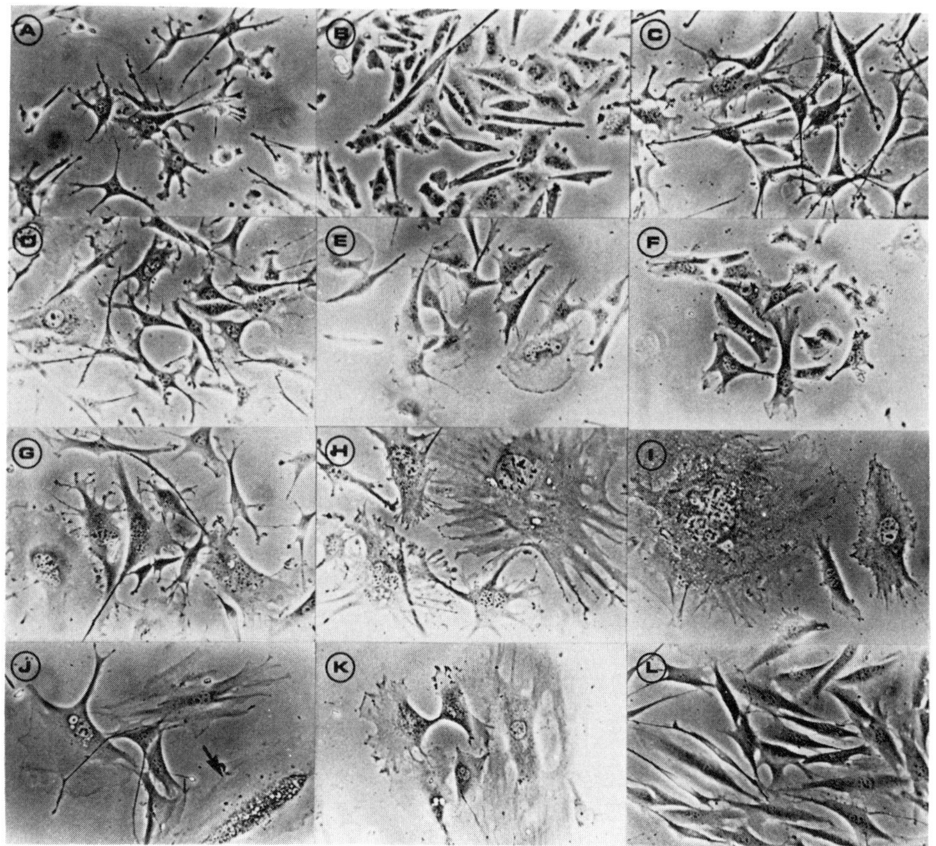

Fig. 1. *Morphology of parent and hybrid cells.* Cultures were grown for 48 hrs at 37°C before fixation in 2.5% glutaraldehyde in PBS. (A) CLID clone A (p30); (B) CHO-EMS 16.4 (p36); (C) Hy 13 (p4); (D) Hy 14 (p4); (E) Hy 11 (p4); (F) Hy 16 (p4); (G) Hy 41 (p4); (H) Hy 51 (p4), (I) Hy 52 (p4); (J), and (K) Hy 12 (p1) and Hy 12 (p5). x300. From Celis *et al.* (15).

ing of the clones isolated as there was a clear change in shape of the cell population between passages (p) 1 and 5. At early passages (Figs. 1J and K) most of the cells were very flat in morphology, resembling senescent fibroblasts and cultures of this hybrid grew very slowly. At later passages, however (Fig. 1L), most of the cells resembled the CHO EMS 16.4 parent shape although they were bigger in size. These cells grow in cultures as well as the CHO EMS 16.4 parent cell.

Table 1. *Properties of parental and cell hybrids*

Cell Line	Mode	Karyotype[a] range	Average no. of chromosomes without centromeric staining[b]	% of cells showing a 'crossed' pattern of microfilament bundles[c]	Tumorigenicity in nude mice: No. of cells injected per mouse[d]	No. of tumours/no. of injected mice	Latency days[e]
CLID clone A	92(p30)	71-101	4±2	52	$1x10^6$	15/15	10
CLID clone A					$6x10^4$	3/3	19
CLID clone A					$1x10^4$	2/4	45
CHO EMS 16.4	20, 19(p36)	18-21	-	1	$1x10^6$	3/21	38
Hy 11	82(p5)	74-84	9±4	21	$1x10^6$	1/6	24
Hy 12	85(p6)	81-90	13±3	12	$1x10^6$	0/5	
Hy 13	93(p7)	73-96	8±1	48	$1x10^6$	2/6	51
Hy 14	86(p6)	72-90	8±2	30	$1x10^6$	5/8	43
Hy 16	97(p6)	88-103	13±1	40	$1x10^6$	8/9	45
Hy 41	87,88(p6)	78-120	7±2	39	$1x10^6$	9/9	29
Hy 51	158(p5)	126-171	7±1	64	$1x10^6$	1/6	37
Hy 52	128(p4)	117-132	3±2	48	$1x10^6$	5/8	24

[a] Based on the analysis of 50 metaphases.
[b] Determined using the Hoechst 33258 staining procedure described by Hilwig and Gropp (14).
[c] Determined from cells (p4) treated with human actin antibodies.
[d] n/n BALB/c/BOM/spf nude mice were inoculated subcutaneously as previously described (11).
[e] Period between inoculation and detection of a small palpable tumor.

From Celis *et al.* (15).

3. CHROMOSOMAL CONSTITUTION OF THE HYBRIDS AND PARENT CELLS

The chromosomal constitution of the parent and hybrid cells are given in Table 1. The presence of CHO chromosomes in the hybrid clones was estimated with the use of the fluorochrome Hoechst 33258 which has been shown to stain preferentially the AT-rich centric heterochromatin of mouse chromosomes (16). CHO chromosomes do not show bright centromeric staining (17) while CLID cells contained on average 4±2 such chromosomes. As shown in Table 1, with the exception of the polyploid hybrid 52 all the clones contained an above-background number of chromosomes without centromeric staining, confirming the hybrid character of the clones. Hybrids 12 (Fig. 2) and 16 contained the highest number of such chromosomes (13±3 and 13±2, respectively) but we did not obtain hybrids having a chromosome number close to that expected of a hybrid keeping the full complement of CHO EMS 16.4 chromosomes. From this observation it is clear that all the hybrids segregated CHO chromosomes. The modal number of chromosomes varied very much among the hybrids (82-158, Table 1). Only hybrids 13, 16, 51 and 52 presented a mode above that of the CLID parent while hybrids 11, 12, 14 and 41 showed a mode below that value. It is likely that due to the wide dispersion of chromosome numbers observed in the parental CLID cells (range 71-101) these latter four hybrids arose from fusions involving CLID cell having a submodal number of chromosomes. Elimination of mouse chromosomes in the hybrids could not be excluded as no detailed chromosome analysis has been performed. Studies are now under way to determine what CHO chromosome(s) are retained in each hybrid.

4. ORGANISATION OF MICROFILAMENT BUNDLES

The organisation of microfilament bundles in the different cell lines permeated with 0.1% Triton X-100 was studied by means of indirect immunofluorescence using human actin antibodies (11, 12) and in

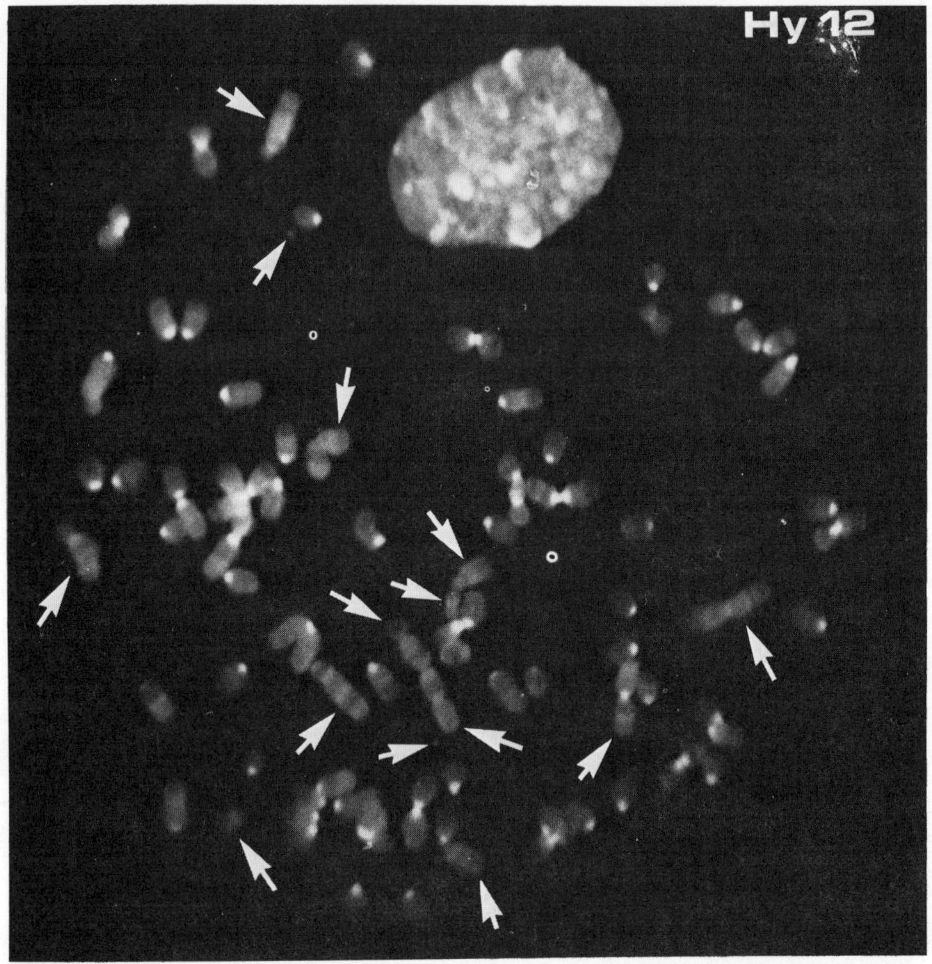

Fig. 2. *Metaphase chromosomes from Hy 12 stained with Hoechst 33258 (4)*. The arrows show chromosomes that do not exhibit differential centromeric fluorescence.

addition, in a few cases, by electron microscopy of whole cells grown directly on support grids (13, 14). Fig. 3 show representative pictures of the microfilament pattern of the parent and some of the hybrids cells as revealed by immunofluorescence. All the hybrids with the exception of Hy 12 presented the crossed pattern observed in the CLID cells (quantitations are given in Table 1). The cells showed microfilament bundles that radiated from or crossed each other at different places in the cell and usually penetrated the cell projections (Fig. 3). In all cases normal patterns of microfilament bundles could be observed in well spread CLID parent or hybrid cells and in some instances we could observe microfilament bundles organized in lattices (11, 18, 19) (Fig. 3, Hy 16), a property that has previously been attributed only to non-neoplastic cells (20). Fig. 4 shows an electron micrograph of microfilament bundles crossing or radiating in Hy 51. Fig. 5 shows such lattices in non-tumorigenic 3T3 B cells. The lattices can be seen above the nucleus and in the cytoplasm of 3T3 B cells.

Cells from early passage cultures of Hy 12 showed a pattern of microfilament bundles similar to that of the stationary well spread normal cells. At later passages, however, most of the cells from this clone resembled the actin pattern of CHO EMS 16.4 cells. Only a small percentage of these cells (see Table 1) showed the crossed pattern of the CLID parent cells.

Analysis of the Triton cytoskeletons by means of electron microscopy (13, 14) revealed abundant microtubules and 100 A^o filaments in all hybrids, indicating that the ability of the cells to produce tumors is not related to a change in the number of these filaments. Similar results indicating that microtubules and 100 A^o filaments are as extensive in transformed as in untransformed cells have been reported by several laboratories (21-27). Fig. 6 shows a representative electron micrograph of a Triton skeleton from hybrid 41 showing microfilament bundles (mfb), microtubules (mt) and 100 A^o filaments (if).

5. TUMORIGENICITY OF THE HYBRIDS IN NUDE MICE

The CLID parental cell line produced 100% tumors when $6x10^4$ cells were injected per nude mouse, while 50% of the animals produced tumors when 10^4 were injected (Table 1). CHO EMS 16.4 cells, however, are low

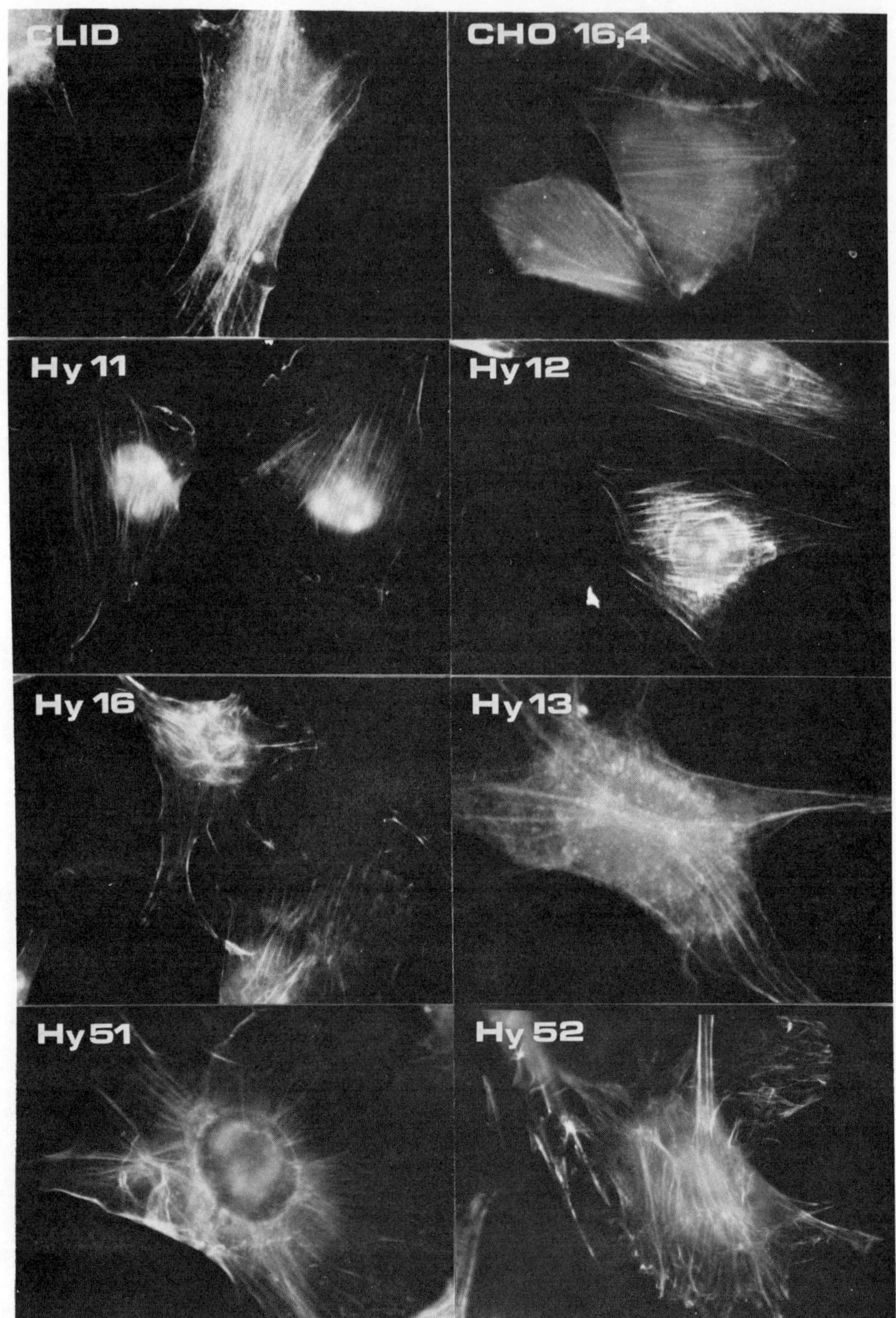
CLID
CHO 16,4
Hy 11
Hy 12
Hy 16
Hy 13
Hy 51
Hy 52

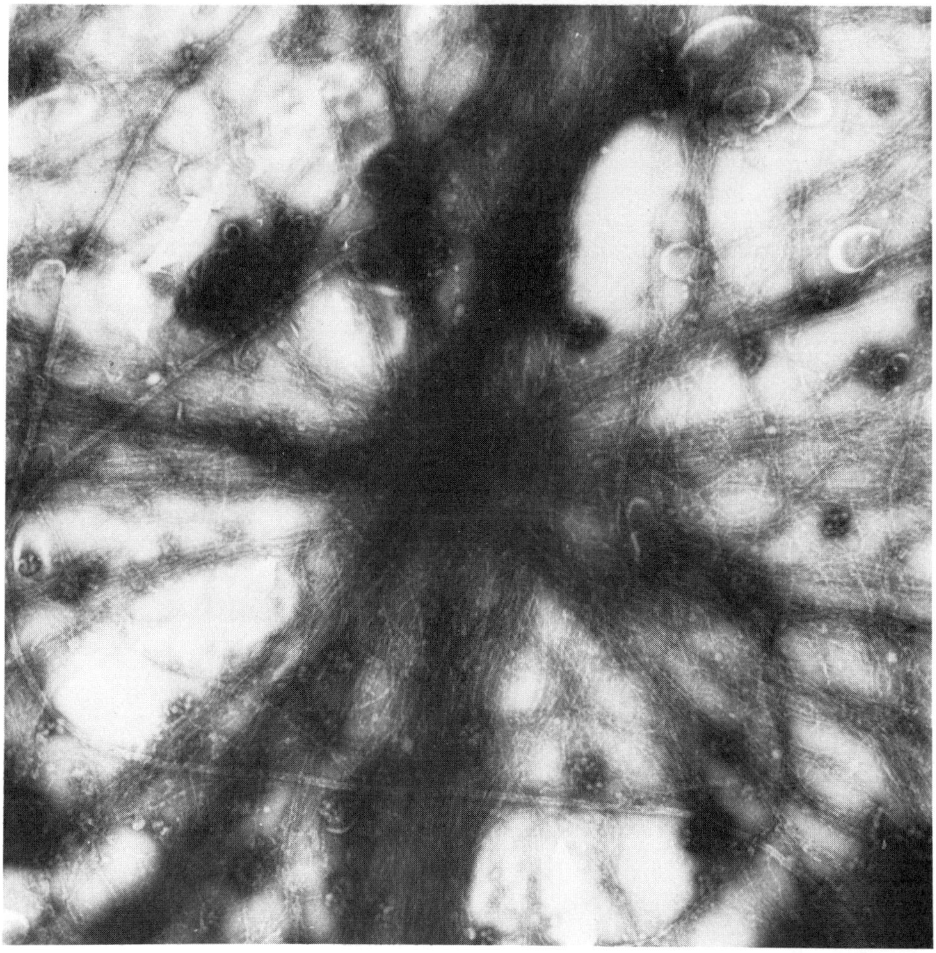

Fig. 4. *Electron micrograph of crossing or radiating microfilament bundles observed in Hy 51.* Triton X-100 treated cells were prepared for electron microscopy as described by Small and Celis (13). From Celis *et al.* (15).

tumorigenic as less than 15% of the animals produced tumors when 10^6 cells were injected. The original CHO cells do not produce tumors when 10^6 cells are injected (11). Only hybrids 14, 16, 41 and 52 con-

Legend for Fig. 3. *Pattern of microfilament bundles in parent cells as well as hybrids.* The cells were permeated with Triton X-100 and treated with human actin antibodies.

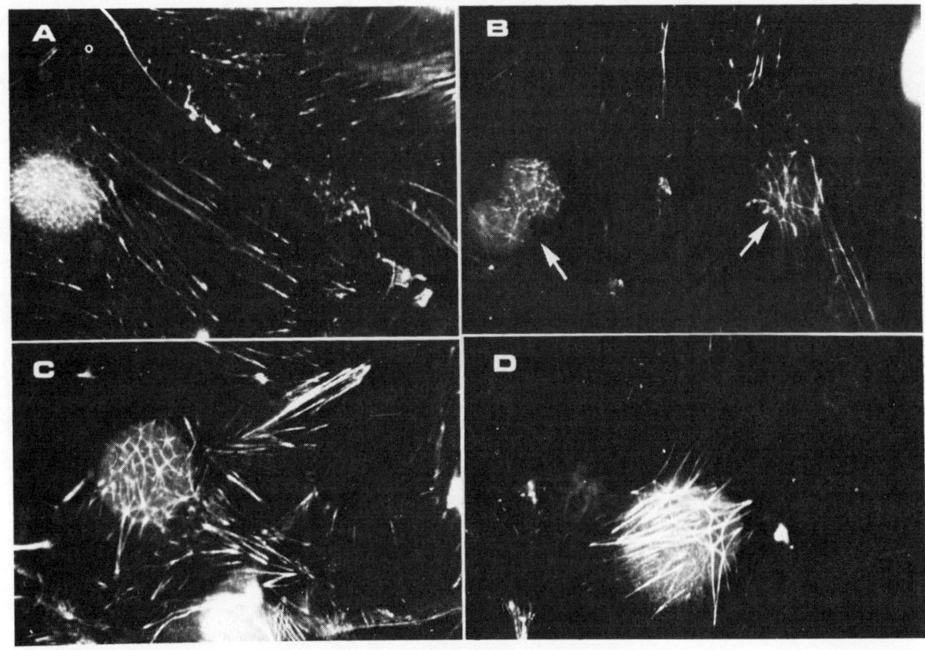

Fig. 5. *Indirect immunofluorescence of actin lattices in 3T3 B cells.* The lattices can be seen above the nucleus and in the cytoplasm.

sistently produced tumors at the site of injection when 10^6 cells were injected per mouse although the latent period in all cases was considerably longer (ranging from 24 to 45 days, Table 1) than that observed in the case of CLID parent (10 days for mice inoculated with 10^6 cells and 19 days for mice injected with $6x10^4$ cells). Hybrid 13 produced tumors in 33% of the animals while hybrids 11 and 51 produced tumors in 16% of the animals. Hybrid 12 did not produce tumors.

6. POLYPEPTIDE SYNTHESIS IN PARENT AND HYBRID CELLS

The hybrid nature of the different clones (Table 1) was further confirmed by high resolution two dimensional gel electrophoretic analysis (28, 29) of total [^{35}S]-methionine labelled polypeptides isolated from the parents as well as from the different hybrid cells. A summary of our preliminary findings is shown in Fig. 7 using the pat-

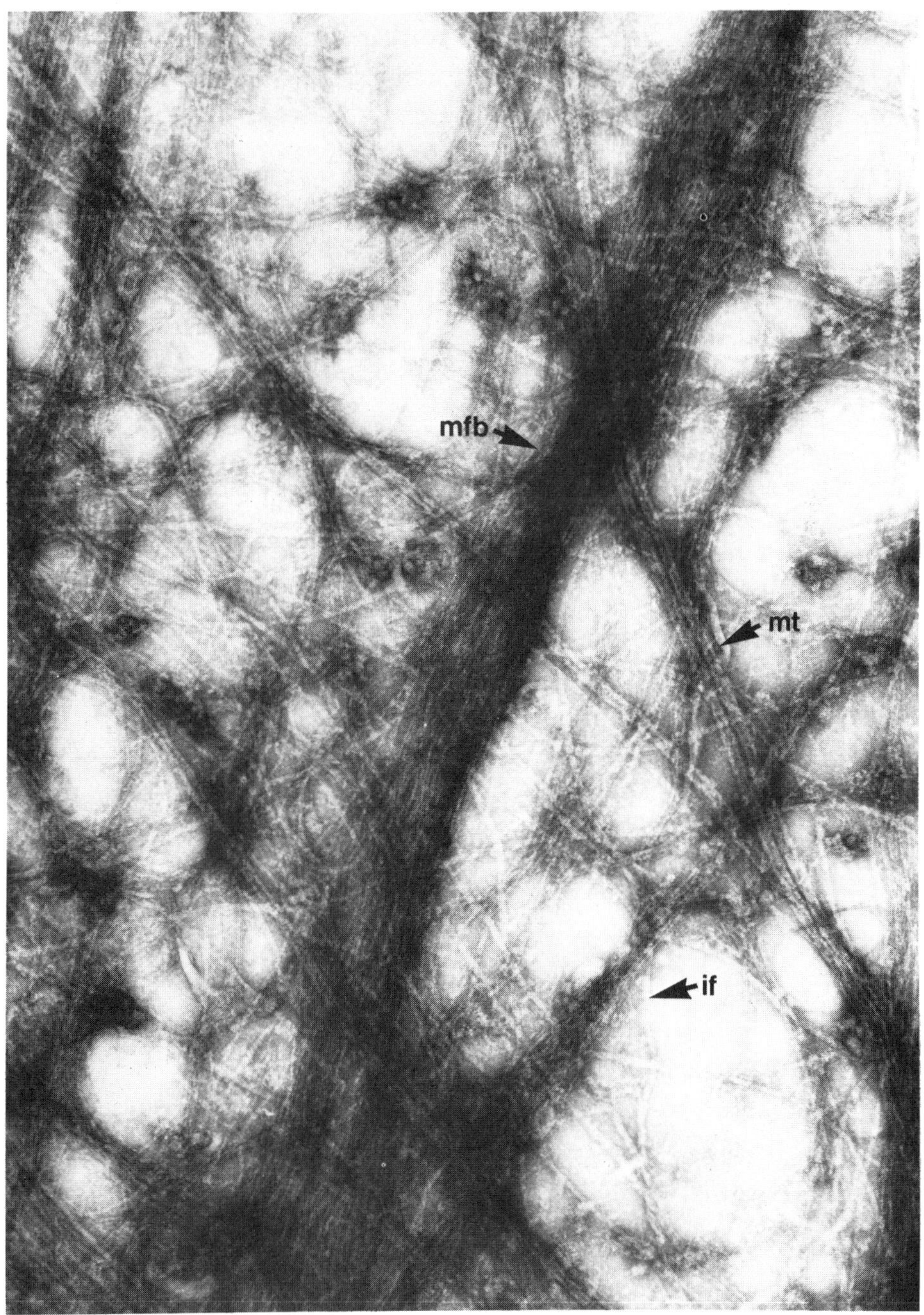

Fig. 6. *Electron micrograph of Triton X-100 extracted Hy 14.* *(if)*= 100 A° filaments; *(mf)*= microfilament bundles and *(mt)*= microtubules.

tern of Hy 11. A complete summary of all the CHO polypeptides found in 6 hybrids is given in Table 2. A total of 750 polypeptides (250 basic(NEPHGE) and 500 acidic (IEF)) were visually compared and in all cases analysed (6 hybrids) the overall polypeptide pattern corresponded to that of the mouse CLID parent. A total of 22 polypeptides (3 basic (NEPHGE) and 19 acidic (IEF)) characteristic of CHO were found in the hybrids (numbered arrows in Fig. 7 , Table 2). Hy 12 contained the highest number of CHO specific polypeptides (19, see Table 2) while no detectable CHO polypeptide was found in Hy 52. This hybrid presents a polypeptide map that is undistinguishable from the parental CLID cell. This result is important as this hybrid contains a background number of chromosomes without centromeric staining (Table 1). About 20 polypeptide spots specific of CHO cells were not detected in the hybrids. Also there are a considerable number of polypeptides that are common to CLID and CHO cells (indicated with small arrow in Fig. 7) but at present it is not possible to determine the origin of these polypeptides in the hybrids. Tryptic peptide analysis of these polypeptides should give valuable information in that direction.

Experiments are now underway to determine if the presence of any CHO specific polypeptides correlates with the retention of a defined CHO chromosome(s). This approach we believe should prove of value in the future to map specific polypeptides to a defined chromosome.

6. DISCUSSION

The results of experiments reported in this article indicate that there is no direct relationship between presence of a "crossed" pattern of microfilament bundles and tumorigenicity, as we have isolated hybrid clones that possessed the "crossed" pattern and yet they did not produce tumors, or their tumorigenicity was low. Thus, from this observation and from previous studies on the organization of microfi-

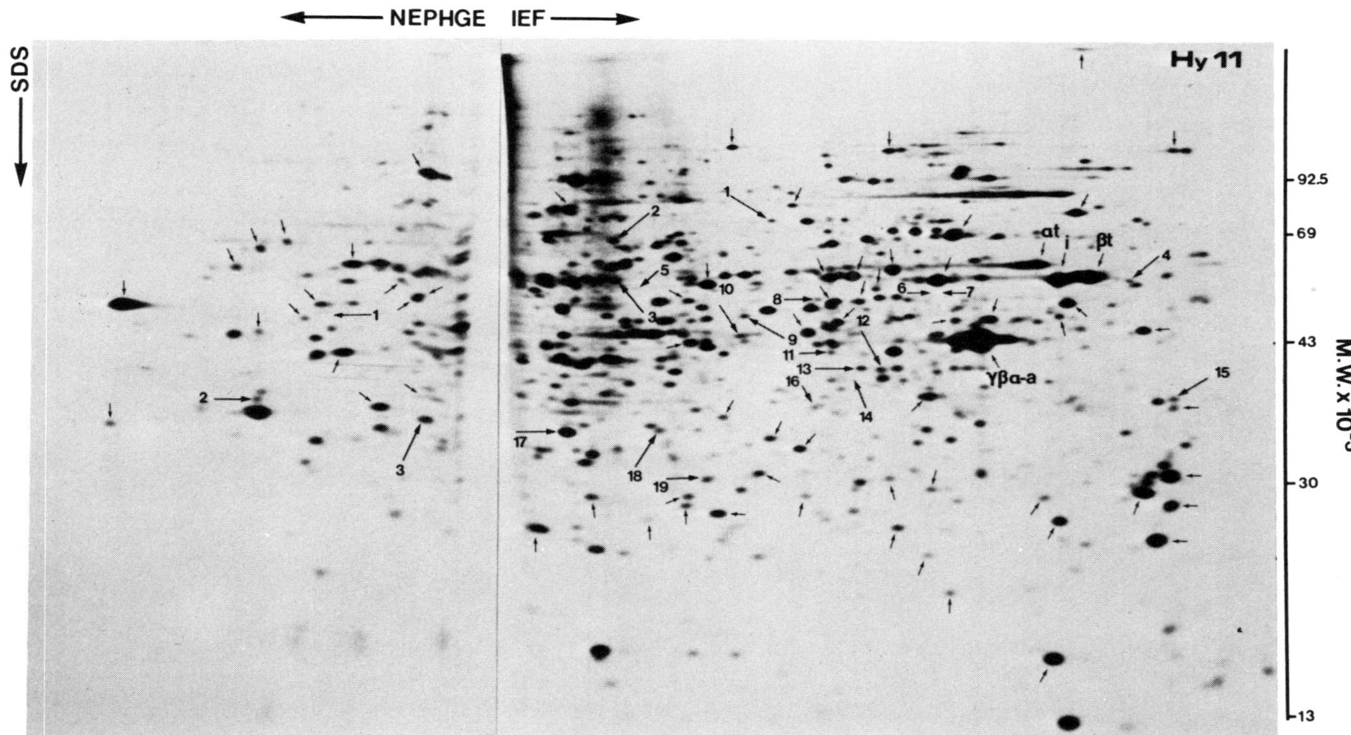

Fig. 7. *Two dimensional gel electrophoresis of total polypeptides from Hy 11*. The numbered spots correspond to CHO specific polypeptides found in the hybrids (see also Table 2). Small arrows indicate polypeptides that are common to CLID and CHO EMS 16.4 cells.

Table 2. *Relative intensity of CHO 16.4 polypeptides in hybrids.*

Polypeptide spot	Parents		Hybrids					
	CHO	CLID	H11	H12	H13	H14	H41	H52
IEF								
1	+++	-	++	+++	++	++	++	-
2	+++	-	++	+	+++	++	++	-
3	+++	-	++	+	++	++	++	-
4	+++	-	++	++	++	-	++	-
5	+++	-	-	-	-	++	++	-
6	+++	-	-	++	-	-	-	-
7	+++	-	-	++	-	-	-	-
8	+++	-	++	++	-	++	-	-
9	+++	-	+	+	+	+	+	-
10	+++	-	+	+	+	+	+	-
11	+++	-	+	-	+	-	-	-
12	+++	-	+	+	+	+	+	-
13	+++	-	+	+	+	+	+	-
14	+++	-	-	+	-	+	+	-
15	+++	-	+	+	+	+	+	-
16	+++	-	-	+	-	-	-	-
17	+++	-	++	++	++	+	++	-
18	+++	-	+	++	+	+	+	-
19	+++	-	++	+	+	-	+	-
NEPHGE								
1	+++	-	-	-	+++	-	-	-
2	+++	-	+	+++	++	+	+	-
3	+++	-	+++	++	+	-	+	-

+++ indicate the intensity of the spot in CHO EMS 16.4. Lower intensities are indicated by ++ or +.

lament bundles in non-virally transformed cells (11) it is clear that alteration or loss of microfilament bundles is not a reliable assay to assess tumorigenicity at the cellular level. A similar lack of correlation between presence of actin cables and tumorigenicity in hybrids of non-virally transformed cells has been reported by Watt *et al.* (30). Recently, Tucker *et al.* (20) have reported that in spontaneously transformed mouse, rat and hamster cells the actin cables were thinner and far fewer in number than those in their non-neoplastic counterparts and proposed that these characteristics were correlated with growth properties of the neoplastic cells. Our results and those of Watt *et al.* (30) indicate that this is not the case for all transformed cells and are further supported by the studies of Willingham *et al.* (31) and Ali *et al.* (32) who have found that the distribution of microfilament bundles is most likely related to adhesiveness to substratum and shape but not to malignant growth properties.

The hybrid nature of the clones was clearly demonstrated by chromosome analysis as well as by high resolution two dimensional gel electrophoresis. From the later analysis it is clear that some of the hybrids contain as much as 50% of the total number of CHO specific polypeptides that could be clearly distinguished from CLID polypeptides. These results are in line with recent experiments of Miller *et al.* (33) who found transcription and processing of both mouse and syrian hamster ribosomal RNA genes in individual somatic cell hybrids.

Even though at present it is not possible to correlate the presence of a CHO polypeptide with the retention of any CHO chromosome it is clear that this type of study could prove of value in the future to map the major cellular polypeptides. Ideally, one will like to study hybrids that have retained single chromosomes or fragments of chromosomes. That this approach is feasible is garanteed by recent results of Kucherlapati and Shin (34) who found that 14 of 17 human isoenzymes markers tested in human x mouse hybrid clones were represented at least one. This result indicates that at least in mouse x human hybrids most human chromosomes can be expressed.

Finally, our results concerning tumorigenicity of the hybrids do not allow us to draw any conclusions about the dominance of recessiveness of malignancy (34-43), as these hybrids segregated hamster chromosomes. Nevertheless, it is clear from our studies that expression or suppression of malignancy in these hybrids is not directly related to the number of hamster chromosome retained but most likely to the type(s) of chromosome retained.

7. ACKNOWLEDGEMENTS

We would like to thank P. Andersen for supplying us with the human actin antibody and O. Jensen for photography. This work was supported by grants from the Danish Natural Science Research Council (to J.E.C.), the Volkswagen Foundation and the Muscular Dystrophy Association, Inc. (to J.V.S.). R.B. is a recipient of an EMBO fellowship.

8. REFERENCES

1) ASH, J.F., VOGT, P.K. and SINGER, S.J. (1976). Reversion from transformed to normal phenotype by inhibition of protein synthesis in rat kidney cells infected with a temperature - sensitive mutant of Rous sarcoma virus. Proc.Natl. Acad. Sci. USA, 73, 3603.
2) BURGER, M.M. (1969). A difference in the architecture of the surface membrane of normal and virally transformed cells. Proc. Natl. Acad. Sci. USA, 62, 994.
3) EDELMAN, G.M. and YAHARA, I. (1976). Temperature sensitive changes in surface modulating assemblies of fibroblasts transformed by mutants of Rous sarcoma virus. Proc. Natl. Acad. Sci. USA, 73, 2047.
4) HILWIG, I. and GROPP, A. (1972). Staining of constitutive heterochromatin in mammalian chromosomes with a new fluorochrome. Exp.

Cell Res., 75, 122.

5) HYNES, R.O. (1973). Alteration of cell surface proteins by viral transformation and proteolysis. Proc. Natl. Acad. Sci. USA, 70, 3170.

6) POLLACK, R., OSBORN, M. and WEBER, K. (1975). Patterns of organization of actin and myosin in normal and transformed cultured cells. Proc. Natl. Acad. Sci. USA, 72, 994.

7) STOKER, M., O'NEILL, C., BERRYMAN, S. and WAXMAN , U. (1968). Anchorage and growth regulation in normal and virus transformed cells. Int. J. Cancer, 3, 683.

8) TODARO, G.J. and GREEN, J. (1963). Quantitative studies of the growth of mouse embryo cells in culture and their development into established lines. J. Cell. Biol., 17, 299.

9) UNKELESS, J.C., TOBIA, A., OSSOWSKI, L., QUIGLEY, J.R., RIFKIN, D.B. and REICH, E. (1973). An enzymatic function associated with transformation of fibroblasts by oncogenic viruses. J. Exp. Med., 137, 85.

10) WANG, E. and GOLDBERG, A.R., (1976). Changes in microfilament organization and surface topography upon transformation of chicken embryo fibroblasts with Rous sarcoma virus. Proc. Natl. Acad. Sci. USA, 73, 4065.

11) CELIS, J.E., SMALL, J.V., ANDERSEN, P. and CELIS, A. (1978). Microfilaments bundles in cultured cells. Expl. Cell Res., 114, 335.

12) ANDERSEN, P., SMALL, J.V. and SOBIESZEK, A. (1976). Studies on the specificity of smooth muscle antibodies. Clin. Exp. Immunol., 26, 57.

13) SMALL, J.V. and CELIS, J.E. (1978). Filament arrangements in negatively stained cultured cells: the organization of actin. Cytobiologie, 16, 308.

14) SMALL, J.V. and CELIS, J.E. (1978). Direct visualization of the 10 nm (100Å) filament network in whole and enucleated cultured cells. J. Cell Sci., 31, 393.

15) CELIS, J.E., SMALL, J.V., KALTOFT, K. and CELIS, A. (1979). Micro-

filament bundles in transformed mouse CLID x transformed CHO cell hybrids. Expl. Cell Res., 120, 79.

16) WEISBLUM, B. and HOENSSLER, E. (1974). Fluorometric properties of the bibenzimidazole derivative Hoechst 33258, a fluorescent probe specific for AT concentration in chromosomal DNA. Chromosoma, 46, 255.

17) FOURNIER, R.E. and RUDDLE, F.H. (1977). Stable association of the human transgenome and host murine chrosome demonstrated with trispecific microcell hybrids. Proc. Natl. Acad. Sci. USA, 74, 3937.

18) LAZARIDES, E. (1976). Actin, α-actinin, and tropomyosin interaction in the structural organization of actin filaments in non-muscle cells. J. Cell. Biol., 68, 202.

19) RATHKE, P.C., SEIB, E., WEBER, K., OSBORN, M. and FRANKE, W.W. (1977). Rod -like elements from actin containing microfilament bundles observed in culture cells after treatment with cytochalisin A (CA). Expl. Cell Res., 105, 253.

20) TUCKER, R.W., SANDFORD, K.K. and FRANKEL, F.R. (1978). Tubulin and actin in paired non-neoplastic and spontaneously transformed neoplastic cell lines *in vitro* fluorescent antibody studies. Cell,
21) 13, 629.
OSBORN, M. and WEBER, K. (1977). The display of microtubules in transformed cells. Cell, 12, 561.

22) DE MEY, J., JONIAU, M., DE BRABANDER, M., MOENS, W. and GEUENS, G. (1978). Evidence for unaltered structure and *in vivo* assembly of microtubules in transformed cell. Proc. Natl. Acad. Sci. USA, 75, 1339.

23) GABBIANI, G., BORGIA, R., CHAPONNIER, C., RUNGGER, E. and WEIL, R. (1978). Cytoskeletal proteins in normal infected and virus transformed cells. Experientia, 34 (7), 940.

24) HYNES, R.O. and DESTREE, A.T. (1978). 10 nm filaments in normal and transformed cells. Cell, 13, 151.

25) RUBIN, R.W. and WARREN, R.H. (1979). Organization of tubulin in normal and transformed rat kidney cells. J. Cell. Biol., 82, 103.

26) WOLIN, S.L. and KUCHERLAPATI, R.S. (1979). Expression of microtubule networks in normal cells, transformed cells and their hybrids. J. Cell Biol., 82, 76.

27) FRANKE, W.W., SCHMID, E., WEBER, K. and OSBORN, M. (1979). HeLa cells contain intermediate-sized filaments of the prekeratin type Expl. Cell Res., 118, 95.

28) O'FARRELL, P.H. (1975). High resolution two dimensional electrophoresis of proteins. J. Biol. Chem., 250, 4007.

29) O'FARRELL, P.Z., GOODMAN, H.M. and O'FARRELL, P.H. (1977). High resolution two dimensional electrophoresis of basic as well as acidic proteins. Cell, 12, 1133.

30) WATT, F.M., HARRIS, H., WEBER, K. and OSBORN, M. (1978). The distribution of actin cables and microtubules in hybrids between malignant and non-malignant cells and in tumors derived from them. J. Cell Sci., 32, 419.

31) WILLINGHAM, M.C., YAMADA, K.M., YAMADA, S.S., POUYSSEGUR, J. and PASTAN, I. (1977). Microfilament bundles and cell shape are related to adhesiveness to substratum and are dissociable from growth control in cultured fibroblasts. Cell, 10, 375.

32) ALI, I.A., MAUTNER, V., LANZA, R. and HYNES, R.O. (1977). Restoration of normal morphology, adhesion and cytoskeleton in transformed cells by addition of a transformation-sensitive surface protein. Cell, 11, 115.

33) MILLER, O.J., DEV, V.G., MILLER, D.A., TANTRAVAHI, R. and ELICEIRI, G.L. (1978). Transcription and processing of both mouse and syrian hamster ribosomal RNA genes in individual somatic cell hybrids. Exp. Cell Res, 115, 457.

34) KUCHERLAPATI, R. and SHIN, S.L. (1979). Genetic control of tumorigenicity in interspecific mammalian cell hybrids. Cell, 16, 639.

35) DEFENDI, V., EPHRUSSI, B., KOPROWSKI, H. and YOSHIDA, M.C. (1967) Properties of hybrids between polyoma transformed and normal mouse cells. Proc. Natl. Acad. Sci. USA, 57, 299.

36) HARRIS, H., MILLER, O.J., KLEIN, G., WORST, P. and TACHIBANA, T.

(1969). Suppression of malignancy by cell fusion. Nature, 233, 363.

37) CROCE, C.M. and KOPROWSKI, H. (1974). Positive control of the transformed phenotype in hybrids between normal and SV40 transformed human cells. Science, 184, 1288.

38) CROCE, C., ADEN, D. and KOPROWSKI, H. (1975). Somatic cell hybrids between mouse peritoneal macrophages and simian virus-40 transformed human cells. II. Presence of human chromosome 7 carrying simian virus-40 genome in cells of tumors induced by hybrid cells. Proc. Nat. Acad. Sci. USA, 72, 1397.

39) AVILES, D., JAMI, J., ROUSSET, J.P. and RITZ, E. (1977). Tumor x host cell hybrids in the mouse: chromosomes from the normal cell parent in malignant hybrid tumors. J. Nat. Cancer Inst., 58, 1391.

40) JONASSON, J. and HARRIS, H. (1977). The analysis of malignancy by cell fusion. VIII. Evidence for the intervention of an extra chromosomal element. J. Cell Sci., 24, 255.

41) JONASSON, J., POVEY, S. and HARRIS, H. (1977). The analysis of malignancy by cell fusion. VII. Cytogenetic analysis of hybrids between malignant and diploid cells and of tumors derived from them. J. Cell Sci., 24, 217.

42) CROCE, C.M. and KOPROWSKI, H. (1978). The genetics of human cancer. Sci. Am., 238, 117.

43) STANBRIDGE, E.J. and WILKINSON, J. (1978). Analysis of malignancy in human cells : malignant and transformed phenotypes are under separate genetic control. Proc. Natl. Acad. Sci. USA, 75, 1466.

GENE TRANSFER IN EUKARYOTES

F.H. Ruddle

Department of Biology and Human Genetics
Kline Biology Tower, Yale University
New Haven, Connecticut 06520, U.S.A.

1. INTRODUCTION

Somatic cell genetics relies on parasexual events in *in vitro* cell populations. The analysis of parasexuality can be used to make inferences on the genetic organization of the test material. The approach is general and can be applied currently to any mammalian species, and to any eukaryote with the future development of appropriate cell culture methods. Parasexuality can be defined more specifically in terms of gene transfer and gene loss mechanisms. Gene transfer mechanisms will be emphasized, because they can be more rigorously defined and controlled in experimental terms.

Gene transfer can be subdivided into four catagories defined in terms of methodology and in terms of the amount of donor genetic material transferred to the recipient. These modes of gene transfer are (1) cell hybridization, (2) microcell mediated gene transfer, (3) chromosome mediated gene transfer, and (4) DNA mediated gene transfer. In the case of cell hybridization whole genomes are transferred and one defines the donor as that parent which subsequently undergoes chromosome loss after cell fusion. Microcell mediated gene transfer (MMGT) represents the fusion of donor microcells containing only one or several chromosomes with genetically intact recipient cells. Thus, in the microcell system, only one or a few chromosomes are transferred to the recipient. Chromosome mediated gene transfer (CMGT) involves the endocytosis of cell free chromosomes by the recipient cells. In this system, only subchromosomal fragments are retained by the recipient. DNA mediated gene transfer (DMGT) deals with the uptake of protein free, extracted DNA by recipient cells. In this case, only relatively small segments of the donor genome are transferred to the recipient cell. For each case, and especially for CMGT and DMGT, it is convenient to designate the transferred donor material as the "transgenome", and the "transformed" recipient cells as the "transgenote". As described in greater detail below, the four methods of gene transfer allow the transfer of transgenomes of different size, thus facilitating genetic analysis at different levels of resolution.

2. CELL HYBRIDIZATION

Cell hybridization effects the transfer of an entire nuclear genome. Hybrids can be readily formed by treating cell populations with membrane fusing agents such as inactivated *Sendai* virus (1, 2). or polyethylene glycol (3). A number of schemes have been developed which permit the efficient selection of heterosynkaryons and the elimination of unfused parental cells and homosynkaryons. The majority of these methods depend on the existence of different recessive, complementing, conditional auxotrophic markers in the contributing parental cells (4-6), but dominant markers may also be used to advantage (7, 8).

Chromosome elimination occurs spontaneously in interspecific hybrids. In hybrid cells, the recipient parent is represented by, at the least, a complete haploid chromosome set whereas the donor chromosome set is partially monosomic. Donor chromosomes are progressively eliminated, but the rate of elimination tends to decrease progressively as a direct function of generation number, and those hybrids which have retained but a few donor chromosomes are generally stable. Factors which determine the direction of segregation are poorly defined but parental chromosomes number, adaptation to growth *in vitro*, epigenetic state, and species origin all appear to play a role. In the case of mouse x hamster hybrids, mouse chromosomes are usually lost. In the case of mouse x human hybrids, human chromosomes are usually, but not invariably, eliminated. The loss of human chromosomes is not absolutely random, and some chromosomes are sometimes preferentially retained (9).

The elimination of donor chromosomes can be regulated experimentally. If a donor chromosome carries a prototrophic gene then, under selective conditions, only cells retaining that gene and its associated chromosome can survive. A good example involves the gene which codes for the enzyme hypoxanthine guanine phosophoribosyltransferase (HGPRT). This gene is X-linked in all mammalian species so far determined. Cells are conditionally dependent of HGPRT activity for survival in medium containing hypoxanthine, aminopterin, and thymidine (HAT medium). Thus, mouse x human hybrid cell populations formed between mouse recipient cells deficient in HGPRT (mo $HGPRT^-$) and human donor cells prototrophic for HGPRT (hu $HGPRT^+$) and grown in HAT medium exhibit a preferential retention of the human X chromosome. Hybrid cells which have retained the human X chromosome can be selected against by exposing the cells to toxic metabolic analogs of hypoxanthine such as thioguanine which are metabolically incorporated into cells possessing HGPRT activity. Thus in the case of the HGPRT system, it is possible to select for and against cells which either possess or lack HGPRT activity.

The cell hybrid system was the first gene transfer system to be developed (10) and to be adapted to the purpose of gene mapping (11, 14). Gene mapping is accomplished by simply correlating the segregating phenotypes (synteny test), correlating the segregation of whole chromosomes with phenotypes (assignment test) or correlating the segregation of parts of chromosomes with phenotypes (regional assignment test). Detailed descriptions of these test procedures have been reviewed elsewhere (6, 9, 15). The cell hybridization-gene transfer system provides a rapid, efficient, and economical procedure for gene mapping. More than 200 genes have been mapped in man in the past decade predominately as a consequence of cell genetics studies. Moreover, the application of regional assignment testing has provided considerable information on the location of genes within chromosomes and the order and spacing of genes along the length of chromosomes. A useful summary of progress in and the current status of the human gene map since the advent of somatic cell genetics is provided by the publications of the Human Gene Mapping Conferences, first held at Yale University, New Haven, in 1973 (16) and then subsequently at Rotterdam (17), Baltimore (18) and Winnipeg (19).

3. MAPPING SILENT GENES

Until recently, somatic cell genetic procedures for gene mapping have relied on gene expression. Differences in the gene product, usually a protein, between donor and recipient have been used to assign the relevant genes to chromosomes. Such a mapping scheme excludes "silent" genes which are not expressed in the parental and derivative hybrid cells used for the somatic cell genetic mapping analysis. Categories of genes and polydeoxynucleotides which are excluded include facultative genes whose expression is restricted to cells of specific epigenic type, regulatory genes, introns, and other nucleotide sequences which play a structural role in gene and chromosome organization such as spacer sequences. Now, with the use of nucleic acid hybridization techniques, the silent genes may be mapped using the methodologies of somatic cell genetics.

Two types of specificities associated with DNA can be used to distinguish donor and recipient genes. The first is nucleotide sequence specificity, and the second is specificity associated with differences in the distribution of restriction endonuclease sites in and around homologous genes originating from donor and recipient cells. Labelled DNA or cDNA probes of the relevant genes are employed to test the two types of specificities. Sequence specificities can be used if the recipient DNA undergoes little or no hybridization with the probe, while the donor gene shows a high level of hybridization. This case obtains for the human hemoglobins. We were able to show that a cDNA probe to human α globin mRNA cross-reacted very weakly with mouse DNA using conventional procedures of liquid hybridization. This situation then made it possible to map the human α globin gene to human chromosome 16 by the hybridization analysis of DNAs extracted from a series of human/mouse cell hybrids (20). Similarly, we were able to show sequence specificities between mouse and human β globin genes. This permitted us to assign the β globin gene to human chromosome 11 (21). In both these systems, the α and β genes were "silent", and the map location of the gene was achieved by directly detecting the presence of the segregating donor gene by nucleic acid hybridization, and then by correlating it with a particular segregating donor chomosome.

The second approach to the mapping of silent genes depends on specificities imparted by the distribution of restriction endonuclease sites. This method makes use of the Southern blotting procedure (22) which has the added advantage of greater sensitivity in comparison with liquid hybridization. Moreover, it is generally a more powerful approach, since differences in the distribution of restriction endonuclease sites are common, whereas sequence differences of sufficient magnitude between homologous gene sequences are less readily realized.

Recently, we have demonstrated the effectiveness of the restriction endonuclease mapping system using two different systems. In both, we have employed cloned recombinant DNA probes. In the first, we have confirmed the assignment of the human β-globin gene to human chromosome 11 by the association of human β-globin gene restriction fragments with the presence of human chromosome 11 in mouse/human hybrids (Huttner, Scangos, and Ruddle, unpublished). In the second, we have assigned the mouse immunoglobin kappa gene to mouse chromosome 6 in an analysis of mouse/Chinese hamster hybrids (23). It has become clear to us from these studies that any cloned DNA sequence can be mapped to a chromosomal site(s) using the somatic genetics approach. Moreover, as we point out elsewhere in this article, the potential resolution of the mapping system is at the level of the gene.

4. MICROCELL MEDIATED GENE TRANSFER

Microcell mediated gene transfer facilitates the transfer of only one or several "donor" chromosomes into a recipient cell (24, 25). The donor parent is treated with mitotic blocking agents which promote the formation of polykaryocytes in which the chromosomes are divided among a number of micronuclei. When these cells are treated with cytochalasin and subjected to centrifugal force, they fragment yielding microcells. Microcells possess a micronucleus containing only one or several intact chromosomes, plus a rim of cytoplasm and an intact plasma membrane. Such cells are viable for only a few hours, but may be rescued by fusion to intact, viable recipient cells. *Sendai* virus and PEG have been successfully used as fusion agents. Selection for microcell hybrids is accomplished by incorporating a conditional auxotrophic marker into the recipient parent, and by purifying the microcells to homogeneity, thus eliminating contaminating intact donor cells. In this kind of system, a donor microcell chromosome bearing the complementing prototrophic gene would invariably be present in all hybrids. Other chromosomes will also be present in all permutations. The advantages of the microcell system are (1) the incorporation of one or only a few chromosomes, thus simplifying the correlation of donor chromosomes with the expression of donor phenotypes; (2) the introduction on only small nuclear and cytoplasmic substances from the donor, thus reducing the possibility of perturbing the epigenetic program of the recipient cell; and (3) control over the direction of chromosome elimination by the selection of the microcell parent. Nevertheless, the donor chromosomes enter the recipient cell intact, and by the same mechanism as cell hybridization. There is little or no breakage or rearrangement of the donor chromosomes. The microcell scheme in contrast to whole cell hybridization effects chromosome segregation prior to fusion.

5. CHROMOSOME MEDIATED GENE TRANSFER

Chromosome-mediated gene transfer was first described by McBride and Ozer (26). Donor cells subjected to mitotic arrest are physically broken, releasing metaphase chromosomes. The chromosomes are mixed with recipient cells, usually in multiplicities of 0.5 to 2 genome equivalents per cell. When conditionally auxotrophic recipient cells (e.g. $HGPRT^-$) are treated with chromosomes from a prototrophic donor, cells of the recipient type that expresss the donor marker can be recovered at a low frequency. Two recent technical improvements, coprecipitation of the chromosomes with calcium phosphate, and post-treatment of the recipient cells with dimethyl sulfoxide, have allowed this frequency to be raised as high as 2×10^{-5} (27). In this system, subchromosomal fragments are transferred to the recipient cell. The fragments range in size from large pieces readily detected by light microscopy (27, 28) to pieces carrying no detectable genetic information beyond the selected prototrophic marker itself. We have coined the term "transgenome" to describe these fragments (29).

The transgenome is typically expressed in an unstable fashion in the recipient cells. That is, in an unstably transformed cell population, between 1% and 10% of the cells lose the ability to express the prototrophic marker in each generation. Loss appear to be an all-or-none phenomenon, in that donor markers that were linked to the prototrophic marker are lost in a concordant fashion (27, 30). Stable sublines can arise in these cell populations that no longer lose the prototrophic marker at a detectable rate (31, 32). In such instances, the transgenome appears to become closely associated with a recipient chromosome in these stable cell lines (25, 33). Indeed, in those cases where a large fragment undergoes stabilization, it can subsequently be detected as a morphologically distinct region of a recipient cell chromosome (27, 28). In this way, the transgenome appears to acquire a centromere function, facilitating its orderly transmission to daughter cells at each mitosis.

The key questions that now arise concerning the transgenome are structural ones: what is the size range of the transgenome; how is it organized in the "unstable" state and in the "stable" state; and what is the molecular basis of stabilization? The recent development of DNA-mediated gene transfer, and its application to genes coding for thymidine kinase (TK), provides a promising means of approaching these questions. Murine cell populations deficient in cytosol TK activity, when treated with live (34) or UV-irradiated (35) Herpes Simplex Virus-1 (HSV-1), give rise to small numbers of cells expressing high levels of TK activity. The TK enzyme expressed by these cells is clearly that encoded by HSV-1 and not the murine enzyme, as judged by its isoelectric point, electrophoretic mobility, immunochemical properties, and ability to phosphorylate iododeoxycytidine (36). Recent studies in our laboratory have shown that one such stable transformant of the Munyon type has a particular mouse chromosome with which the HSV-1 TK phenotype can be correlated (36). This study thereby provides somatic cell genetic evidence for the integration of HSV-1 TK gene at a discrete chromosomal site.

It has been possible to obtain new information on the size of CMGT transgenomes using the integrated HSV TK gene (see section below on DNA mediated gene transfer). In these experiments mouse LM TK(-) cells were transformed with a 3.4 kb BAM 1 defined restriction fragment of HSV-1 (37). Restriction analysis of a stable transformant (clone LH 7) indicated that the donor viral 3.4 kb fragment had integrated into the host chromosome (38). This clone (LH 7) was then used as a donor in a chromosome mediated gene transfer experiment, in which LH 7 chromosomes were transferred into cells of line LM TK(-). The design of this experiment allows one to infer the size limits of the CMGT transgenome by the Southern blotting procedure, using the 3.4 kb HSV-1 TK fragment as a probe. When the DNA of the donor cell LH 7 was cleaved with the restriction enzyme KpmI, the HSV-1 TK gene was found to reside on a cellular restriction fragment of greater than 20 kb. Three of four CMGT lines derived by using LM 7 as a donor had HSV TK fragments indistinguishable from the donor (LHLM 1, 21, and 22) whereas one transformant (LHLM 23) was larger than 20 kb. Additional information was obtained by using restriction endonuclease HmcII which cleaves once within the TK gene. When LH 7 was cleaved with HmcII, a 4.5 kb fragment and a 1.6 kb fragment were produced. Again as with KpmI, three transformants (LHLM 1, 21, and 22) possessed characteristics identical to LH 7. On the other hand LHLM 23 had one band with altered mobility. The data indicated that LHLM 23 had undergone a rearrangement within 1 kb of the original 3.4 kb HSV TK transforming DNA fragment. The CMGT experiments of Miller and Ruddle

(27) and of Klobutcher and Ruddle (28) have shown that the transgenome may be as large as 1 percent of the haploid donor genome based on microscopic measurements of the transgenome. The recent experiments of Scangos *et al.* (37) based on Southern blotting procedures suggest that rearrangements of the donor chromosome can take place within several hundred kb of the selected, prototrophic marker (37). The picture now beginning to emerge indicates that the CMGT transgenomes may span a large size range, extending from 20 kb to 1 x 10^4 kb.

6. DNA MEDIATED GENE TRANSFER

Recently Wigler *et al.* (39) have reported the efficient transfection of murine TK deficient cells with purified HSV-1 DNA. Viral DNA pretreated with restriction endonucleases known to cleave the TK gene (e.g., EcoRI) lost its transforming activity. Endonucleases such as BAM, that did not cleave the gene did not affect activity. Furthermore, a purified 3.4 kb BAM fragment possessed TK transforming activity, and transfected cells at a frequency of 1 colony per 10^6 cells per 40 pg DNA. The same group has reported biochemical evidence for physical integration of the 3.4 kb BAM fragment into host DNA sequences in transformed mouse thymidine kinase deficient host cells (38) and have further shown that integrated single copies of the 3.4 kb HSV TK fragment diluted in recipient mammalian genomes can secondarily transform TK deficient mouse cells. The transformation frequency for secondary transformation ranges from 1 colony per 10^5 to 1 colony per 5 x 10^6 cells per 20 μg cellular DNA. Thus, a specific fragment of the HSV-1 genome can be used for the highly efficient transformation of mammalian cells, and the fate of this fragment can be analyzed biochemically.

In related experiments, Wigler *et al.* (40) have reported successful transformation experiments involving the endogenous TK gene from a number of vertebrate species: namely, chicken, calf, Chinese hamster, mouse and human. Only in the case of human donor TK were experiments described which demonstrated donor specific biochemical properties of the transferred TK. Clearly, an independent confirmation would be highly desirable. The transformation rates extend over a range of ten-fold, but were all impressively high. The lowest was recorded for human DNA which has a value of 1 colony per 10^6 cells per 20 μg/DNA.

The availability of an efficient transformation system for mammalian cells *in vitro* opens up a number of important possibilities. For example, it should now be possible to transfer very small and well-defined regions of donor chromosome segments into recipient cells. Thus, one could analyze the genetic composition of segments containing selectable markers at a very high level of resolution. A second possibility involves the use of DNA mediated transformation as a bioassay for specific genetic segments of complex genomes. In this case, the donor DNA could be fractionated by various biochemical means and the fractions tested for biological activity. The DNA could be purified sequentially through multiple dimensions of separation, as for example, reverse phase chromatography, agar gel electrophoresis, and recombinant DNA cloning. A third possibility lies in the ability to form transgenotes which possess small and highly specified donor transgenomes, either as integrated or independent, episomal-like entities. In sum, the advent of DNA mediated transformation provides a means of performing high resolution gene mapping in higher eukaryotes, purification of genes from complex mammalian genomes, and thè specific genetic modification of mammalian cells. All of these new capabilities should prove invaluable to the genetic analysis of the genetic regulation of differentiated cells in mammalian species, including man.

7. REFERENCES

1) OKADA, Y. (1958). The fusion of Ehrlich's tumor cells caused

by HVJ virus *in vitro*. Biken J., 1, 103

2) HARRIS, H. and WATKINS, J. (1965). Hybrid cells derived from mouse and man: artificial heterokaryons of mammalian cells from different species. Nature, Lond., 205, 640.

3) PONTECORVO, G. (1975). Baltimore Conference: Third International Workshop on Human Gene Mapping. Birth Defects: Orig. Art. Ser. XII: 1976. The National Foundation - March of Dimes, 1976.

4) LITTLEFIELD, J. (1964). Selection of hybrids from matings of fibroblasts *in vitro* and their presumed recombinants. Science, 145, 709.

5) DEMARS, R. (1974). Resistance of cultured human fibroblasts and other cells to purine and pyrimidine analogues in relation to mutagenesis detection. Mutation Res., 24, 335.

6) CREAGAN, R. and RUDDLE, F. (1977). New Approaches to human gene mapping by somatic-cell genetics. In: "Molecular Structure of Human Chromosomes". (ed., J. Yunis), p. 89, Academic Press, New York.

7) BAKER, R., BRUNETTE, D., MANKOWITZ, R., THOMPSON, L., WHITMORE, G., SIMINOVITCH, L. and TILL, J. (1974). Ouabain resistant mutants of mouse and hamster cells in culture. Cell, 1, 9.

8) SIMINOVITCH, L. (1976). On the nature of hereditable variation in cultured somatic cells. Cell, 7, 1.

9) RUDDLE, F. and CREAGAN, R. (1975). Parasexual approaches to the genetics of man. Annu. Rev. Genet., 9, 407.

10) WEISS, M.C. and GREEN, H. (1967). Human-mouse hybrid cell lines containing partial complements of human chromosomes and functioning human genes. Proc. Nat. Acad. Sci. USA, 58, 1104.

11) RUDDLE, F.H. (1969). In: "Problems in Biology: RNA in Development". (ed., E.W. Hanley), University of Utah Press, Salt Lake City, p. 11.

12) RUDDLE, F.H. (1970). Utilization of somatic cells for genetic analysis: possibilities and problems. In: "Symposia of the International Society for Cell Biology", 9, 233, Academic Press.

13) RUDDLE, F.H. (1972). Linkage analysis using somatic cell hybrids. _In_: "Advances in Human Genetics", _3_, 173. (eds., H. Harris and K. Hirschhorn), Plenum Press.

14) RUDDLE, F.H. (1973). Linkage analysis in man by somatic cell genetics. _Nature_, _242_, 165.

15) McKUSICK, V. and RUDDLE, F.H. (1977). The status of gene map of the human chromosomes. _Science_, _196_, 390.

16) BERGSMA, E. (ed.). (1973). New Haven Conference: First International Worskhop on Human Gene Mapping. Birth Defects: Orig. Art. Ser. X: 3, 1974. The National Foundation - March of Dimes, 1974.

17) BERGSMA, D. (ed.). (1974). Rotterdam Conference: Second International Workshop on Human Gene Mapping. Birth Defects: Orig. Art. Ser. XI: 3, 1975. The National Foundation - March of Dimes, 1975.

18) BERGSMA, D. (ed.). (1975). Baltimore Conference: Third International Workshop on Human Gene Mapping. Birth Defects: Orig. Art. Ser. XII: 1976. The National Foundation - March of Dimes, 1976.

19) BERGSMA, D. (ed.). (1977). Winnipeg Conference: Fourth International Workshop on Human Gene Mapping. Birth Defects: Orig. Art. Ser. The National Foundation - March of Dimes. In press.

20) DEISSEROTH, A., NIENHUIS, A., TURNER, P., VELEZ, R., ANDERSON, F., RUDDLE, F., CREAGAN, R. and KUCHERLAPATI, R. (1977). Localization of the hyman α-globin structural gene to chromosome 16 in somatic cell hybrids by molecular hybridization assay. _Cell_, _12_, 205.

21) DEISSEROTH, A., NIENHUIS, A., LAWRENCE, J., GILES, R., TURNER, P. and RUDDLE, F. (1978). Chromosomal localization of human β-globin gene on human chromosome 11 in somatic hybrids. _Proc. Nat. Acad. Sci. USA_, _75_, 1456.

22) SOUTHERN, E. (1975). Detection of specific sequences among DNA fragments separated by gel electrophoresis. _J. Mol. Biol._, _98_,

503.

23) SWAN, D., D'EUSTACHIO, P., LEINWAND, J., SEIDMAN, J., KEITHLEY, D. and RUDDLE, F.H. (1979). Chromosomal assignment of the mouse K Light Chains Genes. Proc. Natl. Acad. Sci. USA, 76, 2735.

24) FOURNIER, R. and RUDDLE, F. (1977a). Microcell-mediated transfer of murine chromosomes into mouse, Chinese hamster, and human somatic cells. Proc. nat. Acad. Sci. USA, 74, 319.

25) FOURNIER, R. and RUDDLE, F. (1977b). Stable association of the human transgenome and host murine chromosomes demonstrated with trispecific microcell hybrids. Proc. Nat. Acad. Sci. USA, 74, 3936.

26) McBRIDE, O. and OZER, H. (1973). Transfer of genetic information by purified metaphase chromosomes. Proc. Nat. Acad. Sci. USA, 70, 1258.

27) MILLER, C. and RUDDLE, F. (1978). Co-transfer of human X-linked markers into murine somatic cells via isolated metaphase chromosomes. Proc. Nat. Acad. Sci. USA, 75, 3346.

28) KLOBUTCHER, L.A. and RUDDLE, F.H. (1979). Phenotype stabilization and transgenome integration in chromosome-mediated gene transfer. Nature, 280, 657.

29) RUDDLE, F. and FOURNIER, R. (1977c). Somatic cell genetic analysis of gene transfer in mammalian cells. In: "Genetic Interaction and Gene Transfer" (ed., C. Anderson), Brookhaven Symposia in Biology, 29, 96.

30) McBRIDE, O., BURCH, J. and RUDDLE, F. (1978). Co-transfer of thymidine kinase and galactokinase genes by chromosome-mediated gene transfer. Proc. Nat. Acad. Sci. USA, 75, 914.

31) DEGNEN, G.A., MILLER, I.L., EISENSTADT, J.M. and ADELBERG, E.A. (1976). Chromosome-mediated gene transfer between closely related strains of cultured mouse cells. Proc. Nat. Acad. Sci. USA., 73, 2838.

32) WILLECKE, K., LANGE, R., KRÜGER, A. and REBER, T. (1976). Cotranfer of two linked human genes into cultured mouse cells.

Proc. Nat. Acad. Sci. USA, 73, 1274.

33) WILLECKE, K., MIERAU, R., KRÜGER, A. and LANGE, R. (1978). Chromosomal gene transfer of human cytosol thymidine kinase into mouse cells. Integration or association of the tranferred gene with non-homologous mouse chromosome. Molec. Gen. Genet., 161, 49.

34) KIT, S., DUBBS, D.R., PIEKARSKI, L.J. and HSU, T.C. (1963). Deletion of thymidine kinase activity from L cells resistant to bromodeoxyuridine. Exp. Cell Res., 31, 297.

35) MUNYON, W., KRAISELBURD, E., DAVIS, D. and MANN, J. (1971). Transfer of thymidine kinase to thymidine kinase less L cells by infection with ultraviolet-irradiated Herpes Simplex Virus. J. Virol., 7, 813.

36) SMILEY, J., STEEGE, D., JURICEK, D., SUMMERS, W. and RUDDLE, F. (1978). A Herpex Simplex Virus 1 integration site in the mouse genome defined by somatic cell genetic analysis. Cell, 15, 455.

37) SCANGOS, G.A., HUTTNER, K.M., SILVERSTEIN, S. and RUDDLE, F.H. (1979). Molecular analysis of chromosome-mediated gene transfer. Proc. Nat. Acad. Sci. USA, 76, 3987.

38) PELLICER, A., WIGLER, M., AXEL, R. and SILVERSTEIN, S. (1978). The transfer and stable integration of the HSV thymidine kinase gene into mouse cells. Cell, 14, 133.

39) WIGLER, M., SILVERSTEIN, S., LEE,L., PELLICER, A., CHENG, Y. and AXEL, R. (1977). Transfer of purified Herpes virus thymidine kinase gene to cultured mouse cells. Cell, 11, 223.

40) WIGLER, M., PELLICER, A., SILVERSTEIN, S. and AXEL, R. (1978). Biochemical transfer and stable integration of the HSV thymidine kinase gene into mouse cells. Cell, 14, 725.

DNA MEDIATED GENE TRANSFER BETWEEN MAMMALIAN CELLS

K. Willecke

Institut für Zellbiologie (Tumorforschung)
Universität Essen, Hufelandstr. 55
D-4300 Essen, Fed. Rep. Germany

1. INTRODUCTION

The experimental transfer and expression of donor genetic material in recipient cells constitutes an assay for the biological function of DNA. If purified DNA can be used for gene transfer, one can possibly study the effects of structural modification, for example by enzymes, heat or X-rays on the biological function of DNA. Since cell culture became a routine method of cell biology, numerous attempts have been reported to demonstrate DNA mediated transfer and functional expression of donor genes in mammalian recipient cells. Most experiments of this kind with mammalian cells have been devised according to the successful DNA mediated gene transfer worked out with bacteria (transformation). In this review the expression "transformation" is only used for DNA mediated gene transfer in bacteria and yeast. Mammalian cell clones which harbour or express a transferred DNA sequence ("transgenome") are called "transferent cells" (1). Since it can be expected that genes coding for neoplastic transformation will eventually also be transferred to mammalian recipient cells by chromosome or DNA mediated gene transfer, it would create unnecessary confusion if the expression "transformation" (in the sense of gene transfer) is also used for mammalian cells.

2. DNA MEDIATED GENE TRANSFER

In discussing recent results and views of DNA mediated gene transfer with mammalian cells it is interesting to compare the conclusions with our present knowledge of transformation in bacteria and yeast because there are a number of parallels in these experimental systems. A recent review on gene transfer in bacteria (2) and two reviews on chromosome mediated gene transfer in mammalian cells have been published (3, 1, see also article by F. Ruddle in this volume). Ottolenghi-Nightingale (19) reviewed the literature on DNA mediated gene transfer in mammalian cells up to 1973. Therefore, in the following review mainly the literature since 1974 is summarized.

In their early studies, Szybalska and Szybalski (5) used spermine to faciliate DNA uptake into human cells. Since then the uptake of DNA, labelled with radioactive thymidine, has been studied with cultured mammalian recipient cells in the presence of several faciliators (6). Ornithine or dimethylsulfoxide have been used for increased uptake of isolated metaphase chromosome (7, 8). Several experimental methods have been worked out for assaying the infectivity of viral nucleic acids, among them the DEAE dextran technique and the calcium technique reviewed by Graham (9). In analogy to bacterial transformation for which divalent cations are required for DNA uptake, Graham and van der Eb (10) coprecipitated viral DNA and calcium phosphate thus enhancing the DNA infectivity. Recently, the calcium method has been improved as the "calcium/dimethylsulfoxide shock" for transfection of human lybphoblastoid cells with herpes simplex virus DNA (11). Calcium ions are probably required both for the formation of precipitate as well as for uptake of DNA into recipient cells. As mentioned below, the calcium technique has become the method of choice for introducing non-viral genes via purified DNA into cultured mammalian recipient cells. The success of the method is critically dependent on the DNA concentration at the time of addition of calcium chloride. At higher DNA concentrations (5 to 20 μg per 10^6 cells) the assay is most efficient. Thus carrier DNA is being added when the biological activity of diluted DNA solutions is assayed.

Bacterial transformation systems (*Bacillus subtilis*, *Pneumoccus*, and *Haemophilus influenzae*) show an unexplained minimal size requirement for the donor DNA, if it is not cleaved by restriction endonucleases (2). This requirement has not been systematically studied with DNA mediated gene transfer in mammalian cells, at least not under conditions where the expression of donor genes in cultured recipient cells has been followed. The preparation of total cellular DNA which has been recently used for biochemically proven gene transfer (12, 13) had a molecular weight of > 40 kb. It was reported that restriction endonuclease digested total cellular DNA can be also used for transfer and expression of mammalian genes (14).

The recent results on biochemically proven DNA mediated transfer of mammalian genes into cultured mammalian cells have all been obtained following the experimental conditions of transfection systems which had been worked out originally for viral nucleic acids, especially for the thymidine kinase gene of Herpes simplex virus HSV-1. This gene had been introduced into the genome of mammalian cells which lacked the enzyme, first by infecting cells with virus inactivated by ultraviolet light (15) or by inoculating cells with fragments of viral DNA (16-18). As recipient cells a human cell line and a mouse cell line LM(TK), defective in thymidine kinase, were used. The latter cell line has never been found to revert to normal mouse thymidine kinase activity. Selection was carried out in medium, containing thymidine, aminoterin and hypoxanthine (HAT) which selects for expression of functional thymidine kinase (TK) or hypoxanthine phosphoribosyl transferase (HGPRT). This medium was developed by Szybalska and Szybalski (5) and has been used extensively in somatic cell genetics after being modified by Littlefield (19). The TK activity expressed after gene transfer in recipient cells has been shown to be virus-specific.

Minson *et al.* (20) showed that other Herpes specific functions can be transferred together with the Herpes TK gene, since one of their transferent cell lines was able to complement the functional defect found in two temperature sensitive mutants of HSV-1. This type of transferent cell line contained one or up to 5 copies of part of the HSV genome. Pellicer *et al.* (21) had used 270 molecules of DNA fragments containing the TK gene per recipient cell and had obtained one clone for every 10^6 recipient cells. Thus it was surprising that the Herpes TK gene could also be transferred to LM(TK^-) cells using high molecular weight total cellular DNA from cells containing only one copy of the TK genome. The maximum frequency of gene transfer observed in this system was 10 colonies, exhibiting Herpes TK, per 10^6 LM(TK) cells per 20 μg of total cellular DNA (12). This frequency was about 40 fold higher than predicted from studies of tranfection with the HSV TK gene, when purified as a 3,4 kb restriction nuclease cleaved fragment of Herpes DNA (21). Minson *et al.* came to similar conclusions (20). They noted that cell clones transfected with fragmented Herpes DNA show uniform levels of Herpes TK activity whereas cell clones transfected with total cellular DNA, harbouring the Herpes TK gene, showed a wide range of Herpes TK activity. In order to explain the relatively high frequency for transfer via total cellular DNA and expression of the Herpes TK gene, Minson *et al.* speculated that an increased rate of integration of virus sequences might result from recombination with homologous host sequences which could be highly reiterated in the recipient chromosomes and which could be flanking the viral genome in the total donor DNA. Again a frequency of 7 colonies per 10^6 cells per 20 μg of DNA was observed. Less colonies were found when the same experiment was carried out with DNA purified from Chinese hamster-, chicken-, calf thymus, or human HeLa cells.

Biochemical proof for interspecies DNA mediated gene transfer was given by Wigler *et al.* (12) only for the transfer of human TK into LM (TK^-) mouse cells. The clones isolated from these experiments contained the human type of TK activity as shown by isoelectric focusing. Willecke *et al.* (30) described an experimental system by which the intraspecies DNA mediated gene transfer of mouse HGPRT into A9 mouse cells, defective in HGPRT, could be biochemically proven. The donor DNA has been isolated from cells which contained an electrophoretic variant of mouse HGPRT. The HGPRT variant had been shown to be probably due to a structural gene mutation in the HGPRT locus on the mouse X chromosome. This variant HGPRT gene has been transferred to A9 mouse cells at a frequency of 0.5×10^{-7}. When placed in non-selective medium the DNA mediated transferent cells gradually lost their ability to express the HGPRT genome at a rate of about 6% per average cell generation. The frequency for isolation of transferent clones, harbouring the variant HGPRT gene, was at least 10 fold lower than reported by Wigler *et al.* (12) for DNA mediated transfer of the TK gene. The difference in frequency could be due to the lower than wild type level of the variant HGPRT activity and to the experimental differences in the methods used for uptake of DNA. Apparently, the technique of Wigler *et al.* (12) is more efficient. This technique has been used to demonstrate the DNA mediated transfer of the adenine phophoribosyltransferase locus (APRT) from Chinese hamster, human or mouse cells into APRT deficient mouse cells (14). These authors also mention the successful DNA mediated transfer of a methotrexate resistant folate reductase gene to wild type cells. Again it was observed that the transferent cells fall into two classes: those that are phenotypically stable when grown in the absence of selective pressure and those that are phenotypically unstable under the same conditions. This finding resembles the results obtained after chromosome mediated gene transfer (1). Wigler *et al.* (14) reported that the total cellular DNA from rabbit liver could be digested with the restriction endonucleases Hin-d III, Kpn I or Xba I and still retained its gene transfer activity for APRT. In our laboratory we had found (M. Klomfass and K. Willecke, unpublished) that human HeLa DNA after fragmentation with the restriction endonuclease BAM-1 could be used for transfer of human TK into LM (TK^-) cells. These results show that fragments of total cellular DNA with defined ends can be used for DNA mediated gene transfer.

Most recently Wigler and coauthors (22) described the cotransfer via isolated DNA of physically unlinked genes. These transferent cells were isolated and identified in an experimental system where one of the genes coded for a selectable marker, for example viral TK. Under these conditions Wigler *et al.* found that either the bacteriophage ΦX 174, the plasmid pBR 322 or the cloned chromosomal rabbit β-globin gene sequences could be transferred together with Herpes TK. The cotransferent cells contained at least one copy of the TK gene and up to 100 copies of the ΦX 174 sequences. The cotransferred sequences were analyzed by hybridization probes. The transfer experiment was carried out with ΦX 174 and viral TK sequences at a molecular ratio of 100 : 1, respectively. The ΦX 174 sequences could only be detected in clones selected for expression of TK. Most of the ΦX - sequences were integrated into cellular DNA since unique restriction fragments were obtaine after cleavage with restriction endonucleases which did not cut the free ΦX - genome. Most of the ΦX - DNA copurified with the high molecular weight fraction and not with extrachromosomal DNA in the Hirt supernatant. This ruled out an extra chromosomal location of the cotransferred ΦX-sequences. In contrast to transferred selectable cellular genes, for which Wigler *et al.* (14) had previously found a loss of 10 to 30% per cell generation, the cotransferred ΦX - sequences were maintained for many generations without loss of translocation of information. Similarly, as found for clones harbouring cotransferred ΦX - sequences, multiple copies per recipient cell were also determined for integrated plasmid pBR 322 sequences. Cell lines have been isolated which contained one or multiple copies of the cotransferred rabbit globin genes. The best explanation of these cotransfer results is given by the assumption that a subpopulation of competent cells for DNA mediated gene transfer exists in the total recipient cell population. Competence of mammalian cells, as defined by the ability of a subpopulation to take up foreign DNA, is not a stable inherited trait (22). In bacteria competence is also not inherited but dependent on the metabolic state of the cell which can for example with *Bacillus subtilis* only be reached after strict nutritional schedule (2). In mammalian cells the competence phenomenon may be experimentally used in the future for introduction and stable integration of any defined gene, provided that the cotransferred gene is presented to the recipient cells in multiple copies relative to the copies of the selectable gene. If this condition can be met the method appears very simple since no ligation of the gene to be cotransferred is required.

Transferent clones which have been isolated after DNA mediated gene transfer tend to lose the transgenome when the selective drug is removed from the culture medium. Assuming that the rate of loss of the transgenome was constant for each generation the HGPRT gene transferred into mouse cells was lost at 6% per cell generation (13), the mouse TK gene transferred into mouse LM (TK^-) cells was lost at about 14% per mean cell generation (M. Klomfass and K. Willecke, unpublished) and up to 27% loss per mouse cell generation was found for the transferred Chinese hamster APRT gene (14). The phenomenon of phenotypic instability had been first discovered with chromosome mediated transfer by McBride and Ozer (7). Later Willecke *et al.* (23) and Degnen *et al.* (4) independently found that phenotypically unstable clones became stable when maintained in selective growth medium for about 30 generations. Degnen *et al.* (4) estimated that stabilization occurred at one in 10^5 transferent cells. Phenotypic stabilization has recently been found in this laboratory for the mentioned mouse cell clone to which the variant HGPRT gene had been transferred by DNA mediated gene transfer (13). After about 80 generations in selective medium these cells were found to be phenotypically stable. So far no experimental results have been reported to prove the notion that phenotypically unstable clones may contain non-integrated mammalian transgenomes. We tried to compare the ability for sequential gene transfer mediated by extrachromosomal DNA purified according to Hirt (25) of Shoyab and Sen (26) from phenotypically unstable and phenotypically stable DNA mediated transferent cells (M. Klomfass and K. Willecke, unpublished). No clones could be detected, however, when extrachromosomal DNA was used for DNA mediated intraspecies gene transfer of mouse HGPRT of TK. This result suggests that the mentioned transgenomes could not be preferentially copurified with extrachromosomal DNA from phenotypcally unstable transferent clones.

As proposed several years ago, phenotypically stable clones should harbour the transgenome covalently integrated in the recipient genome (23). Unfortunately, no molecular probe is available which can be used to analyze the transferred, integrated HGPRT gene by DNA hybridization. Thus we had to use the indirect method of analyzing the segregation pattern of the transgenome in somatic cell hybrids. This method had been used before in order to analyze interspecies chromosome mediated transferent clones which harboured transferred human genomes in mouse recipient cells (27-29). In all cases reported, the human transgenome was found to segregate with non-homologous mouse chromosomes. Thus the transgenome was presumably integrated at a genetic site which was nonlinked to the DNA sequence of the homologous chromosome. So far no indication for preferred integration at specific chromosomal sites has been found. One could argue that inhomologies between the mouse and the human genome might explain that integration of the transferred human gene might not take place at the homologous mouse chromosome. On order to test this hypothesis we fused microcells of DNA mediated tranferent mouse cells which stably expressed the transferred variant mouse HGPRT gene with Chinese hamster cells. Hybrids were isolated which expressed the variant HGPRT gene and appear to harbour only 1 to 3 mouse chromosomes. When counter-selected in medium containing azaguanine and thioguanine, the variant HGPRT activity was lost. If it had been integrated at the homologous position of the defective HGPRT gene copy of the mouse X chromosome, this chromosome should have been segregated from the counter selected hybrids. We should have detected the segregation of the mouse X chromosome from these hybrids by following the segregation of α-galactosidase activity which is coded by a gene flanking the HGPRT gene on the long arm of the mouse X-chromosome. However, we found discordant segregation of the transferred mouse variant HGPRT gene and the mouse α-galactosidase gene from the mentioned hybrid cells. Cosegregation of both genes was only found in microcell hybrids of normal mouse HGPRT revertant calls and the same Chinese hamster cells. This result shows that even after intraspecies gene transfer in the mouse, integration at the homologous genetic site did not occur (Willecke *et al.*, manuscript in preparation). Rosenstrauss and Chasin had also not detected any evidence for homologous mitotic recombination following the separation of linked markers in Chinese hamster somatic cell hybrids (30).

In yeast 3 modes of low-frequency transformation have been described which correspond to 3 different types of integration (31). In addition, autonomous replication of hybrid DNA molecules has recently been shown after high-frequency transformation of yeast (32). Type I and type III transformed yeast cells contain integrations at or near the corresponding site of the recipient genome. Type II integration took place at a chromosomal location genetically unlinked to the homologous region. Thus with regard to integration the results obtained with DNA mediated transferent mammalian cells so far appear to be similar as the type II integration in yeast. Perhaps when more mammalian transferent clones will be analyzed examples of homologous type I or type III integration will be found, too. Alternatively, because of the 200-fold excess of DNA in the mammalian cell compared with the yeast cell, normal homologous integration of the mammalian transgenome may be very rare. Possibly homologies of repetitive sequences in spacers between mammalian genes may be responsible for integration of the mammalian transgenome at chromosomal locations non-linked to the corresponding gene of the recipient cells. Because of this complication fine structure genetic mapping as far as it makes use of homologous recombination cannot be carried out with cultured mammalian cells. Undoubtedly, this question will be reinvestigated when molecular probes for mammalian genes will be available for studying the transgenomes. Until that time the mechanism of recombination in mammalian cells like the mechanism of DNA uptake and the phenomenon of competence, will remain obscure.

When one compares chromosome mediated and DNA mediated mammalian gene transfer it appears that both methods may complement each other with regard to possible application in somatic cell genetics. Transferred genes on mammalian chromosomes or fragments of them can be cytologically recognized under certain conditions and thus the results of gene transfer can be interpreted on terms of gross chromosomal structure (8). This is particularly important for clarification of the role of donor or recipient centromers as possible integration sites and with regard to distribution of transgenomes during mitoses. For all investigations where genes have to be assigned to chromosomes or regions of chromosomes, the modified chromosome dependent gene transfer technique appears to be advantageous.

On the other hand DNA mediated gene transfer allows one to assay the biological function of normal and modified DNA. Particularly when mammalian gene sequences have been ligated or cleaved DNA mediated gene transfer will be the method of choice for studying the biological effects of this manipulation or of cloning mammalian DNA sequences in procaryotic cells. It appears that many new insights into eucaryotic gene expression and better characterizations of dominantly acting genes can soon be expected from further investigation of DNA mediated gene transfer.

3. ACKNOWLEDGEMENTS

I should like to thank my coworkers J. Döhmer, M. Klomfass, R. Mierau, I. Rademacher, and Dr. R. Schäfer who contributed to investigations of DNA mediated gene transfer in our laboratory. Our research was supported by grants of the Deutsche Forschungsgemeinschaft (SFB 102 and Wi 270/6/7/8) to KW.

4. REFERENCES

1) WILLECKE, K. (1978). Results and prospects of chromosomal gene transfer between cultured mammalian cells. Theoret. Appl. Gen., 52, 79.

2) BROOKS LOW, K. and PORTER, D.D. (1978). Modes of gene transfer and recombination in bacteria. Ann. Rev. Genet., 12, 249.

3) MCBRIDE, W.O. and ATHWAL, R.S. (1976). Genetic analysis by chromosome mediated gene transfer. *In Vitro*, 12, 777.

4) OTTOLENGHI-NIGHTINGALE, E. (1974). DNA mediated transformation in mammalian cells. In: Cell Communication. (ed., R.P. Cox), John Wiley and Sons, New York.

5) SZYBALSKA, E.H. and SZYBALSKI, W. (1962). Genetics of human cell

lines IV. DNA-mediated heritable transformation of a biochemical trait. Proc. Nat. Acad. Sc., 48, 2026.

6) FARBER, F.E. and EBERLE, R. (1976). Effects of cytochalasin and alkaloid drugs on the biological expression of herpes simplex virus type 2 DNA. Exp. Cell Res., 103, 15.

7) MCBRIDE, W.O. and OZER, H.L. (1973). Transfer of genetic information by purified metaphase chromosomes. Proc. Nat. Acad. Sc., 70, 1258.

8) MILLER, C.L. and RUDDLE, F.H. (1978). Cotransfer of human X-linked markers into murine somatic cells via isolated chromosomes. Proc. Nat. Acad. Sc., 75, 3346.

9) GRAHAM, F. (1977). Biological activity of tumor virus DNA. Adv. Cancer Res., 25, 1.

10) GRAHAM, F.L. and VAN DER EB, A. (1973). A new technique for the assay of infectivity of human adenovirus 5 DNA. Virology, 54, 536.

11) MILLER, G., WERTHEIM, P., WILSON, G., ROBINSON, J., GEELEN, J. L.M.C., VAN DER NOORDA, J. and VAN DER EB, A.J. (1979). Transfection of human lymphoblastoid cells with herpes simplex viral DNA. Proc. Nat. Acad. Sc., 76, 949.

12) WIGLER, M., PELLICER, A., SILVERSTEIN, S. and AXEL, R. (1978). Biochemical transfer of single-copy encaryotic genes using total cellular DNA as donor. Cell, 14, 725.

13) WILLECKE, K., KLOMFASS, M., MIERAU, R. and DÖHMER, J. (1979). Intraspecies transfer via total cellular DNA of the gene for hypoxanthine phosphoribosyltransferease into cultured mouse cells. Molec. Gen. Genet., 170, 179.

14) WIGLER, M., PELLICER, A., SILVERSTEIN, S., AXEL, R., URLAUB, G. and CHASIN, L. (1979). DNA-mediated transfer of the adenine phosphoribosyltransferase locus into mammalian cells. Proc. Nat. Acad. Sc., 76, 1373.

15) MUNYON, W, KRAISELBURD, E., DAVIS, S. and MANN, J. (1971). Transfer of thymidine kinase to thymidine kinaseless L-cells

by infection with ultraviolet-irradiated herpes simplex virus. J. Virol., 7, 813.

16) BACCHETTI, S. and GRAHAM, F.L. (1977). Transfer of the gene for thymidine kinase to thymidine kinase-deficient human cells by purified herpes simplex viral DNA. Proc. Nat. Acad. Sc., 74, 1590.

17) MAITLAND, N.J. and MCDOUGALL, J.K. (1977). Biochemical transformation of mouse cells by fragments of herpes simplex virus DNA. Cell, 11, 233.

18) WIGLER, M., SILVERSTEIN, S., LEE, L.S., PELLICER, A.,CHENG, Y. C. and AXEL. R. (1977). Transfer of purified herpes virus thymidine kinase gene to cultured mouse cells. Cell, 11, 223.

19) LITTLEFIELD, J.W. (1966). The use of drug-resistant markers to study the hybridization of mouse fibroblasts. Exp. Cell Res., 41, 190.

20) MINSON, A.C., WILDY, P.P., BUCHAN, A. and DARBY, G. (1978). Introduction of the herpes simplex virus thymidine kinase gene into mouse cells using virus DNA or transformed cell DNA. Cell, 13, 581.

21) PELLICER, A., WIGLER, M., AXEL, R.,SILVERSTEIN, S. (1978). The transfer and stable integration of the HSV thymidine kinase gene into mouse cells. Cell, 14, 133.

22) WIGLER, M.,SWEET, R., SIM, G.K., WOLD, B., PELLICER, A., LACY, E., MANIATIS, T., SILVERSTEIN, S. and AXEL, R. (1979). Transformation of mammalian cells with genes from procaryotes and encaryotes. Cell, 16, 777.

23) WILLECKE, K., LANGE, R., KRÜGER, A. and REBER, T. (1976). Cotransfer of two linked human genes into cultured mouse cells. Proc. Nat. Acad. Sc., 73, 1274.

24) DEGNEN, G.E., ADELBERG, I.L. and EISENSTADT, J.M. (1976). Chromosome mediated gene transfer between closely related strains of cultured mouse cells. Proc. Nat. Acad. Sc., 73, 2838.

25) HIRT, B. (1967). Selective extraction of polyoma DNA from in-

fected mouse cell cultures. J. Mol. Biol., 26, 365.

26) SHOYAB, M. and SEN, A. (1978). A rapid method for the purification of extrachromosomal DNA from eucaryotic cells. J. Biol. Chem., 253, 6654.

27) FOURNIER, R.E.K. and RUDDLE, F.H. (1977). Stable association of the human transgenome and most murine chromosomes demonstrated with trispecific microcell hybrids. Proc. Nat. Acad. Sc., 74, 3937.

28) DAVIES, J. and WILLECKE, K. (1977). Segregation of human hypoxanthine phosphoribosyltransferase activity from somatic cell hybrids isolated after fusion of mouse gene transfer cells with Chinese hamster cells. Molec. Gen. Genet., 154, 191.

29) WILLECKE, K., MIERAU, R., KRÜGER, A. and LANGE, R. (1978). Chromosomal gene transfer of human cytosol thymidine kinase into mouse cells. Molec. Gen. Genet., 161, 49.

30) ROSENSTRAUS, M.J. and CHASIN, L.A. (1978). Separation of linked markers in Chinese hamster cell hybrids: mitotic recombination is not involved. Genetics, 90, 735.

31) HINNEN, A., HICKS, J.B. and FINK, G.R. (1978). Transformation in yeast. Proc. Nat. Acad. Sc., 75, 1929.

32) STRUHL, K., STINCHCOMB, D.T., SCHERER, S. and DAVIS, R.W. (1979). High-frequency transformation of yeast: autonomous replication of hybrid DNA molecules. Proc. Nat. Acad. Sc., 76, 1035.

TRANSFER OF DNA INTO PLANT CELLS WITH THE Ti-PLASMID AS A VECTOR

J. Schell[*#] and M. Van Montagu[*]

[*] *Laboratory for Genetics, State University-Gent, Belgium, and*
[#] *Max-Planck-Institut für Züchtungsforschung-Köln, BRD*

1. INTRODUCTION

A. tumefaciens strains induce tumors (crown galls) on a wide range of dicotyledonous plants (1). These tumors contain stably transformed - genetically altered - cells that are selfproliferating and graftable (2).

The capacity to induce tumors is genetically determined by large plasmids: the Ti-plasmids (3). Removal of the Ti-plasmids from oncogenic strains results in the loss of oncogenicity* whereas introduction of Ti-plasmids in non-oncogenic *Agrobacterium* strains produces oncogenic derivatives (4, 5).

Several observations have allowed a fairly precise explanation of this neoplastic transformation. It was demonstrated (6) that Ti-plasmids carry genes that somehow determine the specificity of synthesis of so-called "opines" (7, 8) by crown gall cells. Other Ti-

*Oncogenicity is used here in a broad sense as the capacity (4) of an *Agrobacterium* strain to induce crown gall tumors on normally susceptible host plants.

plasmid genes allow Agrobacteria to use specific opines as sole carbon, nitrogen and energy source (4-7, 9). The correlation between the specificity of opine synthesis in transformed plant cells and the specificity of opine catabolism by the transforming bacteria (8), could thus be explained genetically, provided that one assumed that the Ti-plasmid genes specifying opine synthesis were transferred to the plant cells as a result of - or concomitant with - the transformation event. These observations therefore provided genetic evidence in favour of a model involving the Ti-plasmid in a DNA-transfer from bacterium to plant.

The correctness of this model was demonstrated by hybridisation experiments indicating that a small segment of the Ti-plasmid showed specific homology with DNA extracted from transformed plant cells (10-12). The demonstration that the T-DNA (i.e. the Ti-plasmid DNA segment present in transformed plant cells) is actually responsible for the synthesis of the specific opine by the transformed plant cells and probably also for the maintenance of their tumorous condition, was based on a combination of hybridisation data and genetic mapping of various functions on the Ti-plasmid (11-13). The genetic mapping has also borne out the conclusion that opine synthesis and opine catabolism are determined by distinct genetic loci on the Ti-plasmid (9). All these and other observations can be fitted into a biological model of "genetic colonisation " (11). It is obvious that opine synthesis and catabolism has played a central role in the evolution of Ti-plasmids. Most Ti-plasmids fall into one of three groups depending on whether they code for octopine or nopaline metabolizing enzymes (6, 14, 15) and depending on their host-range (16). These different types of Ti-plasmids are clearly of distinct evolutionary origin since they differ markedly in DNA sequences. Only DNA segments involved in the determination of oncogenicity and conjugational transfer seem to be relatively well conserved in most Ti-plasmids (13, 15).

Furthermore, opines have been found to specifically induce the conjugational transfer properties of Ti-plasmids (17, 18). It is therefore reasonable to assume that Ti-plasmids have evolved as a natural means for *Agrobacterium* to genetically "engineer" or "colonize" plant cells, thus illustrating a new type of a parasitic mode of life. By the transfer of a specific genetic information carried as a defined segment of the Ti-plasmid - the so-called T-DNA - Agrobacteria manage to force proliferating plant cells to synthesize products (opines) that only homologous Ti-plasmid harbouring bacteria can utilize as sole carbon, nitrogen and energy source. In the last couple of years much of the research on the crown gall system has centered around three major problems. This review will briefly report the progress that was achieved with regard to these questions.

2. THE GENETIC AND FUNCTIONAL ORGANISATION OF Ti-PLASMIDS

The general aim of these studies was to provide a definitive proof for the involvement of specific plasmid-borne genes in the determination of the properties of crown gall plant tissues and a first step towards the elucidation of the precise mechanism of tumorous transformation. It was hoped that it would be possible to identify the genes and later the gene products that are directly or indirectly involved in this phenomenon. The approach was to isolate and map mutations inactivating the functions that were supposedly controlled by Ti-plasmid genes. A very efficient way to obtain mutant Ti-plasmids was by insertion of antibiotic resistance transposons (19, 20). No selection for mutant phenotypes has to be devised and a straightforward selection for Ti-plasmids carrying the transposon was sufficient to produce a collection of mutant Ti-plasmids from which most of the desired phenotypes were obtained by screening a few hundred mutants (15, 20).

The location of the site of insertion on a physical map of the

Ti-plasmid was determined by isolating the mutant plasmid on a preparative scale and by analysing the fragmentation pattern of the digest with different restriction endonucleases. The mapping of a given insertion or deletion can be deduced from the restriction fragment(s) which disappear(s) or change(s) mobility. In several cases the mapping was confirmed by analysing heteroduplex molecules formed with a reference plasmid marked by two well mapped insertions under the electron microscope. Recently (21), a more efficient way was developed to analyse large numbers of mutant colonies using the Southern blot hybridisation technique. A filter containing the fragments obtained from a restriction endonuclease digest of the total DNA (chromosomal and plasmid) of the strain to be analysed, was hybridised with the radioactive probes, which consisted of the pure Ti-plasmid DNA and the drug transposon DNA.

A further advantage of transposon insertion mutagenesis is the fact that the site at which the transposon is inserted becomes the starting point for the formation of deletions. Starting with a given pTi::Tn mutant plasmid it was possible, by selection or screening for the loss of one or more plasmid encoded phenotypes, to obtain deletions of varying sizes. The extent of the deletion could then be determined with the same methods as described above for the mapping of insertions.

The physical map on which both the insertion and deletion mutants were localized, had been previously constructed by molecular cloning in pBR322 of large DNA fragments derived from partial Hind III digests of these plasmids. Restriction endonuclease digestion of the different clones and Southern blot hybridisations, established the map order.

A map for Hind III, Hpa I, Sma I, Kpn I, Eco RI, Xba I and Bam I of both an octopine (22a) and a nopaline (23) type to Ti-plasmid was thus constructed.

Table 1. *Localization of some Ti-plasmid encoded functions by transponson insertion mutagenesis.*

Phenotypes		Approximate map position in Md* pTiC58	pTiAch5
Ape	Exclusion of phage Apl (22b,c, 25)	70	9-11
Agr^S	Sensitivity to the pAT-K84 encoded agrocin (25, 26). Only *Agrobacterium* strains harbouring a nopaline plasmid show this phenotype, the other strains are Agr^R.	85-87	---
Arc	Arginine catabolism (27). Is part of a complex, inducible pathway. Deletion mutants constitutive for arginine catabolism (Arc^C) have been isolated (22c, e).	6-7	12
Agc	Agropine catabolism, an octopine tumor specific sugar derivative (28, 22c).	---	50-51
Noc	Nopaline catabolism. An inducible function, possibly under both negative and positive control. Mutants can be grouped in several classes (according to the aspect of colony growth on nopaline as sole nitrogen or sole carbon source). The necessary enzymes are encoded by nopaline Ti-plasmids. Nopaline is an inducer of its own catabolic pathway. Noc constitutive mutants are able to catabolize octopine (7).	6-7 and 11-12	---

*The length of the octopine Ti-plasmid pTiAch5 and of the nopaline Ti-plasmid as measured under the electron microscope (22f) and as obtained from the sum of the fragment lengths from a single restriction endonuclease digest (22a, d), correspond sufficiently well to propose a genome size of 120 Md for pTiAch5 and of 132 Md for pTiC58. A common Sma I site, located in the T-DNA region was chosen as the zero coordinates for both plasmids. All mapping data given refer to distances in Md from this common restriction site.

Table 1 (cont'd)

Phenotypes		Approximate map position in Md* pTiC58	pTiAch5
Nos	Nopaline synthesis in crown gall tumors. This function is encoded by nopaline Ti-plasmids only (6).	0-1	---
Occ	Octopine catabolism. An inducible pathway involving many functions. Octopine is an inducer. Nopaline is not catabolized by the octopine Ti-plasmid encoded enzymes (7, 29).	---	24-26
Tra	Functions responsible for the conjugative phenotype of the plasmid. The transfer genes are repressed in the wild type plasmid. Conditions for induction of transfer have been determined and Tra constitutive mutants have been isolated (30).	70-80 and 14-19	15-20
Onc	Oncogenicity or the capacity for induction of crown galls on at least tobacco, peas and sunflower.	129-132 115 106-108 99-101 74	115-117 97-102 85-90 63-64
Onch	Host range effect on oncogenicity. Tumors are formed on Kalanchoë and/or potatoes, but not on tobacco, peas and sunflower.	128	9 and 105
Orc	Catabolism of ornithine. It can be distinguished from Arc since Arc^+ Orc^-mutants were found (22e).		28

In tables 1 and 2 we have summarized the data for the different Ti-plasmid encoded functions for which mutations were obtained and mapped. It appears from these studies that the Ti-plasmids have been assembled functionally starting from a number of different building blocks. Although little information is as yet available on the number

Table 2. *Localization of some Ti-plasmid encoded functions by deletion mapping.*

Approximate coordinates of the deletions in Md		Mutant phenotype
pTiC58	Δ 99 - 13	Onc^- Noc^- Orc^- Ape^-
	Δ 64 - 131	Onc^- Agr^R Ape^- tra^-
	Δ 35 - 110	Onc^- Agr^R Ape^- tra^-
	Δ 4 - 16	Noc^- Orc^C
	Δ 3 - 16	Noc^- Orc^-
	Δ 3 - 12	Noc^- Arc^C
pTiAch5	Δ 105 - 17	Onc^- Ape^-
	Δ 85 - 118	Onc^-

The "viability" of these deletion plasmids suggests that the origin of replication must be in the region 16 to 35.

of different genes required for the determination of a particular phenotype, it is nevertheless possible to make some generalizations.

(i) Oncogenicity functions

As indicated in Fig. 1 the Onc mutations were found to be distributed over the entire Ti-plasmid. These findings underline that there is probably a diversity of functions involved in determining consecutively the contact between the bacteria and the plant (31-33), the transfer of the Ti-plasmid via a plant receptor structure, the transfer of a Ti-plasmid DNA to the plant nucleus, the restructuring of the T-DNA into a replicating structure and finally the expression of functions that interfere with the plant cell metabolism so as to create the tumor cell phenotype.

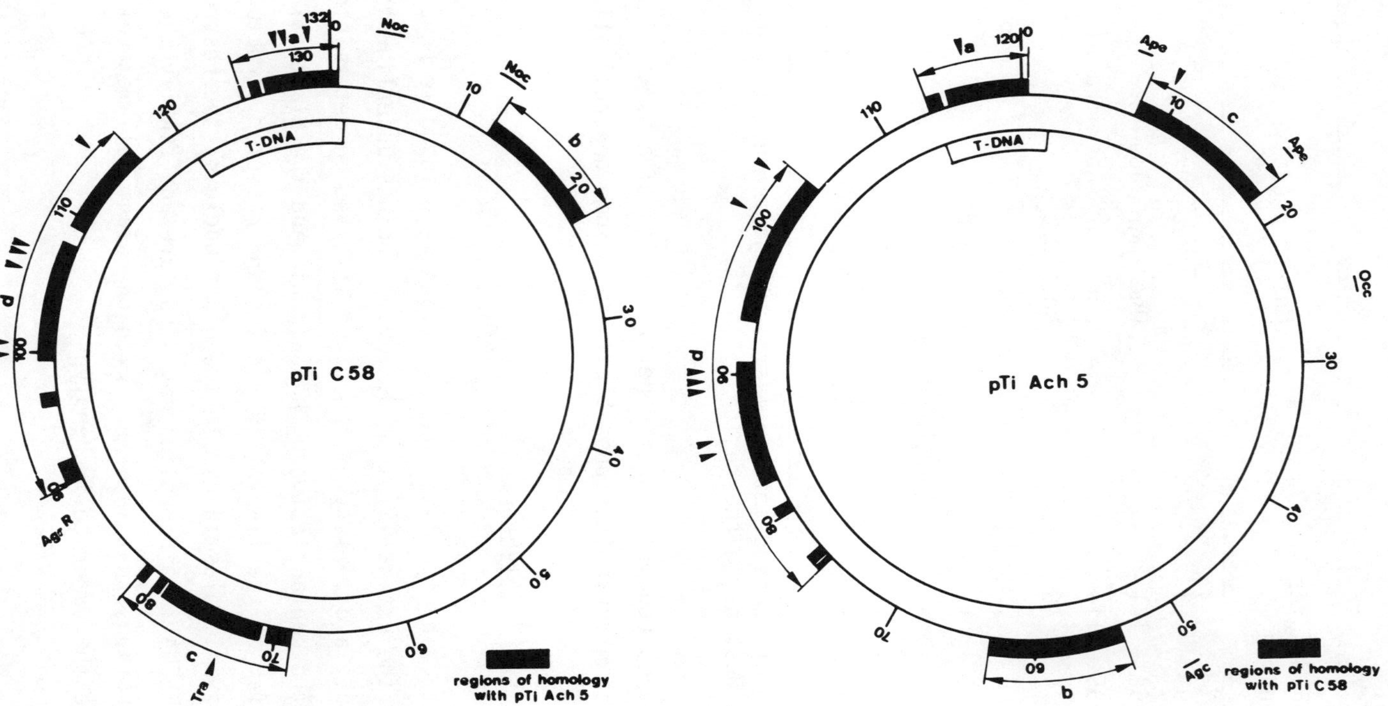

Fig. 1. *Functional organization of an octopine (pTiAch5) and a nopaline (pTiC58) plasmid.* The length of the plasmids (in Md) is indicated along the outer circle and is used as map coordinates. A Sma I restriction site in a segment common to both plasmids is chosen as zero point. The sequences common to both types of Ti-plasmid are indicated by a heavy line and are labeled a to d. The sites of transposon insertions resulting in Onc$^-$ phenotypes are indicated by an arrow.

By definition the Onc mutants which map within the T-DNA identify those genes supposedly involved in the establishment and/or maintenance of the tumorous growth of the plant cells; in nopaline plasmids these genes span roughly 5 Md. It is striking to note that this region also corresponds to the major area of homology between nopaline and octopine Ti-plasmids. To date there is no biochemical information about the products of this region. It is, however, well established that the Onc region of the T-DNA is actively transcribed in the plant cell (34, 22g). Interestingly, some Onc mutants (both within and outside of the T-DNA region) suggest a host specific interaction. For example, some mutants affect functions which are dispensible for tumor formation on Kalanchoë but not on other plants. There is no information about the products encoded by Onc regions outside of the T-DNA except that several of these DNA fragments cloned in *E. coli* synthesize proteins in minicells.

(ii) Opine biosynthesis

Ti-plasmid insertion mutants producing an $Onc^{+}Nos^{-}$ phenotype were isolated (11, 12, 15, 20). Agrobacteria carrying such mutant Ti-plasmids induce tumors in which no nopaline synthesis can be detected. It is important to stress that these mutations were found to map within a particular fragment of the T-DNA region of the Ti-plasmids (see further), thus providing evidence for the direct and active involvement of this DNA segment in the control of opine synthesis in transformed plant cells. Furthermore, these observations demonstrated that opine synthesis and determination of tumorous growth must be functionally independent but are controlled by DNA segments adjacent to one another on the T-DNA.

(iii) Opine catabolism

The functions involved in providing *Agrobacterium* with the capacity to use octopine or nopaline as sole nitrogen and/or sole carbon source can be analyzed due to the availability of a large set of insertion and deletion mutants in these functions (20, 22i). Furthermore, these regions of the Ti-plasmid have been isolated and propagated by molecular cloning techniques. Cloned DNA fragments have been used to study the expression of these regions in *Agrobacterium* (22i, j). Preliminary results point to the existence of a rather complex operon structure probably containing both negative and positive controlling elements. For the octopine plasmid pTiB6 there clearly is a common element in the regulation of octopine catabolism and conjugal transfer (7, 29). These mapping data have also borne out the conclusion that opine synthesis and opine catabolism are determined by distinct genetic loci on the Ti-plasmid.

When taken together with hybridisations studies (15, 22d), comparing various segments of octopine and nopaline Ti-plasmids (see Fig. 1), these genetic studies have clearly indicated that the genes allowing Agrobacteria to catabolize opines appear to have determined the evolution of these plasmids and hence of the rown gall phenomenon. It is interesting to note that these genes do not appear to have a single origin but must instead be of diverse origins since little or no homology was found in these genes between octopine and nopaline type plasmids.

3. T-DNA, ITS SIZE, LOCALISATION AND POSSIBLE ASSOCIATION WITH PLANT DNA

When it became obvious that the opine synthesizing capacity expressed by the transformed plant cells, was actually a trait determined by the *Agrobacterium* Ti-plasmid, it was evident to consider the possibility that a segment of the Ti-plasmid became part of the transformed plant genome. A first indication was obtained by solution DNA hybridisation studies. Some restriction fragments of the octopine plasmid pTiB6806 did indeed show an accelerated rate of reassociation after addition of DNA from a particular tobacco crown gall tumor (10). A more complete picture was obtained when Southern gel blotting hybridisations were performed with the crown gall DNA. Total tumor DNA was digested with a variety of restriction enzymes and used to drive the hybridisation of nick translated cloned fragments of the Ti-plasmid (11, 12, 22h). Some generalizations may be advanced from this approach. In the case of all tumors induced by the nopaline plasmids pTiT37 and pTiC58 the T-DNA corresponds to one large 15.6 Md continuous segment of the Ti-plasmid. Cloned fragments representing the whole of the Ti-plasmid were used as radioactive probes in this Southern gel blotting hybridisations. Only fragments overlapping with the thus defined T-DNA region showed positive and reproducible hybridisations. The T-DNA is not integrated in plastid DNA (M.-D. Chilton, personal communication) but appears to be located in the nucleus (22k). Several copies of the T-DNA can be present as seen in Fig. 2 where border fragments of the T-DNA were used as probes in hybridisations to Southern blots of tumor DNA. In this tumor line one can observe that there are at least three different right borders and three different left borders. The molecular weights of these fragments suggest that they are composed of T-DNA linked to some other DNA, possibly plant DNA.

As can be seen in Fig. 3 an Eco RI digest of a cloned tobacco teratoma T37 Crown-gall DNA indicated the presence of two distinct "right end border" composite fragments of ±9.0 and 6.0 Md, respectively. Both these composite fragments were recently cloned (22m), using bacteriophage lambda as the initial cloning vector. A careful analysis by Southern blot hybridisations of restriction endonuclease fragments derived from these cloned composite fragments is summarized in Fig. 4. As can be seen the 6.0 Md fragment indeed consisted of the "right end" border of the T-DNA linked to a very small sequence of DNA not present as such in Ti-plasmid. The 9.0 Md fragment gave unexpected results. Indeed it not only contained the expected "right

COMPOSITE FRAGMENTS REPRESENTING THE BORDERS BETWEEN T-DNA AND PLANT DNA

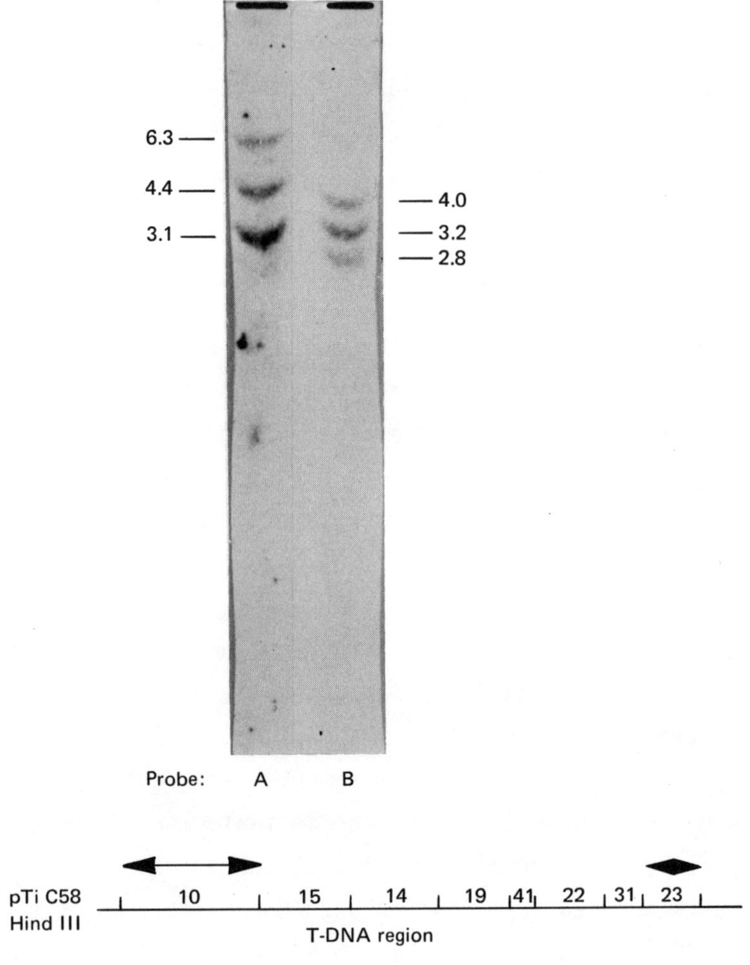

Fig. 2. *A "genomic blot" of Wisconsin 38 tobacco crown gall DNA, digested with Hind III restriction endonuclease, was hybridised to the nick-translated T-DNA border fragments H-10 (lane A) and H-23 (lane B).* The autoradiogram demonstrates the existence of at least three border fragments.

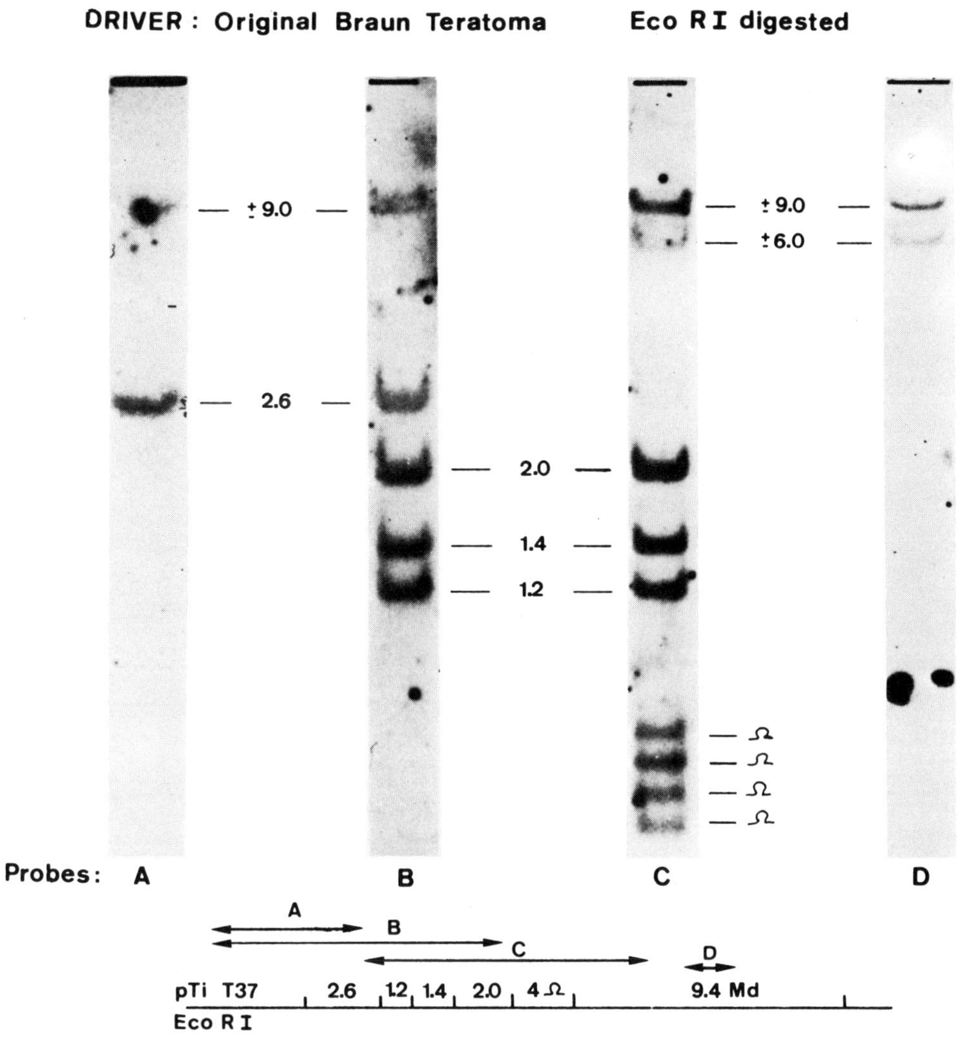

Fig. 3. *A "genomic blot" of cloned T37 tobacco teratoma from Dr. A. Braun's collection, digested with Eco RI was hybridised to nick-translated T-DNA fragments A, B, C, D.*

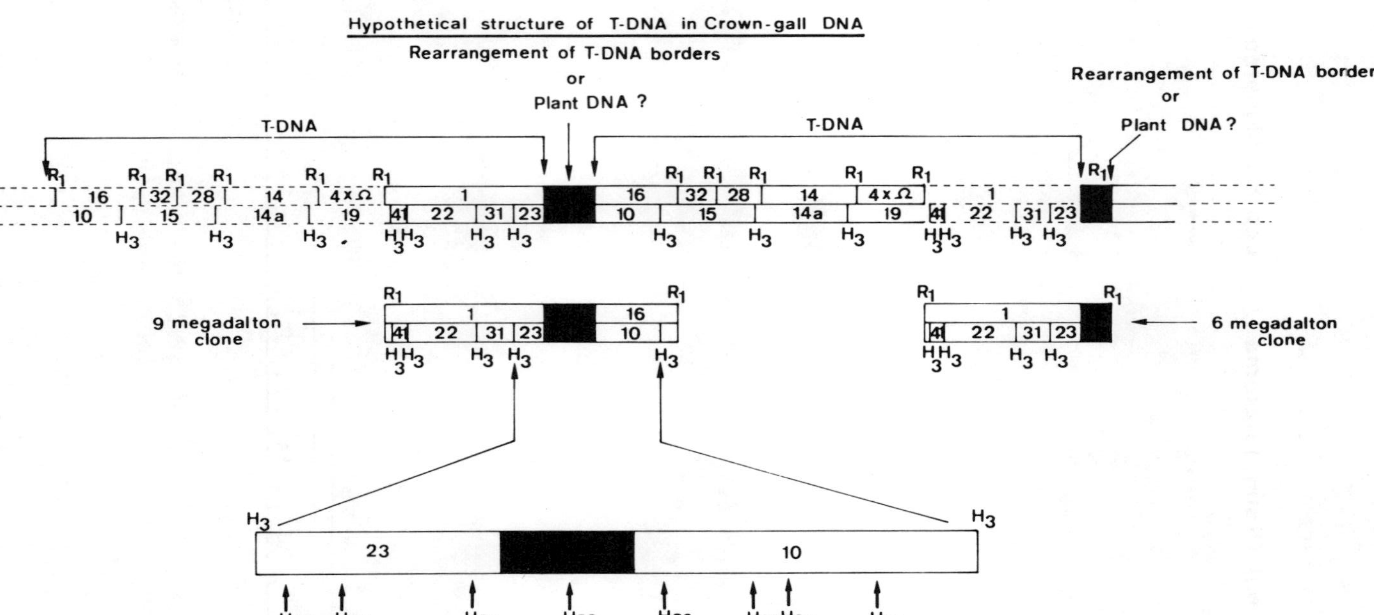

Fig. 4. *Model of T-DNA in plants.*
In solid lines the arrangement of the internal restriction endonuclease fragment of the T-DNA is illustrated. It is important to note that this arrangement of T-DNA fragments is identical both in the Ti-plasmid DNA and in the DNA of tobacco crown gall. Underneath the structure of the T-DNA Eco RI "right end" border composite fragments of ±9.0 and 6.0 Md is illustrated. These composite fragments were isolated from T37 tobacco crown gall DNA by molecular cloning.

end" border of the T-DNA (the Hind III fragments 23, 31, 22 and 41) but also part of the "left end" border (part of Hind III fragment 10). Furthermore, a sequence of about 0.3 Md was found that could not be detected as such either in the Ti-plasmid Hind III fragment 23 or in the Hind III fragment 10.

Two different models could account for these observations:

1° The T-DNA forms an independent replicon, "right end" and "left end" borders of the T-DNA are joined, rearrangements (e.g. partial duplications) of the DNA of the border sequences have occurred and explain the fragments that do not occur as such in the T-DNA segment of the Ti-plasmid DNA.

2° The T-DNA is integrated in some plant DNA so that at least two T-DNA segments are present as a tandem but separated by a 0.3 Md sequence of plant DNA.

Work is in progress to distinguish between these two possibilities.

Nothing much is presently known about the mechanism by which the T-DNA is either integrated or rearranged to form an independent replicon in the plant nucleus. A number of observations, however, indicate that the "ends" of the T-DNA are somehow involved. Within the resolution of our analysis (restriction fragment mapping) we found the T-DNA ends of both octopine and nopaline Ti-plasmids to be identical in several independent crown gall lines initiated on tobacco, petunia and arabidopsis. Furthermore, inserts of transposons within a segment of the T-DNA region, non-essential for tumor formation, yield transformed cell lines with a T-DNA which has the same "ends" as found in crown gall containing wild-type T-DNA. The insert in this DNA is located at precisely the same site within the T-DNA region as in the mutated Ti-plasmid with which the tumor line was initiated.

By genetic means (insertion and deletion mutants) it was established that the T-DNA consists of at least three different functional units. A central segment of about 5.0 Md is conserved in all types of Ti-plasmids. Mutations in this segment invariably result in the loss of capacity to produce plant tumors (20).

To either side of this conserved DNA segment, we found DNA sequences that are different in different types of Ti-plasmids (22d). Mutations in these non-conserved segments of the T-DNA do not result in the loss of capacity to induce tumors. Mutations in what has been called the right side of the T-DNA (± 1.5 Md), do, however, result in Ti-plasmids that induce tumors in which no opine synthesis occurs, thus identifying the DNA sequence involved in opine synthesis.

Possible aberrant phenotypes of plant tumors induced with Ti-plasmids with a mutation in the "left" end of the T-DNA, have not yet been carefully studied.

4. CAN THE Ti-PLASMID BE USED AS A HOST VECTOR SYSTEM FOR PLANTS?

With the realization that Ti-plasmids are in fact a natural host vector system able to promote transfer, integration and expression of "foreign" DNA in plants, we asked whether or not the properties of this system could be used to introduce, at will, foreign DNA sequences in various plants. Recently (11, 12, 15) we were able to report that this was indeed the case. The general strategy used was to incorporate, by *in vivo* recombination, a bacterial transposon, Tn7 into the 1.5 Md segment of the T-DNA that codes for opine synthesis. Subsequently, we were able to demonstrate that tobacco tumor lines induced with such Tn7 harbouring Ti-plasmids, did indeed contain a T-DNA consisting of the whole of the T-DNA (15 Md) of the wild type plasmid together with the whole of the Tn7 DNA (9.5 Md) still inserted in its original site in the T-DNA. Whether or not the T-DNA is transcribed in these plant cells, has not yet been established.

An important question is whether or not plant cells containing a T-DNA segment can be used to breed new plants. Recent observations (35) have demonstrated that whole plants can be regenerated from transformed teratoma cultures. In these studies tobacco teratoma derived tumor shoots were isolated and grafted to cut stem tips of normal tobacco plants of a morphologically distinct cultivar. This way, shoots were obtained that developed quite normally and ultimately flowered and set viable seed. It was found that the leaves of these grafts were normally organized but were still transformed in the sense that, when such specialized cells were isolated and planted on a basic culture medium, they grew as crown gall cells and synthesized nopaline. These tissues were studied by Southern blotting hybridisations and it was found that they still contained T-DNA from the TiT37 plasmid (22, 25) (and M.P. Gordon, personal communication). In fact, we were able to demonstrate that the T-DNA segment found in tissues derived from organized leaves of the teratoma grafts, was the same as the T-DNA segment found in the original teratoma tissues with which the grafts were initiated. No gross rearrangement of the T-DNA had therefore occurred during the differentiation of tumor cells to organized plant cells. It was thus demonstrated that it is possible to create new plants containing a specific DNA segment using the Ti-plasmid as a host vector.

These promising results will now be followed by experiments where non-transposon DNA and possibly plant genes are inserted into the T-DNA by *in vivo* recombination.

5. ACKNOWLEDGEMENTS

The authors wish to thank their collaborators (22) for providing the information presented in this article. This work was supported by grants from the "Kankerfonds van de A.S.L.K." and from the "Fonds voor Wetenschappelijk Geneeskundig Onderzoek" (no. 3.0052.78).

6. REFERENCES

1) DE CLEENE, M. and DE LEY, J. (1976). The host range of Crown gall. Bot. Rev., 42, 389.
2) BRAUN, A.C. and WHITE, P.R. (1943). Bacterial sterility of tissues derived from secondary crown gall tumors. Phytopathology, 33, 85.
3) ZAENEN, I., VAN LAREBEKE, N., TEUCHY, H., VAN MONTAGU, M. and SCHELL, J. (1974). Supercoiled circular DNA in crown-gall inducing *Agrobacterium* strains. J. Mol. Biol., 86, 109.
4) VAN LAREBEKE, N., ENGLER, G., HOLSTERS, M., VAN DEN ELSACKER, S., ZAENEN, I., SCHILPEROORT, R.A. and SCHELL, J. (1974). Large plasmid in *Agrobacterium tumefaciens* essential for crown-gall inducing ability. Nature, 252, 169.
5) WATSON, B., CURRIER, T.C., GORDON, M.P., CHILTON, M.-D. and NESTER, E.W. (1975). Plasmid required for virulence of *Agrobacterium tumefaciens*. J. Bacteriol., 123, 255.
6) BOMHOFF, G., KLAPWIJK, P.M., KESTER, C.H.M., SCHILPEROORT, R.A., HERNALSTEENS, J.P. and SCHELL, J. (1976). Octopine and nopaline synthesis and breakdown genetically controlled by a plasmid of *A. tumefaciens*. Mol. Gen. Genet., 145, 177.
7) PETIT, A. and TEMPÉ, J. (1978). Isolation of *Agrobacterium* Ti-plasmid regulatory mutants. Molec. Gen. Genet., 167, 147.
8) PETIT, A., DELHAYE, S., TEMPÉ, J. and MOREL, G. (1970). Sur les guanidines des tissus de crown gall. Mise en évidence d'une relation biochimique spécifique entre les souches d'*Agrobacterium* et les tumeurs qu'elles induisent. Physio. Vég., 8, 205.
9) KLAPWIJK, P., HOOYKAAS, P., KESTER, H., SCHILPEROORT, R.A. and

RÖRSCH, A. (1976). Isolation and characterization of *Agrobacterium tumefaciens* mutants affected in the utilization of octopine, octopinic acid, and lysopine. J. Gen. Microbiol., 96, 155.

10) CHILTON, M.-D., DRUMMOND, H.J., MERLO, D.J., SCIAKY, D., MONTOYA, A.L., GORDON, M.P. and NESTER, E.W. (1977). Stable incorporation of plasmid DNA into higher plant cells: the molecular basis of crown gall tumorigenesis. Cell, 11, 263.

11) SCHELL, J., VAN MONTAGU, M., DE BEUCKELEER, M., DE BLOCK, M., DEPICKER, A., DE WILDE, M., ENGLER, G., GENETELLO, C., HERNALSTEENS, J.P., HOLSTERS, M., SEURINCK, J., SILVA, B., VAN VLIET, F. and VILLARROEL, R. (1979). Interactions and DNA transfer between *A. tumefaciens,* the Ti-plasmid and the plant host. Proc. R. Soc. Lond. B., 204, 251.

12) SCHELL, J. (1978). The use of the Ti-plasmid as a vector for the introduction of foreign DNA into plants. Proc. IVth Int. Conf. Plant Path. Bact., I.N.R.A.-Angers, 115.

13) DEPICKER, A., VAN MONTAGU, M. and SCHELL, J. (1978). Homologous DNA sequences in different Ti-plasmids are essential for oncogenicity. Nature, 275, 150.

14) MONTOYA, A., CHILTON, M.-D., GORDON, M.P., SCIAKY, D. and NESTER, E.W. (1977). Octopine and nopaline metabolism in *Agrobacterium tumefaciens* and crown-gall tumors cells: role of plasmid genes. J. Bacteriol., 129, 101.

15) VAN MONTAGU, M. and SCHELL, J. (1979). The Ti-plasmids of *A. tumafaciens*. In: "Plasmids of medical environmental and commercial importance" (eds., K. Timmis and A. Pühler), Elsevier/North Holland Medical Press, Amsterdam, 71.

16) TOMASHOW, M., PANAGOPOULOS, C., GORDON, M.P. and NESTER, E.W. (1979). Host range of *A. tumefaciens* is determined by the Ti-plasmid, in press.

17) KERR, A., MANIGAULT, P. and TEMPÉ, J. (1977). Transfer of virulence *in vivo* and *in vitro* in *Agrobacterium*. Nature, 265, 560.

18) GENETELLO, C., VAN LAREBEKE, N., HOLSTERS, M., DEPICKER, A.,

VAN MONTAGU, M. and SCHELL, J. (1977). Ti-plasmids of *Agrobacterium* as conjugative plasmids. Nature, 265, 561.

19) BREVET, J., KOPECKO, D.J., NISEN, P. and COHEN, S.N. (1977). Promotion of insertions and deletions by translocating segments of DNA carrying antibiotic resistance genes. In: "DNA, insertion elements, plasmids, and episomes". (ed., A.I. Bukhari, J.A. Shapiro and S.L. Adhya), Cold Spring Harbor Laboratory, N.Y., 169.

20) HOLSTERS, M., SILVA, B., VAN VLIET, F., GENETELLO, C., DE BLOCK, M., DHAESE, P., DEPICKER, A., INZE, D., ENGLER, G., VILLARROEL, R., VAN MONTAGU, M. and SCHEll, J. (1979). The functional organization of nopaline *A. tumefaciens* plasmid pTiC58. Submitted to Plasmid.

21) DHAESE, P., DE GREVE, H., DECRAEMER, H., SCHELL, J. and VAN MONTAGU, M. (1979). Rapid mapping of transposon insertion and deletion mutations in the large Ti-plasmids of *A. tumefaciens*. Submitted to Nucleic Acids Research.

22) Unpublished work of the authors' laboratory:
a) DE VOS, G., *et al.*, in preparation.
b) HERNALSTEENS, J.P., *et al,*, in preparation.
c) DE GREVE, H., *et al.*, in preparation.
d) DEPICKER, A., *et al.*, in preparation.
e) DE BLOCK, M., *et al.*, in preparation.
f) ENGLER, G., *et al.*, in preparation.
g) SEURINCK, J., *et al.,* in preparation.
h) DE BEUCKELEER, M., *et al.*, in preparation.
i) VAN HAUTE, E., *et al.*, in preparation.
j) LEEMANS, J., *et al.*, in preparation.
k) WILLMITZER, L., *et al.*, in preparation.
m) O'FARRELL, P., *et al.*, in preparation.

23) DEPICKER, A., DE WILDE, M., DE VOS, G., DE VOS, R., VAN MONTAGU, M. and SCHELL, J. (1979). Molecular cloning of overlapping segments of the nopaline Ti-plasmid pTiC58 as a means to restriction endonuclease mapping. Submitted to Plasmid.

24) ELLIS, J.G., KERR, A., VAN MONTAGU, M. and SCHELL, J. (1979). *Agrobacterium:* genetic studies on agrocin 84 production and the biological control of crown gall. Physiol. Plant Path., in press.

25) VAN LAREBEKE, N., GENETELLO, C., HERNALSTEENS, J.P., DEPICKER, A., ZAENEN, I., MESSENS, E., VAN MONTAGU, M. and SCHELL, J. (1977). Transfer of Ti-plasmids between *Agrobacterium* strains by mobilization with conjugative plasmid RP4. Molec. Gen. Genet., 152, 119.

26) ENGLER, G., HOLSTERS, M., VAN MONTAGU, M., SCHELL, J., HERNALSTEENS, J.P. and SCHILPEROORT, R.A. (1975). Agrocin 84 sensitivity: a plasmid determined property in *Agrobacterium tumefaciens*. Molec. Gen. Genet., 138, 345.

27) ELLIS, J., KERR, A., TEMPÉ, J. and PETIT, A. (1979). Arginine catabolism: a new function of both octopine and nopaline Ti-plasmids of *Agrobacterium*. Molec. Gen. Genet., 173, 263.

28) FIRMIN, J.L. and FENWICK, R.G. (1978). Agropine - a major new plasmid-determined metabolite in crown gall tumors. Nature, 276, 842.

29) KLAPWIJK, P.M., SCHEULDERMON, T. and SCHILPEROORT, R.A. (1978). Co-ordinated regulation of octopine degradation and conjugative transfer of Ti-plasmids in *Agrobacterium tumefaciens*: Evidence for a common regulatory gene and separate operons. J. Bacteriol., 136, 775.

30) PETIT, A., TEMPÉ, J., KERR, A., HOLSTERS, M., VAN MONTAGU, M. and SCHELL, J. (1978). Substrate induction of conjugative activity of *Agrobacterium tumefaciens* Ti-plasmids. Nature, 271, 570.

31) LIPPINCOTT, B.B., WHATLEY, M.H. and LIPPINCOTT. J. (1977). Tumor induction by *Agrobacterium* involves attachment of the bacterium to a site on the host plant cell wall. Plant Physiol., 59, 388.

32) MATTHYSSE, A., WYMAN, P. and HOLMES, K. (1978). Plasmid-dependent attachment of *Agrobacterium tumefaciens* to plant tissue

culture cells. Infect. Immun., 22, 516.

33) WHATLEY, M.H., MARGOT, J.B., SCHELL, J., LIPPINCOTT, B.B. and LIPPINCOTT, J.A. (1978). Plasmid and chromosomal determination of *Agrobacterium* adherence specificity. J. Gen. Microbiol., 107, 395.

34) GURLEY, W.B., KEMP, J.D., ALBERT, M.J., SUTTON, D.W. and CALLIS, J. (1979). Transcription of Ti-plasmid derived sequences in three octopine-type crown gall tumor lines. Proc. Natl. Acad. Sci. USA., 76, 2828.

35) TURGEON, R., WOOD, M.N. and BRAUN, A.C. (1976). Studies on the recovery of Crown gall tumor cells. Proc. Natl. Acad. Sci. USA, 73, 3562.

EXPRESSION OF MESSENGER RNAs INJECTED INTO *XENOPUS LAEVIS* OOCYTES

G. Marbaix and G. Huez

Laboratoire de Chimie Biologique
Département de Biologie Moléculaire
Université Libre de Bruxelles
B-1640 Rhode St-Genèse, Belgium

1. INTRODUCTION

The genetic information carried by eukaryotic messenger RNAs can be translated to polypeptides either in cell-free protein synthesizing systems or after microinjection into living cells.

Cell-free or *in vitro* systems are, in brief, constituted of cellular lysates or homogenates from which membranes, nuclei and mitochondria have been removed by low speed centrifugation. To date, the wheat-germ (1) and the reticulocyte (2) systems are the most widely utilized. In the case of the reticulocyte lysate, a micrococcal nuclease pre-treatment is used (2) to degrade the endogenous messenger RNA. In other cases, a pre-incubation of the system is performed to get rid of these mRNAs. The main advantage of *in vitro* protein synthesizing systems is that their background incorporation of labelled amino acids into proteins is low. The translation efficiency of an added preparation of messenger RNA can thus be measured simply by looking at the stimulation of this incorporation. Analysis of the translation products is also simplified by the almost complete absence of endogenous protein synthesis. One has to notice here that generally, mRNA samples to be tested in cell-free systems must be relatively devoid of ribosomal RNA contaminants which hinder translation. Further characteristics of the *in vitro* systems will be given hereafter by comparison with the *in vivo* system constituted by *Xenopus laevis* oocytes.

Microinjection of messenger RNA into living cells was almost simultaneously initiated with muscle cells (3) and with frog (*Xenopus laevis*) oocytes and eggs (4, 5). It was supposed that, if there was no species - nor cell type - incompatibility between the translation machinery of these cells and a messenger RNA preparation from another type of cell and (or) species, translation of the injected mRNA would occur.

The messenger RNA which has been used in the first study of oocytes microinjection was rabbit globin mRNA isolated and purified according to methods developed in our laboratory (6, 7, 8). A first evidence for the translation of added globin mRNA in a reticulocyte lysate system had just been obtained at that time (9).

2. *XENOPUS* OOCYTE MICROINJECTION PROCEDURE

Full-grown oocytes of the South African frog *Xenopus laevis* (10, 11) are enormous cells of approximately 1 to 1.2 mm in diameter which can withstand the injection of a 50 nl volume of an aqueous RNA solution. This frog is commercially available and can supply oocytes all the year long: this is the reason why its oocytes are preferred to those of other amphibians for mRNA microinjection studies. Oocytes or eggs from other amphibians may, however, be used (11a).

Clusters of oocytes taken from the ovaries of *Xenopus* females can be kept in Barth (12) saline medium (modified according to Gurdon (13)) for a few days at 19°C. In the microinjection technique that we use, the biggest oocytes of these clusters are isolated using watchmaker's forceps but the follicle cells which surround them are generally not removed. Oocytes are then placed in small half-spherical inserts made in the bottom of a plastic dish filled with modified Barth medium and injected under immersion. Micropipettes 15 to 20 μm in diameter are made from 2 μl commercial capillaries using an automatic microforge. The volume of solution to be delivered is measured by looking at the displacement of the meniscus in the capillary using a binocular equipped with a micrometric scale.

The oocytes may then be incubated for several hours or several days at 19°C in a small volume of modified Barth medium (50 to 100 μl for 10 oocytes) containing the radioactive amino acid used to label the synthesized proteins.

3. TRANSLATION OF RABBIT GLOBIN mRNA IN *XENOPUS* OOCYTES: A TYPICAL EXAMPLE

All details about this study as well as further information are given elsewhere (4, 5, 14, 15 and 16).

An aqueous solution of 9S rabbit reticulocyte RNA which was at that time with good reasons presumed (6, 7, 8, 9) to be globin mRNA was microinjected as previously described into a batch of several oocytes. The RNA concentration was 400 μg/ml and the injected volume was 50 nl per oocyte; haemin was also included in the injected solution. Another batch of cells was injected with injection medium devoid of RNA as a control. The two sets of oocytes were then incubated for 15 hrs in modified Barth medium containing [^{3}H]-histidine (50 Ci/mMole and 100 μCi/ml). At the end of the incubation, the two batches of oocytes were washed in Barth solution and separately homogenized in a buffer containing carrier rabbit haemoglobin (10 mg/ml). Cell debris and yolk platelets were removed by low speed centrifugation and the supernatants were analyzed by molecular filtration on Sephadex G-100 columns prepared in homogenization buffer.

The result of this analysis is shown in Fig. 1. In the elution profile corresponding to control oocytes (A), one observes a peak of excluded radioactive material which corresponds to endogenously synthesized proteins and a peak of retarded material corresponding to free [^{3}H]-histidine. No radioactivity peak is observed in the region where rabbit haemoglobin is eluted from the column. On the contrary, in the profile corresponding to oocytes injected with 9S RNA (B) an appreciable amount of radioactive material is eluted in a region which perfectly coincides with that of haemoglobin. Part of this material was submitted to polyacrylamide gel electrophoresis and shown to migrate exactly as rabbit haemoglobin (5). We thus concluded that the protein material whose synthesis is determined by 9S RNA injection into frog oocytes behaves like rabbit haemoglobin as far as its molecular weight and electric charge are concerned.

Further analyses were performed to definitely establish whether this material is rabbit haemoglobin. It was shown that it can be dissociated into two polypeptides which behave like α and β rabbit globin chains when chromatographed on a carboxymethyl-cellulose column (5). Finally, a definitive identification of the polypeptides synthesized in frog oocytes under the direction of 9S reticulocyte RNA to α and β rabbit globin chains was established by the characterization of tryptic peptides obtained from the supposed rabbit haemoglobin made in *Xenopus* cells. These peptides were indeed shown to be identical to those obtained by tryptic digestion of genuine α and β rabbit globin (15).

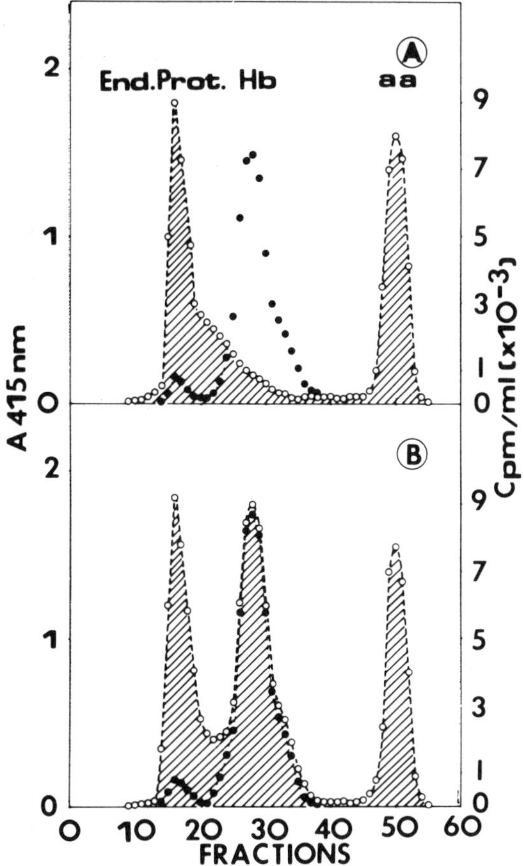

Fig. 1. *Molecular filtration profiles on Sephadex G100 columns of proteins synthesized by oocytes injected either with control buffer (A) or with a rabbit globin mRNA solution (B).* After microinjection, oocytes were incubated with [^{3}H]-histidine for 15 hrs. At the end of the incubation, oocytes were washed and homogenized in Tris-glycine buffer 0.05 M pH 8.9 (1 ml for 10 oocytes) containing rabbit haemoglobin (10 mg/ml). Cellular debris and yolk platelets were removed by centrifugation and supernatants analyzed on Sephadex columns made in Tris-glycine buffer. This is a typical result from the initial work of J.B. Gurdon, C.D. Lane and G. Marbaix. —●— Absorbance at 415 nm (carrier haemoglobin); ---- 0 ---- Radioactivity.

These results, when first published (5, 15), confirmed and extended those of Lockard and Lingrel (9) who had brought the first convincing indication that the 9S reticulocyte RNA fraction contains globin mRNA. This work using the frog oocyte injection system indeed brought the most complete characterization of α and β globin chains synthesized in an heterologous translation system under the direction of 9S reticulocyte RNA.

4. CHARACTERIZATION OF THE *XENOPUS* OOCYTE TRANSLATION SYSTEM

Useful general information can be found in Refs. 4, 17, 18, 19, 20 and 21.

(i) Lack of species - and cell type-specificity of the *Xenopus* oocyte system

We have seen that the cellular system constituted by *Xenopus* oocytes is able to translate the mRNAs coding for rabbit haemoglobin which are messages from a differentiated mammalian cell. There thus does not seem to exist any cell type - nor species - specificity restriction when the translation machinery of frog oocytes is confronted with a messenger RNA from a differentiated tissue of another vertebrate. Numerous examples of this lack of specificity have been obtained since this first observation was made. Messenger RNAs from various specialized tissues of several animals, vertebrates (22, 23, 24, 25, 26, 27, 28, 28a) or not (29) as well as viral RNAs (30, 31, 32) have been successfully translated in *Xenopus* oocytes*. These cells are even able to translate vegetal (cellular (33, 34) and viral (35, 35a, 36, 37)) and myxomycete (38) messages*.

An example of plant viral mRNA translation is given at Fig. 2. This result was obtained in collaboration with Tineke Rutgers and Lous van Vloten-Doting from Leiden (37). Aqueous solutions of genomic RNAs 1, 2, 3 and of RNA 4 of the multicompoment Brome Mosaic

---

*The given list of mRNAs translated in oocytes is not intended to be complete.

Virus have been injected into *Xenopus* oocytes (50 nl per cell at 1 mg/ml). After incubation at $19^{o}C$ for 15 hrs with [^{3}H]-leucine in the medium, the oocytes were homogenized in Tris-glycine buffer, yolk platelets were removed by low speed centrifugation and the synthesized proteins were analyzed by SDS-polyacrylamide gel electrophoresis followed by fluorography of the dried gel. The results of this experiment show that the four viral RNA species are translated into 4 polypeptides having molecular weights of 125,000, 112,000, 34,000 and 23,000, respectively. The product coded for by RNA 4 is the coat protein. Function(s) of the other polypeptides is (are) still unknown.

The demonstration that the frog oocyte translation machinery can accommodate all kinds of eukaryotic mRNAs tested was a very important fact. This constituted a powerful argument against a supposed role of tissue-specific translation factors in differentiation.

On the other hand, translation of prokaryotic messages (which lack a cap) like f2 , MS_2 or Qβ phage RNAs into frog oocytes has not been detected up to now (4, and our unpublished results in collaboration with W. Fiers and C. Weissmann). This is probably due to the rapid degradation of mRNAs lacking a "cap" in oocytes (39). It was indeed recently shown that *in vitro* capped prokaryotic mRNAs can be efficiently translated in a eukaryotic cell-free system (40). Synthetic polynucleotides are not translated in *Xenopus* oocytes (41) and are rapidly degraded (42), with the exception of polyadenylic acid which is stable.

(ii) <u>Fidelity of injected message translation in oocytes</u>

We shall consider two different levels of fidelity. First, we may ask whether the translation machinery of the oocyte makes erroneous amino acid replacements during translation of a message iso-

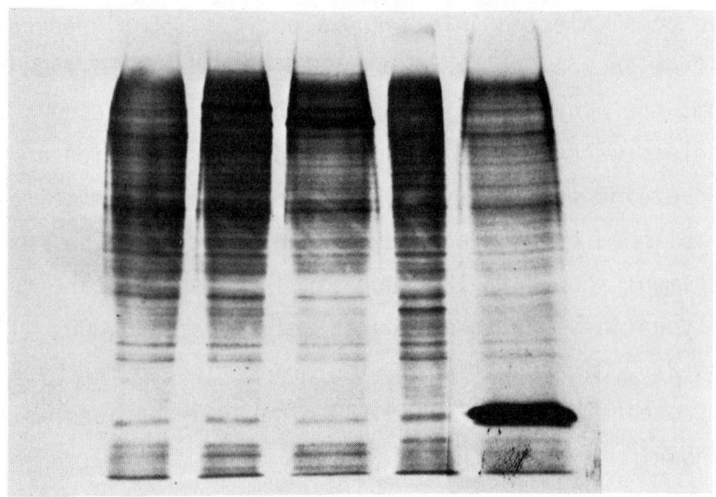

Fig. 2. *Fluorograph of a SDS-electrophoresis gel of proteins synthesized by control oocytes and by oocytes injected with either RNAs 1, 2, 3 or 4 of Brome Mosaic Virus.* After injection, cells were incubated with [^{3}H]-leucine for 15 hrs. At the end of the incubation, oocytes were washed and homogenized. Cellular debris and yolk platelets were removed by centrifugation. An aliquot of each supernatant was boiled with SDS and 2-mercaptoethanol and then applied to the gel. From left to right: control uninjected oocytes, oocytes injected with RNA_1*, with RNA_2*, with RNA_3 and with RNA_4. These results were obtained in collaboration with T. Rutgers and L. van Vloten-Doting (37).
*Preparations of RNA_1 and RNA_2 were cross-contaminated.

lated from a different species and (or) tissue? From the initial complete study concerned with the translation of rabbit globin mRNA in frog oocytes (5, 15), we have good reasons to assume that if such errors happen, they are extremely infrequent. Furthermore, in all examples of foreign message translation inside oocytes, it has never been possible to suspect such replacements and, on the contrary, the oocyte translation products always behave like the genuine proteins.

Another possibility is to obtain incomplete translation products of injected messages in *Xenopus* oocytes. This often happens with *in vitro* systems. These are indeed cell-free extracts inevitably contaminated by proteolytic and nucleolytic enzymes. In these systems, translation of a given unique message often gives rise, especially when a high molecular weight mRNA is used, to multiple incomplete translation products due to mRNA (and) protein degradation. This does not seem to occur in frog oocytes. When a messenger RNA preparation is injected into these cells, the message molecules are progressively integrated into the oocyte translation machinery and translation occur in normal, physiological, cellular conditions. Furthermore, partially degraded mRNA molecules are probably rapidly hydrolyzed like injected ribosomal RNA or synthetic polynucleotides (42). Incompleted or wrong protein products are probably also eliminated.

A main advantage of the *in vivo* oocyte system as compared to *in vitro* systems thus comes from this important property: oocytes are normal living cells. One may thus hope to observe the synthesis of correct physiological translation products when a given mRNA preparation is injected into them. Some examples will be given now.

The high molecular weight Tobacco Mosaic Virus (TMV) genomic RNA has been shown to be translated to a single 140,000 Daltons polypeptide unrelated to the virus coat protein when injected into *Xenopus* oocytes (35). Even if the function of this polypeptide is not yet established, this unique translation product much more probably corresponds to a physiological entity than the multiple synthesized polypeptides previously observed in *in vitro* systems. The same kind of result has been observed when the high molecular weight RNA_1 and RNA_2 of Brome Mosaic Virus have been injected into frog oocytes (37) (see Fig. 2), each genomic RNA being translated to a single high molecular weight polypeptide.

The ability of the oocyte system to translate large messenger RNAs to well-defined products helped to solve the problem of thyroglobulin quaternary structure determination. It was indeed shown that the 33S mRNA coding for this protein was translated in frog oocytes to a 300,000 Daltons polypeptide (43). As thyroglobulin has a molecular weight of 660,000, it was concluded that it has a dimeric structure.

The fidelity of the oocyte system is also proven by the fact that injected mRNAs are translated to biologically active products. This is the case, for example, of mouse β-glucuronidase (44) and human or mouse interferons (25, 45, 46) mRNAs.

(iii) Translation efficiency of the oocyte system

When a messenger RNA preparation is injected into *Xenopus* oocytes, its maximum rate of translation is of course not immediately reached. Some time is needed for the diffusion of the message molecules in the cytoplasm and for their association with the various factors required for translation. Contrarily to what was first believed (14), there is no spare translational capacity in oocytes and the injected mRNA has to compete with the endogenous messages for translation (47). A steady-state of constant translation rate of exogenous mRNA is reached after 7 to 20 hrs (48, 49, 50) provided that this mRNA species is stable.

At low concentration of injected mRNA (smaller than 10 ng per oocyte for globin mRNA), a linear relationship is observed between this concentration and the translation rate; at higher concentration, a sort of "saturation" is reached (14, 51).

The translation efficiency of rabbit β-globin mRNA at 19°C in *Xenopus* oocytes was estimated to be of 30 β-globin molecules synthesized per hour and per mRNA molecule (16). This figure concerns the early steady-state of translation and is approximately half the rate observed in reticulocytes at the same temperature (52). When oocytes age during their *in vitro* incubation, their translation efficiency progressively decreases; however, as far as a stable mRNA is injected, its translation may proceed from 4 to 15 days depending on the batch of cells which is used (16). Reinitiation on an injected β-globin mRNA molecule may thus occur from around 2,000 to around 6,000 times in *Xenopus* oocytes whilst it occurs a few times only in *in vitro* systems. These last systems are indeed active for one or two hrs only. It is worth noting here that a mRNA preparation does not need to be pure for efficient translation in oocytes: total cellular RNA may even be used (53).

Rabbit β-globin mRNA is one of the most efficiently translated messages when injected into frog oocytes. For example, translation of α-globin message occurs with a much lower yield; however, injection of haemin at the same time as α-globin mRNA makes its translation as efficient as that of β-globin mRNA (54). Nothing is known yet concerning the mechanisms of this control. Several other mRNA species are also translated with a relatively low yield in *Xenopus* oocytes. This is the case of thyroglobulin mRNA (43) and of the 35S genomic RNAs of retroviruses (31, 32), for example. In these cases, the translation products can only be detected in oocytes homogenates by antibody precipitation.

5. USE OF FROG OOCYTES FOR THE STUDY OF THE ROLE OF THE POLYADENYLATE SEGMENT OF EUKARYOTIC MESSENGER RNAs

It is not the purpose of this section to bring a comprehensive survey of the present knowledge concerning all aspects of the 3'-OH polyadenylate segment (Poly(A)) of eukaryotic messenger RNAs. This can be found in recent (55, 56) and less recent (57-60) reviews. What we want to remind here is that the frog oocyte system allowed to clearly prove a role of this poly(A) stretch in the mechanisms which ensure the stability of some eukaryotic messenger RNAs. A detailed report of the results which will be reported hereafter has been published recently (61).

From the work of several groups, it was known that 3'-OH poly(A) is not required for the translation of messenger RNAs (62, 63, 64). This was shown by comparing the efficiencies of translation of native and of enzymatically deadenylated preparations of mRNAs in cell-free protein synthesizing systems. These efficiencies were found to be similar. However, in the case of a particularly good *in vitrc* system working for more than one hour and a half, it was noticed that the protein synthesis directed by messenger RNA lacking poly(A) levelled off sooner than that directed by native mRNA (64). Cell-free protein synthesizing systems were anyway certainly not the most adequate to detect a possible effect of poly(A) on the stability of the message. These systems are indeed short-lived, they generally work for 30 to 90 minutes and each message molecule is but translated a few times. We thus decided to use the long-lived *in vivo* system constituted by *Xenopus* oocytes to compare the stability of native and poly(A)-free rabbit globin mRNA. This study was made possible by a fruitful cooperation with the group of Professor U.Z. Littauer in Rehovot where Hermona Soreq developed a very specific method for the removal of the 3'-OH poly(A) segment of messenger RNAs (64, 65).

(i) Experimental studies

The stabilities of native and deadenylated globin mRNAs were thus compared after their injection into frog oocytes. Stabilities were first estimated by measurement of globin synthesis in the injected cells different times after injection (48). Later on, the amount of globin mRNA present in cells was directly measured by molecular hybridization with a radioactive complementary DNA probe synthesized on rabbit globin mRNA as a template using reverse transcriptase from Avian Myeloblastosis Virus (66). These experiments showed that native globin mRNA is very stable and efficiently translated for several days in frog oocytes (this had been already shown

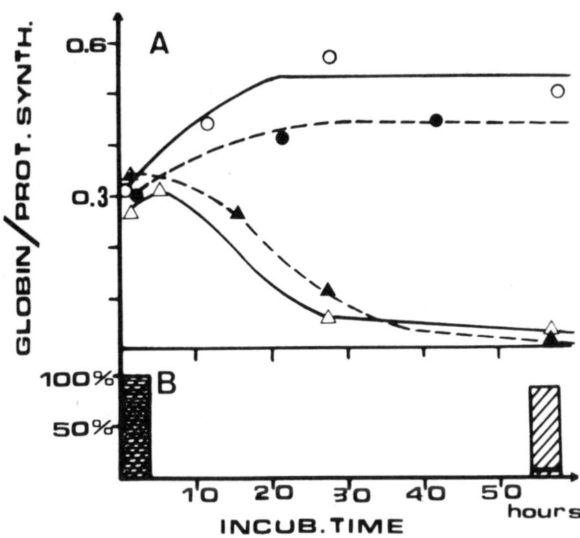

Fig. 3. A. *Stability of various globin mRNA preparations injected into frog oocytes as measured by their capacity to direct globin synthesis.* O = native mRNA; Δ = deadenylated mRNA; ▲ = mRNA containing a poly(A) segment with less than 20 A residues; ● = deadenylated and then readenylated mRNA. B. *Stability of native* (▨) *and deadenylated* (▤) *globin mRNA preparations into frog oocytes as measured by molecular hybridization with a* [^3H] *complementary DNA probe*. From Ref. 84, with required authorizations.

in Ref. 16) whilst poly(A)-free message works but for a short period of time and is rapidly degraded (see Fig. 3).

An objection to this conclusion was that the polynucleotide phosphorylase treatment required to remove the poly(A) sequence could have affected another part of the message molecule which really would be responsible for the stability. It was thus necessary to show that readdition of a new polyadenylate segment to a previously deadenylated message molecule is sufficient to restore its stability. This could be done thanks to the collaboration of René Devos from Professors W. Fiers and R. Gillis laboratories in Ghent. Poly(A) was readded at the 3'-OH end of poly(A)-free globin mRNA using an

ATP : RNA adenyltransferase from *E. coli* (67) and this "reconstituted" mRNA was indeed shown to be as stable as native poly(A)-containing mRNA (68). The poly(A) segment itself is thus necessary to ensure the stability of globin mRNA. It is of course not known whether it is sufficient!

We then asked the question: "How is the stability of globin mRNA related to the length of the poly(A) stretch?" We thus tested the stability of several batches of globin mRNA with decreasing sizes of poly(A) sequences after their injection into frog oocytes. These globin mRNA preparations with well-defined poly(A) lengths had been prepared in Professor Littauer's laboratory. The answer we obtained was: "There is not proportionality between stability and poly(A) length but, when reduced to a threshold value of 10 to 20 adenylate residues, the poly(A) stretch does not ensure stability any more" (69). This observation can be correlated with that of Perry and Kelley who observed that, *in vivo*, messenger RNAs with long poly(A) stretches are not more stable than mRNAs with short poly(A) stretches (70). To conciliate these facts with the fact that poly(A) shortens when mRNAs physiologically age (71-75), one has to conclude that as long as poly(A) has a sufficient size, message stability is ensured but also that poly(A) is stochastically degraded by endonucleolytic cleavage.

The oocyte microinjection system and the possibility to add a labelled poly(A) segment at the 3' end of a message molecule offered the opportunity to directly determine the way the 3'-OH poly(A) sequence of a messenger RNA is degraded in a living cell, namely in *Xenopus* oocytes. We thus prepared two samples of globin mRNA carrying a radioactive poly(A) stretch. The first one contained around 45 [^{3}H]-labelled adenylate residues added at the 3' end of the unlabelled poly(A) segment of native globin mRNA. The second preparation contained but 0.6 (mean value) labelled adenylate residue added at the end of native globin mRNA. The two labelled mRNA samples were injected into different sets of oocytes and the TCA-precipitable radioactivity still present in cells was measured after increasing periods of incubation. It was observed that the degradation kinetics of labelled poly(A) sequences was the same in both cases (61). The most straightforward interpretation of this result is that the poly(A) segment is not degraded by an exonucleolytic process but by a stochastic endonucleolytic cleavage as indirectly deduced above.

The studies about the role of poly(A) that we reported up to now have been made using rabbit globin mRNA only. It was important to see whether the concept of stabilization of eukaryotic mRNAs by 3'-OH polyadenylation is general. An interesting case is that of HeLa cells histone mRNAs which are naturally devoid of poly(A). We obtained these message molecules from Dieter Gallwitz in Marburg and we studied their stability after injection into oocytes as well as the effect of 3'-OH polyadenylation on this stability. Stabilities of both native and polyadenylated mRNA preparations were estimated by measurement of histones synthesis in the injected cells different times after microinjection (76). One can see at Fig. 4 that synthesis of four histones is clearly detected in oocytes injected with both message fractions. This synthesis begins to decrease 7 hrs after injection in the case of oocytes injected with native message whilst it increases during the first 19 hrs and is still very high more than 43 hrs after injection if polyadenylated histone mRNA is used. It is thus clear that the addition of a 40 adenylic residues long poly(A) segment at the 3'-OH end of the four naturally poly(A)-free mRNAs coding for H_3, H_{2b}, H_{2a} and H_4 human histones functionally stabilises these messages (76). These results thus extend our previous conclusion obtained from experiments using native and deadenylated globin mRNA.

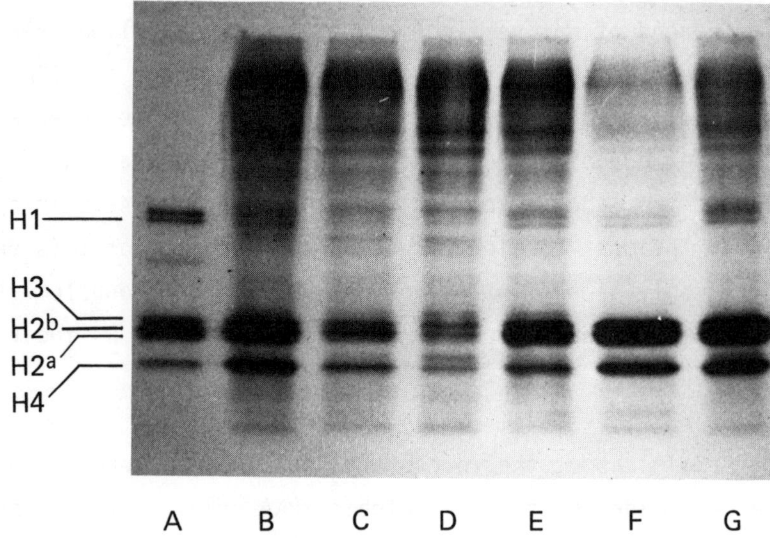

Fig. 4. *Fluorograph of a SDS-polyacrylamide gel electrophoresis of proteins from oocytes injected with either native histone mRNA from HeLa cells (channels b-d) or this mRNA fraction previously polyadenylated (channels e-g).* At different times after microinjection, sets of oocytes from each batch were incubated with [^{3}H]-lysine for several hrs period. a = reference ^{14}C HeLa cells histones. Incubation periods: b; e, 0-7 hrs; c-f, 7-19 hrs; d, g, 43-60 hrs. From Ref. 76, with required authorizations.

(ii) <u>Conclusions and discussion about the role of poly(A)</u>

From our above reported work, we conclude that one role for the 3'-OH poly(A) segment of eukaryotic messenger RNAs is to ensure their stability in the cytoplasm during translation. It is known that human globin mRNA (77), human placental lactogen mRNA (78), *Xenopus* liver vitellogenin and albumin mRNAs (4) and carp proinsulin mRNA (T. Rapoport, personal communication) are translated for long periods of time after their injection into frog oocytes. These results about several polyadenylated mRNAs are thus in perfect agreement with ours. On the other hand, a recent report (79) concerning the stability of human interferon mRNA injected into *Xenopus* oocytes claims that deadenylation of this message does not modify its stability which is already quite low for the native polyadenylated molecule. However, in this paper, the authors estimated the stability of the mRNA preparations by looking at the kinetics of interferon accumulation inside the oocytes only. As it is known that the synthesized interferon is secreted outside these cells after injection of interferon mRNA (46), it thus seems that these results have to be reconsidered.

The molecular mechanism by which the poly(A) segment ensures its protective function is still unknown. One may suppose that the 78,000 Daltons protein specifically associated with the polyadenylate sequence of eukaryotic mRNAs (80) plays some role in this protection. From what we presently know, we may assume that given mRNA species are provided, after their synthesis, with poly(A) segments which will stochastically shorten later by endonucleolytic cleavage. When such a cleavage happens to occur in the proximal region of the poly(A), leaving a too short residual poly(A) sequence at the 3'-OH end of the mRNA molecule, this molecule is rapidly degraded (69) by a mechanism that we have shown to require translation (81).

The presence of a long enough 3'-OH poly(A) segment is required to ensure the stability of some species of mRNA but this necessary condition could not be sufficient. Another structure in the mRNA molecule is perhaps also required. It is indeed worth to report here that polyadenylation of the RNA_4 of Alfalfa Mosaic Virus which codes for the coat protein and which is not naturally adenylated does not increase at all the stability of this message when injected into frog oocytes (our unpublished observations in collaboration with L. van Vloten-Doting and T. Rutgers). On the other hand, it is not excluded that mRNA-stabilizing mechanisms other than the poly(A)-associated one might exist in eukaryotic organisms. One may also think that the poly(A) segment could fulfil other functions in eukaryotic mRNA metabolism.

6. THE "CAP" OF EUKARYOTIC mRNAs AND FROG OOCYTES

Most eukaryotic messenger RNAs (a few viral mRNAs are the exception) carry a peculiar structure called "cap" at their 5'-end. This "cap" consists of 7-methylguanosine post-transcriptionally added to the mRNA nuclear precursor and linked by a 5' to 5' bond to the first 5' nucleotide of the transcribed RNA molecule. Numerous studies using *in vitro* protein synthesizing systems have generally shown (there are several conflicting reports) that this structure most probably plays an important role in the initiation of eukaryotic mRNAs translation (40, 56, 82).

Since they are concerned with *in vivo* situations, two studies using the frog oocyte system have brought interesting results concerning the role of the "cap" in mRNA translation. A first work (39) shows that the presence of a "cap" or even 5'-blocking of mRNA with unmethylated guanosine protects reovirus mRNA against degradation after injection into *Xenopus* oocytes. A second work (83) shows that the presence of a "cap" structure is required for injected globin mRNA translation to occur in oocytes. In this last study, the authors have not checked whether the "decapped" globin mRNA they injected was rapidly degraded: this could explain their observation. It is thus worth to keep in mind that a role for the "cap" might be to protect mRNA against degradation. However, this does not seem to be the unique function of this structure since, from the work of Furuichi *et al.* (39), 5'-blocking of mRNA with unmethylated guanosine is sufficient to protect it against 5'-exonucleolytic degradation whilst initiation of translation furthermore requires methylation to give the complete "cap".

7. POST-TRANSLATIONAL MODIFICATIONS OF ALIEN POLYPEPTIDES SYNTHESIZED IN mRNA-INJECTED OOCYTES

It was noticed very soon that the translation products of mRNAs injected into *Xenopus* oocytes undergo in these cells the same post-translational modifications that they normally undergo in their native cells. Some examples are: N-acetylation of terminal methionine in calf lens epithelium αA_2 crystallin (22), phosphorylation of trout testis protamines (unpublished results of T. Wu, S. Gilmour, G. Dixon and J.B. Gurdon quoted in Refs. 18 and 20), of *Xenopus* liver vitellogenin (49) and glycosylation of immunoglobulins (85, 86). Another type of post-translational processing of injected mRNAs translation products which occurs in frog oocytes is the cleavage either of a precursor polypeptide to several proteins (this is the case for the structural proteins of several viruses (30-32, 87) and for yolk platelets proteins (49)) or of a "signal" hydrophobic peptide (88, 89) whose role is to guide into the lumen of the endoplasmic reticulum proteins made for export or storage in cytoplasmic vesicles (this is the case for immunoglobulin light chain (90), albumin, milk proteins (91), promellitin (29), proinsulin (92) and placental lactogen (78)). Subcellular compartmentation of albumin and globin made in *Xenopus* oocytes under the direction of injected messenger RNAs even occurs (91). Furthermore, interferon, a protein which is normally exported from the producer cell is most probably exported from frog oocytes when synthesized under direction of injected mRNA (46).

It thus appears that post-translational events which normally occur in a wide variety of differentiated cells from various animals can also occur in the oocyte of *Xenopus laevis*, a cell which is not naturally designed to encounter these foreign polypeptides. This means either that most post-translational modifications of proteins are not due to specialized enzymatic equipments of differentiated tissues or that the informational RNA for the synthesis of the specialized enzymes has been injected into oocytes at the same time as the mRNA coding for the considered protein. This last hypothesis can be eliminated for most situations with the exception of the formation of some types of viral proteins (31, 32, 87) (see later).

The conclusion is thus: "This lack of cell-type specificity of modifying enzyme systems suggests that the existence of modified proteins in a cell is determined by the availability of amino acid sequences (and we shall add: or (and) secondary or (and) tertiary structures) on which enzymes act and not by the availability of the enzymes themselves". (J.B. Gurdon (18)).

An interesting comparison of the oocyte and an *in vitro* translation system concerning some post-translational modifications of mRNA translation products was given by Mous *et al.* (93).

(i) Complete processing of the precursor polypeptide to Avian Myeloblastosis Virus (AMV) virion structural proteins in *Xenopus* oocytes

Useful information concerning the mechanism of production of Avian Myeloblastosis Virus (a retrovirus) virion structural proteins has been obtained using the frog oocyte system. This will be given now with some details as an example of what can be learned using this system. Detailed information can be found in Refs 31 and 94.

When injected into frog oocytes, the 35S genomic RNA of AMV is translated to the precursor for the group - specific antigens of the virus ("gag" proteins, constitutive of the inner core of the virion). Furthermore, if a "pulse-chase" experiment is performed with AMV 35S RNA injected oocytes, one observes that this Pr 76 precursor is progressively processed to the final p27, p19 and p12/15 virion constitutive proteins. As shown in the original work (31), it is clear that all final products of the processing of Pr 76 as well as the cleavage intermediate polypeptides are made in the oocyte as they are in the infected cells which normally harbor the virus (95).

In order to learn more about the origin (viral or cellular) of the enzymatic activities involved in the cleavage of the Pr 76 pre-

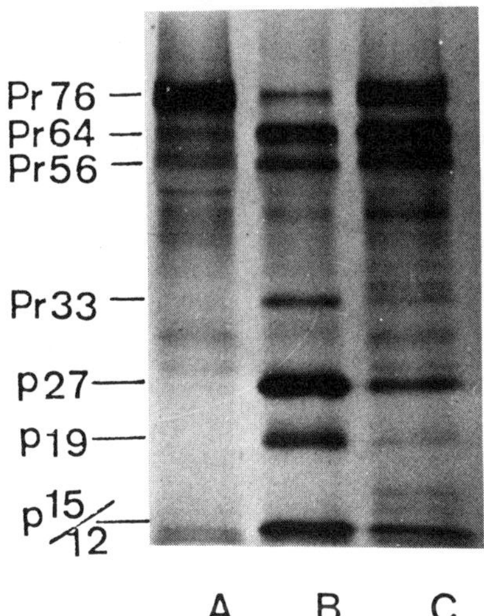

Fig. 5. *Fluorograph of a SDS-electrophoresis gel of immunoprecipitates of Avian Myeloblastosis Virus (AMV) proteins made in oocytes.* Immunoprecipitation was done with a polyvalent antiserum raised against AMV. (A) Viral proteins from oocytes injected with 35S AMV genomic RNA and incubated for 4 hrs at 19°C in Barth medium containing [^{35}S]-methionine. (B) Viral proteins resulting from a "chase" in oocytes preinjected with viral RNA: labelled proteins from oocytes treated as at (A) were injected in other oocytes which had been previously injected with viral RNA 24 hrs before and not labelled. These oocytes were then further incubated for another 48 hrs period in an unlabelled medium. (C) Viral protein resulting from a "chase" in oocytes not preinjected with viral RNA (see B). From Ref. 94, with required authorizations.

cursor polypeptide, the following experiment was then performed. Oocytes were injected with 35S RNA from AMV. They were subsequently incubated with [^{35}S]-methionine for a short period of time (4 hrs). In these conditions, enough labelled Pr 76 is synthesized while no significant processing of this polypeptide has time to occur. After this incubation, the oocytes were homogenized and the extract was dialyzed in order to eliminate the free labelled amino acid. Part of this homogenate was then injected into two separate batches of oocytes. The oocytes from one of these batches had received an injection of AMV RNA 24 hrs before and had been incubated without radioactive amino acid for this period of time. The other batch was constituted of control uninjected oocytes also incubated for 24 hrs without labelled amino acid. After injection of the extract containing the labelled Pr 76, the two sets of oocytes were incubated for another 48 hrs period in an unlabelled medium. At the end of this period, the oocytes were homogenized and their content of labelled viral proteins analyzed by gel electrophoresis after immunoprecipitation. The result of this experiment is given at Fig. 5. It is clear that the processing of the Pr 76 precursor is by far more pronounced in the oocytes which were allowed to synthesize viral proteins before the injection of the extract containing the labelled Pr 76.

From the results presented above, it can be concluded that a virus-encoded protein is involved in the cleavage of the Pr 76 precursor and that there is no need for the injection of a "viral processing factor" together with the viral RNA to obtain a perfect cleavage of this precursor. Whether this viral polypeptide is itself the specific processing protease or whether it activates (or modifies) a cellular enzyme present in the host infected cell is still unknown. It is also not clear whether this viral polypeptide is identical to one of the virion structural proteins. There are, however, some arguments in favour of this possibility (94, 96). The most probable hypothesis is that the "viral processing factor" is synthesized as a part of the Pr 76 polypeptide. It would then be generated from this precursor either autocatalytically, or by the action of an oocyte cellular enzyme. If such an enzyme does exist in frog oocyes, one must notice that it does not show any specificity for the precursor "gag" polypeptide of the avian retroviruses. It has indeed been shown that the genomic viral RNA from the bovine leukemia virus can be translated in frog oocytes and that the complete processing of its "gag" precursor to the virion structural proteins also occurs in these cells (32).

8. AMINOACYLATION OF TRANSFER RNAs AND OF TURNIP YELLOW MOSAIC VIRUS RNA INJECTED INTO *XENOPUS* OOCYTES

It is not the purpose of the present paper to review this field of research. However, due to the direct role of transfer RNAs in translation, it is worth to briefly report here a few observations about the fate of these molecules when injected into frog oocytes.

It was first observed that contrarily to ribosomal RNA and synthetic polynucleotides (except poly(A)), transfer RNA is not degraded after injection into *Xenopus* oocytes (42). Later, Gatica *et al.* observed that yeast phe-tRNA is acylated when injected into these cells (97); the acylating capacity of *Xenopus* oocyte was estimated to be sufficient to acylate more than a hundred times its transfer RNA endogenous content. Furthermore, it was shown that the oocyte is able to add the terminal -C-A nucleotides to yeast phe-tRNA lacking these residues (98). Injected aminoacyl tRNAs were also shown to be really utilized in oocyte protein synthesis (99). The same type of observations was made for *E. coli* val-tRNA and for Turnip Yellow Mosaic Virus RNA (100) which had been shown to behave like a transfer RNA *in vitro*.

9. CONCLUSIONS: ADVANTAGES OF THE FROG OOCYTE TRANSLATION SYSTEM

Gurdon *et al.*, in the conclusion of their original work (4) perfectly summarize most of the advantages of the *Xenopus* oocyte translation system. They write: "For the study of messenger RNA and its translation, the microinjection of *Xenopus* eggs and oocytes has three special merits. First, the translation of purified mRNA is undertaken in a normal living cell, and is therefore less likely to be affected by artefacts than a cell-free system. Second, injected oocytes are capable of translating mRNA with a high efficiency for long periods. Finally, *Xenopus* oocytes seem to show very little species specificity with respect to the type of mRNA which they can translate. It seems possible that all kinds of eukaryotic and animal virus mRNA may be capable of translation in *Xenopus* oocytes. The large size, resistance to microinjection, and easy availability of *Xenopus* oocytes has relieved us of the incentive to test the translational usefulness of eggs and oocytes from other animals species (4)". All this still holds true. One may add that mainly due to their fragility, frog eggs are no more used when one simply needs to test mRNA translation, that messenger RNAs do not need to be purified to be translated in oocytes, and that even vegetal virus RNAs have been translated in these cells. A further advantage of the oocyte system is that it performs various types of post-translational modifications of translation products. It thus permits the study of the mechanisms of these processes.

In the present paper, we brought some information about the *Xenopus* oocyte translation system. Let us add that in another part of this book, the reader will learn that the oocyte nucleus (the big "germinal vesicle") can be used as an *in vivo* transcription system for injected genes. Post-transcriptional processing of the injected genes transcription products as well as transfer of produced mRNAs to the cytoplasm also occur in these nuclei.

So, besides their role in the perpetuation of the *Xenopus laevis* species, *Xenopus* oocytes constitute a unique system for the study of all steps of the genetic information transfer from the genes themselves to terminal biologically active proteins.

10. ACKNOWLEDGEMENTS

We thank Professor H. Chantrenne for his interest in our work and for stimulating discussions. We are very much indebted to all colleagues and friends who participated in experiments described in the present review. Part of the work reported here was supported by the Belgian State (Actions Concertées) and by the "Fonds Cancérologique de la Caisse Générale d'Epargne et de Retraite". G.M. and G.H. are fellows of the "Fonds National Belge de la Recherche Scientifique"

11. REFERENCES

1) MARCUS, A, EFRON, D. and WEEKS, D.P. (1974). The wheat embryo cell-free system. Methods in Enzymology, 30, 749.
2) PELHAM, H.R. and JACKSON, R.J. (1976). An efficient mRNA-dependent translation system from reticulocyte lysates. Eur. J. Biochem., 67, 247.
3) GRAESSMANN, A. and GRAESSMANN, M. (1971). The formation of melanin in muscle cells after the direct transfer of RNA from Harding-Passey melanoma cells. Hoppe-Seyler's Z. Physiol. Chem. 352, 527.
4) GURDON, J.B., LANE, C.D., WOODLAND, H.R. and MARBAIX, G. (1971). Use of frog eggs and oocytes for the study of messenger RNA and its translation in living cells. Nature, 233, 177.
5) LANE, C.D. MARBAIX, G. and GURDON, J.B. (1971). Rabbit Haemoglobin synthesis in frog cells: the translation of reticulocyte 9S RNA in frog oocytes. J. Mol. Biol., 61, 73.
6) MARBAIX, G. and BURNY, A. (1964). Separation of the messenger RNA of reticulocyte polyribosomes. Biochem. Biophys. Res. Comm., 16, 522.
7) CHANTRENNE, H., BURNY, A. and MARBAIX, G. (1967). The search for the messenger RNA of hemoglobin. Progress in Nucleic Acid Research and Molecular Biology, 7, 173.
8) HUEZ, G., BURNY, A., MARBAIX, G. and LEBLEU, B. (1967). Release of messenger RNA from rabbit reticulocyte polyribosomes at low concentration of divalent cations. Biochim. Biophys. Acta, 145 629.
9) LOCKARD, R.E. and LINGREL, J.B. (1969). The synthesis of mouse

hemoglobin β-chains in a rabbit reticulocyte cell-free system programmed with mouse reticulocyte 9S RNA. Biochem. Biophys. Res. Comm., 37, 204.

10) DEUCHAR, E. (1975). "*Xenopus*, the South African clawed frog". John Wiley and sons, London.

11) GURDON, J.B. (1967). African clawed frog. In: "Methods in developmental Biology", (eds., F.H. Wilt and N.K. Wessells), Crowell Co., New York, 75.

11a) BRACHET, J., HUEZ, G. and HUBERT, E. (1973). Microinjection of rabbit haemoglobin messenger RNA into amphibian oocytes and embryos. Proc. Natl. Acad. Sci. U.S.A., 70, 543.

12) BARTH, L.G. and BARTH, L.J. (1959). Differentiation of cells of the *Rana pipiens* gastrula in unconditioned medium. J. Embroyol. Exp. Morph., 7, 210.

13) GURDON, J.B. (1968). Changes in somatic cell nuclei inserted into growing and maturing amphibian oocytes. J. Embryol. Exp. Morph., 20, 401.

14) MOAR, V.A., GURDON, J.B., LANE, C.D. and MARBAIX, G. (1971). Translational capacity of living frog eggs and oocytes, as judged by messenger RNA injection. J. Mol. Biol., 61, 93.

15) MARBAIX, G. and LANE, C.D. (1972). Rabbit haemoglobin synthesis in frog cells: II. Further characterization of the products of translation of reticulocyte 9S RNA. J. Mol. Biol., 67, 517.

16) GURDON, J.B., LINGREL, J.B. and MARBAIX, G. (1973). Message stability in injected frog oocytes: long life of mammalian α and β globin messages. J. Mol. Biol., 80, 539.

17) GURDON, J.B. (1973). The translation of messenger RNA injected in living oocytes of *Xenopus laevis*. In: "Karolinska Symposia on Research Methods in Reproductive Endocrinology, 6th Symposium", 225.

18) GURDON, J.B. (1974). Molecular Biology in a living cell. Nature, 248, 772.

19) GURDON, J.B. (1974). "The Control of gene expression in animal

development". Clarendon Press, Oxford.

20) LANE, C.D. and KNOWLAND, J. (1975). The injection of RNA into living cells: the use of the frog oocytes for the assay of mRNA and the study of the control of gene expression. In: "The biochemistry of Animal Development" (ed., R. Weber), Academic Press, New York, 3, 145.

21) GURDON, J.B. (1977). Egg cytoplasm and gene control in development. Proc. R. Soc. Lond. B., 198, 211.

22) BERNS, A.J., KRAAIKAMP, M. BLOEMENDAL, H. and LANE, C.D. (1972). Calf crystallin synthesis in frog cells: the translation of lens-cell 14S RNA in oocytes. Proc. Natl. Acad. Sci. U.S.A., 69, 1606.

23) SMITH, M., STAVNEZER, J., HUANG, R.C., GURDON, J.B. and LANE, C.D. (1973). Translation of messenger RNA for mouse immunoglobulin light chains in living frog oocytes. J. Mol. Biol., 80, 553.

24) CHAN, L., KOHLER, P.O. and O'MALLEY, B.W. (1976). Translation of ovalbumin mRNA in *Xenopus laevis* oocytes. J. Clin. Invest., 57, 576.

25) REYNOLDS, F.H. Jr, PREMKUMAR, E. and PITHA, P.M. (1975). Interferon activity produced by translation of human interferon messenger RNA in cell-free ribosomal systems and in *Xenopus* oocytes. Proc. Natl. Acad. Sci. U.S.A., 72, 4881.

26) BEATO, M. and RUNGGER, D. (1975). Translation of the messenger RNA for rabbit uteroglobin in *Xenopus* oocytes. FEBS Lett., 59, 305.

27) LANCLOS, K.D. and HAMILTON, T.H. (1975). Translation of hormone-induced messenger RNA in amphibian oocytes. Proc. Natl. Acad. Sci. U.S.A., 72, 3934.

28) HEW, C.L. and YIP, C. (1976). The synthesis of freezing-point-depressing protein of the winter flounder *Pseudopleuronectus americanus* in *Xenopus laevis* oocytes. Biochem. Biophys. Res. Comm., 71, 845.

28a) NICKOL, J.M., LEE, K.L., HOLLINGER, T.G. and KENNEY, F.T. (1976). Translation of messenger RNA specific for tyrosine aminotransferase in oocytes of *Xenopus laevis*. Biochem. Biophys. Res. Comm., 72, 687.

29) KINDAS-MÜGGE, I., LANE, C.D. and KREIL, G. (1974). Insect protein synthesis in frog cells: the translation of honey-bee promelitin messenger RNA in *Xenopus* oocytes. J. Mol. Biol., 87, 451.

30) LASKEY, R.A., GURDON, J.B. and CRAWFORD, L.V. (1972). Translation of encephalomyocarditis viral RNA in oocytes of *Xenopus laevis*. Proc. Natl. Acad. Sci. U.S.A., 69, 3665.

31) GHYSDAEL, J., HUBERT, E., TRAVNIČEK, M., BOLOGNESI, D.P., BURNY, A., CLEUTER, Y., HUEZ, G., KETTMANN, R., MARBAIX, G., PORTETELLE, D. and CHANTRENNE, H. (1977). Frog oocytes synthesize and completely process the precursor polypeptide to virion structural proteins after microinjection of Avian Myeloblastosis Virus RNA. Proc. Natl. Acad. Sci. U.S.A., 74, 3230.

32) GHYSDAEL, J., KETTMANN, R. and BURNY, A. (1979). Translation of Bovine Leukemia Virus virion RNA in heterologous protein synthesizing systems. J. Virol., 29, 1087.

33) VAN DER DONK, J.A. (1975). Translation of plant messengers in egg cells of *Xenopus laevis*. Nature, 256, 674.

34) SCHRODER, J., KREUZALER, F. and SCHMOCK, J. (1977). Translation of plant-specific messenger RNAs in living animal cells. FEBS Lett., 81, 10.

35) KNOWLAND, J. (1974). Protein synthesis directed by the RNA from a plant virus in a normal animal cell. Genetics, 78, 383.

35a) KONDO, M., MARBAIX, G., MOENS, L., HUEZ, G., CLEUTER, Y. and HUBERT, E. (1975). Synthesis of viral coat protein in *Xenopus* oocytes injected with Brome Mosaic Virus RNA, 10th FEBS Meeting, Paris, Abstract 352.

36) VAN VLOTEN-DOTING, L., BOL, J., NEELEMAN, L., RUTGERS, T.,VAN DALEN, D., CASTEL, A., BOSCH, L., MARBAIX, G., HUEZ, G., HUBERT, E. and CLEUTER, Y. (1977). *In vivo* and *in vitro* translation of the RNAs of Alfalfa Mosaic Virus. In: "Nucleic Acids

and Protein Synthesis in Plants". (eds., L. Bogorad and J.H. Weil), Plenum Publishing Corporation, New York, 387.

37) RUTGERS, T., VAN VLOTEN-DOTING, L., MARBAIX, G., HUEZ, G., HUBERT, E. and CLEUTER, Y. (1977). Translation of the RNAs of Brome Mosaic Virus in *Xenopus* oocytes, 11th FEBS Meeting, Copenhagen, Abstract A 2-5, 205.

38) DICOU, E., HUEZ, G., MARBAIX, G. and BRACHET, P. (1979). Synthesis of *Dictyostelium discoideum* secretary proteins in *Xenopus laevis* oocytes. FEBS Lett., 104, 275.

39) FURUICHI, Y., LA FIANDRA, A. and SHATKIN, A.J. (1977). 5'-terminal structure and mRNA stability. Nature, 266, 235.

40) PATERSON, B.M. and ROSENBERG,M.(1979).Efficient translation of prokaryotic mRNAs in a eukaryotic cell-free system requires addition of a cap structure. Nature, 279, 692.

41) WOODLAND, H. and AYERS, S. (1974). Effects on protein synthesis of injecting synthetic polyribonucleotides into living cells. Biochem. J., 144, 11.

42) ALLENDE, C.C., ALLENDE, J.E. and FIRTEL, R.A. (1974). The degradation of ribonucleic acids injected into *Xenopus laevis* oocytes. Cell, 2, 189.

43) VASSART, G., REFETOFF, S., BROCAS, H., DINSART, C. and DUMONT, J.E. (1975). Translation of thyroglobulin 33S messenger RNA as a means of determining thyroglobulin quaternary structure. Proc. Natl. Acad. Sci. U.S.A., 72, 3839.

44) LABARCA, C. and PAIGNE, K. (1977). mRNA directed synthesis of catalytically active mouse β-glucuronidase in *Xenopus* oocytes. Proc. Natl. Acad. Sci. U.S.A., 74, 4462.

45) CAVALIERI, R.L., HAVELL, E.A., VILČEK, J. and PESTKA, S. (1977). Synthesis of human interferon by *Xenopus laevis* oocytes: two structural genes for interferons in human cells. Proc. Natl. Acad. Sci. U.S.A., 74, 3287.

46) LEBLEU, B., HUBERT, E., CONTENT, J., DE WIT, L., BRAUDE, I.A. and DE CLERCQ, E. (1978). Translation of mouse interferon mRNA

in *Xenopus laevis* oocytes and in rabbit reticulocyte lysates. Biochem. Biophys. Res. Comm., 82, 665.

47) LASKEY, R.A., MILLS, A.D., GURDON, J.B. and PARTINGTON, G.A. (1977). Protein synthesis in oocytes of *Xenopus laevis* is not regulated by the supply of messenger RNA. Cell, 11, 345.

48) HUEZ, G., MARBAIX, G., HUBERT, E., LECLERCQ, M., NUDEL, U., SOREQ, H., SALOMON, R., LEBLEU, B., REVEL, M. and LITTAUER, U.Z. (1974). Role of the poly(A) segment in the translation of globin mRNA in *Xenopus* oocytes. Proc. Natl. Acad. Sci. U.S.A., 71, 3143.

49) BERRIDGE, M.V. and LANE, C.D. (1976). Translation of *Xenopus* liver messenger RNA in *Xenopus* oocytes: vitellogenin synthesis and conversion to yolk platelets proteins. Cell, 8, 283.

50) ASSELBERGS, F.A.M., VAN VENROOIJ, W.J. and BLOEMENDAL, H.(1979). Messenger RNA competition in living *Xenopus* oocytes. Eur. J. Biochem., 94, 249.

51) MARBAIX, G. and GURDON, J.B. (1972). The effect of reticulocyte ribosome "factors" on the translation of haemoglobin messenger RNA in living frog oocytes. Biochim. Biophys. Acta, 81, 86.

52) HUNT, T., HUNTER, T. and MUNRO, A. (1969). Control of haemoglobin synthesis: rate of translation of the messenger RNA for the α and β chains. J. Mol. Biol., 43, 123.

53) CAMPBELL, P. N., MC ILREAVY, D. and TARIN, D. (1973). The detection of the messenger ribonucleic acid for the α-lactalbumin of guinea pig milk. Biochem. J., 134, 345.

54) GIGLIONI, B., GIANNI, A.M., COMI, P., OTTOLOENGHI, S., and RUNGGER, D. (1973). Translational control of globin synthesis by haemin in *Xenopus* oocytes. Nature New Biol, 246, 99.

55) KARPETSKY, T.P., BOGUSKI, M.S. and LEVY, C.C. (1979). Structure, properties and possible biological functions of polyadenylic acid. Subcellular Biochem., 6, 1.

56) REVEL, M. and GRONER, Y. (1978). Post-transcriptional and trans-

lational controls of gene expression in eukaryotes. Ann. Rev. Biochem., 47, 1079.

57) GREENBERG, J.R. (1975). Messenger RNA metabolism of animal cells. J. Cell Biol., 64, 269.

58) LEWIN, B. (1975). The relationship between heterogenous nuclear RNA and messenger RNA. Cell, 4, 11.

59) BRAWERMAN, G. (1976). Characteristics and significance of the polyadenylate sequence in mammalian mRNA. Progress in Nucleic Acid Research and Molecular Biology, 17, 118.

60) SHAFRITZ, D.A. (1977). Messenger RNA and its translation. In: "Molecular Mechanisms of Protein Biosynthesis" (eds., H. Weissbach and S. Petska), Academic Press, N.Y., 555.

61) MARBAIX, G., HUEZ, G., SOREQ, H., GALLWITZ, D., WEINBERG, E., DEVOS, R., HUBERT, E. and CLEUTER, Y. (1979). Role of the polyadenylate segment in the stability of eukaryotic messenger RNAs. In: "Gene Functions - 12th FEBS Meeting, Dresden, 1978", (ed., S. Rosenthal). Pergamon Press, Oxford, 427.

62) BARD, E., EFROM, D., MARCUS, A. and PERRY, R.P. (1974). Translational capacity of deadenylated mRNA. Cell, 1, 101.

63) WILLIAMSON, R., CROSSLEY, J. and HUMPHRIES, S. (1974). Translation of globin mRNA from which the poly(A) has been removed. Biochemistry, 13, 703.

64) SOREQ, H., NUDEL, U., SALOMON, R., REVEL, M. and LITTAUER, U.Z. (1974). *In vitro* translation of poly(A)-free globin mRNA. J. Mol. Biol., 88, 233.

65) SOREQ, H. and Littauer, U.Z. (1977). Purification and characterization of polynucleotide phosphorylase from *E. coli*. J. Biol. Chem., 252, 6885.

66) MARBAIX, G., HUEZ, G., BURNY, A., CLEUTER, Y., HUBERT, E., LECLERCQ, M., CHANTRENNE, H., SOREQ, H., NUDEL, U. and LITTAUER, U.Z. (1975). Absence of poly(A) segment in globin mRNA accelerates its degradation in *Xenopus* oocytes. Proc. Natl. Acad. Sci. U.S.A., 72, 3065.

67) SIPPEL, A.E. (1973). Purification and characterization of ATP: RNA adenyltransferase from *E. coli*. Eur. J. Biochem., 37, 31.

68) HUEZ, G., MARBAIX, G., HUBERT, E., CLEUTER, Y., LECLERCQ, M., CHANTRENNE, H., DEVOS, R., SOREQ, H., NUDEL, U. and LITTAUER, U.Z. (1975). Readenylation of poly(A)-free globin mRNA restores its stability *in vivo*. Eur. J. Biochem., 59, 589.

69) NUDEL, U., SOREQ, H., LITTAUER, U.Z., MARBAIX, G., HUEZ, G., LECLERCQ, M., HUBERT, E. and CHANTRENNE, H. (1976). Globin mRNA species containing poly(A) segments of different lengths. Eur. J. Biochem., 64, 115.

70) PERRY, R.P. and KELLEY, D.E. (1973). Messenger RNA turnover in mouse L cells. J. Mol. Biol.,79, 681.

71) BRAWERMAN, G. (1973). Alterations in the size of the poly(A) segment of newly-synthesized mRNA of mouse ascites cells. Mol. Biol. Rep., 1, 7.

72) SHEINESS, D. and DARNELL, J.E. (1973). Poly(A) segment in mRNA becomes shorter with age. Nature New Biol., 241, 265.

73) MERKEL, C.G., KWAN, S.P. and LINGREL, J.B. (1975). Size of the poly(A) region of newly synthesized globin mRNA. J. Biol. Chem., 250, 3725.

74) NOKIN, P., HUEZ, G., MARBAIX, G., BURNY, A. and CHANTRENNE, H. (1976). Molecular modifications associated with ageing of globin mRNA *in vivo*. Eur. J. Biochem., 62, 509.

75) NOKIN, P., BURNY, A., HUEZ, G. and MARBAIX, G. (1976). Globin messenger RNA from anaemic rabbit spleen: size of its polyadenylate segment. Eur. J. Biochem., 68. 431.

76) HUEZ, G., MARBAIX, G., GALLWITZ, D., WEINBERG, E., DEVOS, R., HUBERT, E. and CLEUTER, Y. (1978). Functional stabilization of HeLa cell histone mRNAs injected into *Xenopus* oocytes by 3'-OH polyadenylation. Nature, 271, 572.

77) MANIATIS, G.M., RAMIREZ, F. CANN, A., MARKS, P.A. and BANK, A. (1976). Translation and stability of human globin mRNA in *Xenopus* oocytes. J. Clin. Invest., 58, 1415.

78) MOUS, J., PEETERS, B., VAN BELLEGEM, H. and ROMBAUTS, W. (1979). Translation of biologically active messenger RNA from human placenta in *Xenopus* oocytes. Eur. J. Biochem., 94, 393.

79) SEHGAL, P.B., SOREQ, H. and TAMM, I. (1978). Does 3'-terminal poly(A) stabilize human fibroblast interferon mRNA in oocytes of *Xenopus laevis*?. Proc. Natl. Acad. Sci. U.S.A., 75, 5030.

80) BLOBEL, G. (1973). A protein of molecular weight 78,000 bound to the poly(A) region of eukaryotic mRNAs. Proc. Natl. Acad. Sci. U.S.A., 70, 924.

81) HUEZ, G., MARBAIX, G., BURNY, A., HUBERT, E., LECLERCQ, M. CLEUTER, Y.,CHANTRENNE, H., SOREQ, H. and LITTAUER, U.Z. (1977). Degradation of deadenylated rabbit α-globin mRNA in *Xenopus* oocytes is associated with its translation. Nature, 266, 473.

82) SHATKIN, A.J. (1976). Capping of eukaryotic mRNAs. Cell, 9, 645.

83) LOCKARD, R.E. and LANE, C.D. (1978). Requirements for 7-methyl-guanosine in translation of globin mRNA *in vivo*. Nucl. Acids. Res., 5, 3237.

84) MARBAIX, G., HUEZ, G. and SOREQ, H. (1977). What is the role of poly(A) on eukaryotic messengers? Trends Biochem. Sci., 2, N 106.

85) JILKA, R.L., CAVALIERI, R.L., YAFFE, L. and PESTKA, S. (1977). Synthesis and glycosylation of the MOPC-46B immunoglobulin kappa chain in *Xenopus laevis* oocytes. Biochem. Biophys. Res. Comm., 79, 625.

86) DECOEN, N.J. and BRINGER, A.E. (1977). Fucose incorporation into oocyte-synthesized rat immunoglobulins. FEBS Lett., 79, 191.

87) KATZ, R.A., MANIATIS, G.M. and GUNTAKA, R.V. (1979). Translation of Avian Sarcoma Virus RNA in *Xenopus laevis* oocytes. Biochem. Biophys. Res. Comm., 86, 447.

88) BLOBEL, G. and SABATINI, D.D. (1971). Ribosome-membrane interaction in eukaryotic cells. In: "Biomembranes". (ed., L.A. Manson), Plenum Publishing Corporation, New York, 2, 193.

89) BLOBEL, G. and DOBBERSTEIN, B. (1975). Transfer of proteins

across membranes. J. Cell Biol., 67, 835.

90) MACH, B., FAUST, C.F. and VASSALI, P. (1973). Different sizes of the product of the 14S immunoglobulin light chain mRNA translated *in vitro* and in amphibian oocytes. Mol. Biol. Rep., 1, 3.

91) ZEHAVI-WILLNER, T. and LANE, C. (1977). Subcellular compartmentation of albumin and globin made in oocytes under the direction of injected messenger RNA. Cell, 11, 683.

92) RAPOPORT, T.A., THIELE, B.J., PREHN, S., MARBAIX, G., CLEUTER, Y., HUBERT, E. and HUEZ, G. (1978). Synthesis of carp proinsulin in *Xenopus* oocytes. Eur. J. Biochem., 87, 229.

93) MOUS, J., PEETERS, B., ROMBAUTS, W. and HEYNS, W. (1977). Synthesis of rat prostatic binding protein in *Xenopus* oocytes and in wheat germ. Biochem., Biophys. Res. Comm., 79, 1111.

94) HUEZ, G., GHYSDAEL, J., TRAVNIČEK, M., BURNY, A., CLEUTER, Y., KETTMANN, R., MARBAIX, G. and PORTETELLE, D. (1979). Post-translational processing of oncornavirus proteins. In: "Processing and Turnover of Proteins and Organelles in the Cell - 12th FEBS Meeting, Dresden, 1978". (eds., S. Rapoport and T. Schewe) Pergamon Press, Oxford, 3.

95) VOGT, V., EISENMAN, E. DIGGELMANN, H. (1975). Generation of Avian Myeloblastosis Virus structural proteins by proteolytic cleavage of a precursor polypeptide. J. Mol. Biol., 96, 471.

96) VON DER HELM, K. (1977). Cleavage of Rous sarcoma viral polypeptide precursor into internal structural proteins *in vitro* involves viral protein p16. Proc. Natl. Acad. Sci. U.S.A., 74, 911.

97) GATICA, M., TARRAGO, A., ALLENDE, C.C. and ALLENDE, J.E. (1975). Aminoacylation of transfer RNA microinjected into *Xenopus laevis* oocytes. Nature, 256, 675.

98) SALARI, A., GATICA, M. and ALLENDE, J.E. (1977). *In vivo* repair of the 3'-terminus of transfer RNA injected into amphibian oocytes. Nucl. Ac. Res., 4, 1873.

99) GATICA, M. and ALLENDE, J.E. (1977). Aminoacyl transfer from phenylalanyl-tRNA microinjected into *Xenopus laevis* oocytes. Biochem. Biophys. Res. Comm., 79, 352.

100) JOSHI, J., HAENNI, A.L., HUBERT, E., HUEZ, G. and MARBAIX, G. (1978). *In vivo* aminoacylation and "processing" of Turnip Yellow Mosaic Virus RNA in *Xenopus laevis* oocytes. Nature, 275, 339.

59) [illegible], K. and [illegible] (1981). [illegible] transferase [illegible] [illegible] Biochem. Biophys. Res. Comm. [illegible]

60) [illegible], A., [illegible] and M[illegible] (1981). [illegible] yellow mosaic virus RNA in [illegible] protoplasts. [illegible] 27[illegible], 25[illegible]

SURROGATE GENETICS IN THE FROG OOCYTE

A. Kressmann and M.L. Birnstiel

Institut für Molekularbiologie II
der Universität Zürich
Hönggerberg, 8093 Zürich, Switzerland

1. INTRODUCTION

About 20 years ago Jacob and Monod introduced the concept of the operon. Their idea that a single regulatory sequence, the operon, controlled and co-ordinated the expression of several structural genes opened up the way for our present day understanding of gene expression in prokaryotes. Rightly or wrongly,this concept dominates present day research on the elucidation of gene structure in eukaryotes. Consequently, now that many eukaryotic genes have been cloned and partially or completely sequenced the DNA base sequences have been rigorously searched for structures equivalent to the prokaryotic operator, terminator or replicator signals.

Some promising structures which might be analogous to those in bacteria have indeed been found. Thus comparative sequence analysis has suggested that genes transcribed by polymerase II have a DNA signal similar to the Pribnow box (1 and D.S. Hogness, personal communication). Furthermore, DNA sequences highly similar to the bacterial attenuator sequences which govern termination of transcription have been found near the 3' ends of the histone genes (2).

However, specific functions can only be assigned to such sequences once their biological activity has been demonstrated. The classical genetical approach which has been so successful in elucidating regulatory DNA signals in prokaryotes cannot easily be applied to eukaryotes, so that an alternative method, called "Surrogate Genetics" has been developed (3). In this alternative scheme the putative regulatory sequences are modified, deleted or inverted and the altered gene units introduced into a living cell so that the expression of these genes can be evaluated. Once the "phenotype" of the structural alteration has been recognized, it is then possible to deduce what role is played by specific regulatory DNA sequences.

There are now several ways in which cloned and modified DNA can be introduced into living cells. One method is the mechanical microinjection of DNA into nuclei of tissue culture cells (see this volume). Alternatively, cells can be transformed using deproteinized eukaryotic DNA (4), plasmid recombinant DNA or by means of viruses carrying eukaryotic chromosomal genes (5). In many of these systems it is necessary to have a selective marker in order to isolate cells which have received foreign DNA and to distinguish them from those that have not. For mechanical injection of DNA by means of thin capillary pipettes it is clear that the task becomes easier the larger the cell nucleus. The oocytes and eggs of the amphibian *Xenopus laevis* which are exceptionally large cells are therefore particularly suited to injection techniques.

In this paper, we give a detailed account of our oocyte nucleus injection technique which involves the centrifugation of the oocyte to render the location of the oocyte nucleus visible. The results show that not only are the oocytes capable of transcribing injected template DNAs at high rate, but in some cases with an astonishingly high fidelity. The application of the technique to the study of *in vitro* modified genes i.e. experiments involving Surrogate Genetics, is also discussed.

(i) *Xenopus laevis* oocytes

By all criteria the amphibian oocyte is a remarkable cell. With a diameter of 1-1.5mm it is 10^5-10^6 times larger in volume than a normal cell. The development of each oocyte in the ovaries of *Xenopus laevis* extends over several months (6). During this period components are assembled which allow rapid development from the egg to embryo, up to the blastula stage, without much intervention of the activity of the cell nuclei. A large amount of maternal mRNA accumulates (7). In this regard, it has been calculated that the endogenous RNA synthesis of the oocyte nucleus is more rapid, by 2-3 orders of magnitude than that found in a tissue culture cell (8). At maturity, the occyte contains an excess of RNA polymerases, which would suffice for 10^4-10^5 somatic cells (9). The oocyte also contains 40ng histone proteins (10), a histone mass equivalent to 5000 diploid *Xenopus* nuclei. The mature oocyte contains a cytoplasm not unlike that of an ordinary tissue culture cell in composition and is therefore capable of translating, because of its size, exceedingly large quantities of exogenous mRNA (reviewed in 11).

From this short summary covering some of the pecularities of the amphibian oocyte it is clear that these cells not only synthesize RNA rapidly but that they also contain an excess capacity of macromolecules such as histones, RNA polymerases and a protein synthesizing apparatus which can be deployed for the rapid expression of injected DNA templates both at the level of RNA and protein. Since in oocyte injection experiments 10^7-10^8 cloned gene units are usually transferred to a single oocyte nucleus, the gene dosage of that particular gene is of course unusually high, it is perhaps not too surprising that not all genes are faithfully expressed.

(ii) Injection of DNA into nuclei of *Xenopus laevis* oocytes

Transcription of DNA, injected into oocytes and unfertilized eggs of *Xenopus laevis*, was first investigated by A. Colman (12). In these early studies calf thymus DNA as well as synthetic desoxy-polynucleotides were used as templates. Newly synthesized RNAs were scored by determining the incorporation of RNA precursors and their sedimentation characteristics were determined by sucrose gradient centrifugation. It was first reported by J.E. Mertz and J.B. Gurdon, that transcription is most efficient when the DNA is placed within the oocyte nucleus (13), while, by comparison, injection of DNA into the cytoplasm of eggs or oocytes yields considerably less or no transcription of the foreign template. The oocytes used for injection experiments (stage 5) are full of yolk platelets which give the vegetal pole of the oocytes its typical light colouring. The animal pole is covered by a brown pigment. The oocyte nucleus usually resides within the pigmented animal half of the oocyte. Although at stage 5 the nucleus is relatively large with a diameter of about 0.2mm and should therefore be easily penetrated by the injection needle, this is nevertheless a difficult task because the oocyte is opaque and the nucleus hidden from view.

J.B. Gurdon had previously developed an elegant but technically demanding method of injecting HeLa nuclei into the Germinal Vessicle (nucleus) of *Xenopus* oocytes (14). In this method, the injection needle is held in a vertical position and aimed at the apex of the animal pole. The tip of the needle is then moved towards the center of the oocyte. At the same time, the oocyte is squeezed with a pair of forceps. As the needle penetrates the oocyte the nucleus lying on the central animal-vegetal axis will be pierced by the needle. About 50-80% of all nuclei can be injected successfully in this way. We have developed an easier and faster technique which we will summarize in detail below.

The technique of microinjection was introduced to our laboratory by C. Malacinski and E. Triplett in 1975/76. It became clear during these early experiments that the DNA had to be injected into the oocyte nucleus which proved to be difficult for us. Now, classical embryologists have shown that centrifugation of oocytes and eggs leads to a stratification of the contents of these cells. The real break-through came for us in 1976 when we noticed that by the same procedure the location of the *Xenopus* oocyte nuclei could be made visible (15). We were able to demonstrate by serial sectioning of centrifuged oocytes that in oocytes aligned with the animal pole upwards the nucleus migrates towards the animal pole under the influence of centrifugal force. This movement is accompanied, fortuitously, by a displacement of pigment granules within the animal hemisphere. A brown ring of variable intensity (depending on the centrifugal force applied) is formed which is concentric with the cell nucleus. The brown pigment ring serves as an easy target since injection just below the oocyte surface in the dead center of this ring leads inevitably to nuclear penetration.

2. MATERIALS AND METHODS

(i) Removal of oocytes from the frog

Oocytes are taken from *Xenopus laevis* females which are not quite fully grown (ca. 150 g). Best results are obtained from females which have been acclimatized in the lab for several weeks and have been stimulated with 100 U Pregnyl (N.V. Organon Oss, Holland) two weeks prior to removal of the oocytes. For the removal of the oocyte the frog is narcotized in 1 l of MS 222 (Sandoz) at a concentration of 3-3.5g/l. After 10 minutes exposure to the drug the frog remains anaesthesized for 1/2 to 1 hr. The frog is placed, on its back, on a wet cloth. An incision of about 1 cm long, slightly offset from the ventral middle line, is made into the skin. From now on all operations are performed aseptically. The peritoneum and the muscle tissue are cut open. A small portion of the ovary is pulled out with forceps and removed with a pair of scissors. The clump of oocytes is immediately transferred to a petri dish containing modified Barth medium (16). The rest of the ovary is pushed back into the body cavity. The peritoneum and the muscle tissue are sewn up and then the skin closed off, using cat gut. The operated frog is put back into a container filled with water to which a few drops of mercurochrom have been added. The oocytes are kept at $+18^{o}C$ and can be used for at least two days.

(ii) Preparation and centrifugation of oocytes

Oocytes of stage 5 and 6 (Ref.6) are separated from the ovary with a platinum or steel wire loop. The oocytes are each covered with an envelope of follicle cells and the whole structure is referred to as an oocyte in the subsequent text. 50-150 oocytes at a time are placed onto a nylon net (gauge 0.8mm, thickness of each fiber approx. 0.3mm; scrynel NY 850 HD, Zürcher Beuteltuchfabrik AG, Moosstr.2, 8803 Rüschlikon, Switzerland) which has been previously glued to the bottom of a petri dish with a few drops of chloroform and is covered in modified Barth medium. All operations are carried out aseptically.

Free oocytes are manipulated using a Pasteur pipette whose tip has been broken off to yield a wide lumen, the rough edges having been smoothed by touching the pipette to a flame. The oocytes are orientated roughly on the net in such a way that the brown animal pole is upwards. Using long forceps the petri dish and its contents are placed in an MSE Coolspin centrifuge rotor bucket (i.e. a centrifuge which will hold 500ml tissue culture bottles) and centrifuged for 10 minutes at 18°C at 1300-1800 rpm. This corresponds to approx. 400xg.

Oocytes differ considerably in their consistancy from frog to frog. It is advisable to carry out a small series of tests to determine the best centrifugation conditions. Centrifugation is considered optimal when the dark pigment ring has just begun to appear. During the centrifugation the oocytes are forced into the meshes of the nylon net and remain firmly fixed. When the centrifuge has come to a standstill the oocytes will present themselves with pigment rings facing the injector. Oocytes can be kept at this stage for at least 1 hr prior to injection (and possibly much longer) as the nucleus does not move back rapidly into the cytoplasm. The centrifugation of the oocyte does not impair the capacity to synthesize RNA (35).

(iii) Injection apparatus (Fig.1)

Glass capillaries (GC 100 F 4, Clark Electromedical Instruments, England) are pulled with a glass micro-electrode puller (PN-3 Narishige Scientific Instruments Laboratory Ltd. Japan). The end of the needle is broken to a diameter of 10-20µm, as determined in a light microscope with an appropriate standardizing occular. To obtain the desired diameters, the needle is held at an angle of about 30^{0} against a glass plate while being observed under a binocular microscope and is scraped gently along its tapered end with Tungsten wire. Occasionally small fragments at the tip of the needle break off. Needles with the

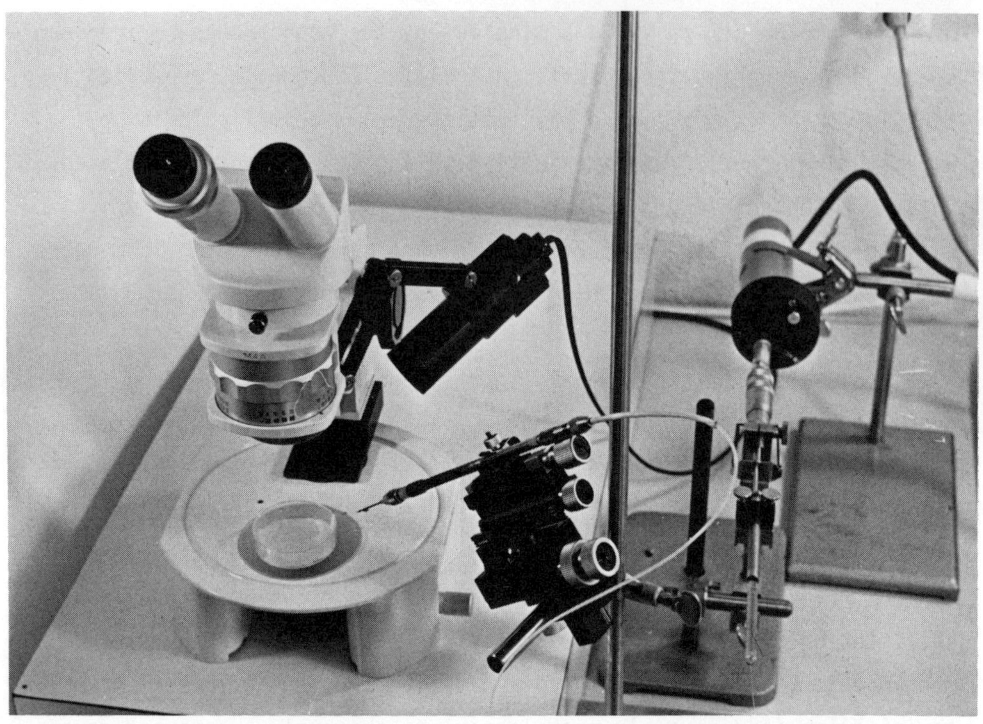

Fig. 1. *Instrumentation for oocyte injection.*

correct diameter and a slanting pointed end (although it may be quite jagged) are selected. The needle is filled with paraffin oil from its non-tapered end by means of a 1ml tuberculine syringe. It is fixed onto a simple micromanipulator (MM 33, Gebr. Märzhäuser, Germany) via a needle holder and connected by teflon tubing (an elastic plastic cannot be used because of the slack introduced by it), also filled with paraffin oil, to a 5μl syringe (Hamilton 85 NE). The syringe is driven by a foot operated motor via a micrometer screw to give a flow rate of 0.2μl/minute. Such a motor can be simply constructed from a Barbecue spit-turning motor. A constant injection volume is maintained by keeping the needle in each oocyte for a fixed time during continuous liquid flow.

(iv) Injection solutions

Injection medium usually contains 1-5μg of DNA and 50-100uCi (α^{32}P)-GTP (Amersham, London) specific activity 100-400 Ci/mMol) in 10μl injection buffer (10mM Tris HCl pH 7.5 and 80mM NaCl). The minimum volume that can be handled is about 2μl. All DNAs should be thoroughly purified by two consequential CsCl gradient centrifugations using optical grade CsCl. The DNA is dissolved in 10mM Tris HCl pH 7.5 (containing no EDTA) and precipitated with ethanol (0.3M NaAc pH 5.5; 2.5 Vol. ethanol) overnight at -20^{0}C. The DNA is pelleted, washed with ice-cold 80% ethanol, dried under vacuum and redissolved in injection buffer. The desired amount of radioactive precursor is lyophylized and is taken up with the DNA-containing injection buffer.

(v) Injection

1-3μl of injection solution is delivered from a teflon tipped micro capillary and placed on a piece of parafilm. From now on all operations are observed under the binocular microscope. The injection needle is introduced into the drop with the aid of the micromanipulator. The solution is sucked into the needle by turning the micrometer screw slowly. The hydraulic system must be free of air bubbles, so that when suction is applied, the miniscus within the needle rises immediately.

The needle attached to the micromanipulator is aimed at the oocytes at an angle of about 60-70^{0}. The oocytes are aligned relative to the tip of the needle by manoeuvring of the petri dish. The tip of the needle is introduced into the dead center of the brown ring, just below the surface of the oocyte. 20nl of the injection medium (i.e. 2-10ng DNA together with 0.1-0.2μCi (α^{32}P)-GTP are injected into each oocyte nucleus. The injection volume can be controlled by starting and stopping the foot operated motor. The method that we prefer is to leave the electric motor running all the time and to count the seconds that the needle remains within the oocyte. This method has the great advantage that the volume per oocyte is extremely reproducible (within 5%) and that the needle will not be plugged up by yolk. This method is also less sensitive to any slack or impedence within the hydraulic system. The first method is more economical of course.

Any uninjected oocytes are removed from the nylon net by a jet of medium delivered from a Pasteur pipette. The medium is then exchanged in the petri dish. The oocytes are incubated at 18^{0}C (temperatures of 23^{0}C must not be exceeded) for the desired time. As a routine procedure we inject the DNA on the first day and the radioactive label on the second. In this case the (α ^{32}P)-GTP injection is directed to the cytoplasm. For this second injection, the oocytes do not need to be recentrifuged since they remain fixed within the mesh. If an oocyte adheres to the needle upon injection, the needle can be pulled back out of the buffer and oocyte will detach from the needle as soon as it comes into contact with the buffer surface.

(vi) RNA extraction

Injected and incubated oocytes are removed from the nylon mesh by a jet of medium, as described above, and the oocytes showing an unequal distribution of pigment are rejected. The remaining oocytes are washed in Barth's medium. They can be frozen and kept for indefinite time at -70^{0}C. 30-100 oocytes are placed in a 15ml corex tube and resuspended in 1-2.5ml buffer (10mM Tris HCl, pH 7.5, 1.5mM MgCl, 10mM NaCl, 1mg/ml Proteinase K) and homogenized immediately by pushing a loosely fitting pistil into the corex tube. As soon as possible, the solution is made 2% SDS (final concentration), the solution is incubated for 30 minutes at room temperature and vortexed from time to time. The turbid liquid is made to 0.3M NaAC and extracted three times with phenol/chloroform 1:1, then three times with chloroform alone to remove any phenol. At this stage the solution can be treated with DNase after addition of 10-20mM $MgCl_2$ (a white precipitation may form which can be centrifuged off). For this step 10μg/ml RNase-free DNase are added. After 30 min incubation at 37^{0}C proteinase K is added to 10μg/ml and the nucleic acids are prepared by repeated phenol/chloroform extraction. We find that DNase treatment is not required for most analyses and usually it is omitted. The RNA solution is now clear and colourless. The RNA is recovered by ethanol precipitation, redissolved in 0.2% SDS at a final RNA concentration of 2μg/μl and can be kept frozen at -20^{0}C indefinitely.

(vii) Injection technique for unfertilized eggs of *Xenopus laevis*

Xenopus laevis females, two weeks previously stimulated by an intramuscular injection of 100 U of Pregnyl (N.V. Organon Oss, Holland) are induced to lay unfertilized eggs within 8-10 hrs by an injection of 200-250 U of Pregnyl into the dorsal lymph space (17). The eggs are collected by squeezing the posterior of the frog held over a 50mm petri dish containing 5ml of Barth solution. After the Barth solution has been removed, the eggs are treated for 2 min with a 3% cysteine-HCl/0.1% Papain (African Papaya, Calbiochem, San Diego, California) 0.2 NaOH solution and then washed five times with 2ml fresh Barth solution. The eggs are placed onto a nylon net, animal pole upwards, fixed to the bottom of a 50mm petri dish (see above).

3. CHROMATIN ASSEMBLY OR DEGRADATION OF INJECTED DNAs

DNA injected into the cytoplasm of oocytes does not penetrate the nucleus and is degraded. Supercoiled covalently closed DNA (form I) is first converted to relaxed, but still covalently closed molecules (form Ir) by a nicking-closing activity. Afterwards it is degraded to nicked circular DNA (form II), then full length linear DNA (form III) and finally to shorter linear molecules by endonucleolytic cleavages (18,19). When injected into the nucleus, DNA form I is first relaxed to the form Ir, then new supercoil turns are added. The DNA is conserved in this form. SV40 DNA can be finally found in a chromatin-like structure very similar to authentic SV40 minichromosomes (19). The same results are obtained for other circular DNAs such as 5S ribosomal DNA (20) and ribosomal RNA genes (21). Injected nicked circular DNA (form II) is ligated within the nucleus and processed as described for the Ir form. DNA form III is thought not to be assembled into nucleoprotein complexes, but is degraded (19), presumably by exonucleases since circular DNA is conserved. However, type III DNA survives within the nucleus long enough for transcripts to be detected (see later).

4. DNA SYNTHESIS AND DNA REPLICATION

During oogenesis of the *Xenopus laevis* oocyte no nuclear DNA is synthesized, whereas 2-3 hrs after egg fertilization genomic DNA replicates and DNA synthesis is observed (22). Micro-injection of purified DNAs into unfertilized egg cytoplasm stimulates incorporation of (^{3}H) thymidine into DNA (23). R.A. Laskey and J.B. Gurdon claimed that *Xenopus laevis* egg cytoplasm contains an enzyme complex capable of replicating covalently closed circular DNA from polyoma virus but not DNA of bacterial origin (24). Supercoils of recombinant plasmid containing rDNA from *Xenopus laevis* which had been incubated with cell-free unfertilized egg extracts were converted to early and late Cairns structures, suggesting again that the egg cytoplasm is capable of replicating eukaryotic DNA (25). More recently, cloned histone genes of *Psammechinus miliaris* were injected into unfertilized egg cytoplasm (R. Clerc, unpublished results). Although incorporation of labelled DNA precursors into DNA proceeded rapidly, DNA sequences serving as origin of DNA replication could not be identified nor was it possible to confirm that eukaryotic DNA is a better template for DNA synthesis than prokaryotic DNA.

5. TRANSCRIPTION

(i) Genes transcribed by polymerase III

The transcriptional activity of genes coding for 5S rRNA of *Xenopus laevis* and *borealis* (20,26-29) and coding for tRNAs of *Xenopus laevis* (15,30-32), of the nematode *C.elegans* (33) and of yeast (34) have been studied in the frog oocyte. All these genes either as chromosomal DNA (20,26) or cloned in prokaryotic vectors (15,20,27-34) are expressed efficiently within the oocyte nucleus. The transcription is faithful with respect to the length of the product, strand selectivity and hybridization properties. Where the RNA was characterized by fingerprinting the primary structure of the *in vivo* product and that synthesized in the oocyte was found to be identical (26,30,31). A portion of the 5S RNA was shown to carry a tetraphosphate 5' end indicating that the 5S RNA is probably a primary transcript (27). A small proportion of RNA molecules exhibited read-through at the 3' end. This is also observed *in vivo* and may therefore reflect a genuine property of 5S DNA transcription. Transcription of 5S or tRNA genes within the oocyte shows a sensitivity towards α amanitin typical for polymerase III (20,

33,35). That transcription in the oocyte can be quite selective is shown by the fact that a DNA clone containing three repeat units of the *Xenopus borealis* 5S genes, showed differential transcription of these units within the oocyte (28). Similarly $tDNA^{met}_{1}$ unit consisting of eight genes for seven different tRNAs (S.G. Clarkson, unpublished results) also yield different levels of transcripts for some of these genes. In all these experiments the 5S and at least two 4S RNA genes were found to be expressed monocistronically.

That DNAs coding for tRNAs from such sources as *Xenopus*, nematodes and yeast are all transcribed in the oocyte shows the universality of the transcription process catalyzed by the oocyte polymerase. However, there are distinct differences in the rates of transcription. tRNA genes of yeast are transcribed sluggishly, although direct comparisons are difficult since different isocoding tRNA species were studied. The highest transcription rates are observed with cloned tRNA genes of *Xenopus laevis* where a rate of 30 transcripts per hour/gene is obtained. Processing of tRNA shows a similar universality across the species. Such processing includes nucleolytic cleavages, splicing and modification. Most interestingly these steps also occur in yeast $tRNA^{tyr}$ which contains an intervening sequence within the structural gene. Although this intron is present in a foreign DNA the oocyte is nevertheless capable of splicing the precursor accurately (34).

(ii) Genes transcribed by polymerase II

Although nuclear injection of DNA started with studies on the transcription of SV40 (13,36) and histone DNA (15), the application of the oocyte injection technique to the study of these genes has yielded results more slowly than with 5S and tRNA genes. Quite generally it is observed that polymerase II genes are expressed at a much lower rate than 5S and tRNA genes and only a portion of the transcripts appears to be faithful mRNA. A series of other genes injected into the oocyte have produced no faithful product whatsoever.

The histone genes (37,38) are transcribed efficiently when injected into the oocyte nuclei, as much as 25% of all RNA being derived from this foreign template. We observe that covalently circular DNA is a much better template than linear DNA (35). Also supercoiled histone DNA is a much better template than supercoiled plasmid-histone DNA recombinants. Although the cloned histone DNA we use contains all five types of histone genes only the H2A and the H2B are efficiently expressed at both the RNA and the protein level. The mRNAs, as determined by S1 mapping, contain true 5' and 3' ends. The anticoding strand of the histone DNA is also transcribed to a certain extent, so that not all transcripts of injected histone DNA are faithful. Interestingly, polydisperse RNA and RNA derived from the anticoding strand is sequestered within the oocyte nucleus and only RNA derived from the codogenic strand and of discrete size are admitted to the cytoplasm (35).

(iii) Genes transcribed by polymerase I

Plasmid recombinants containing the ribosomal gene unit of *D. marginalis* and *X. laevis* were injected into oocytes and the transcriptional complexes were spread and examined under the electron microscope (21,39). A small portion of the gene units reproduces the typical Miller picture of rDNA "Christmas trees". Interestingly, the chromatin structure differed for the plasmid and the rDNA spacer sections of the recombinant molecules. Other rDNA molecules show an abnormal pattern of transcription. This is a situation not unlike that found for sea urchin histone DNA where some faithful and unfaithful transcripts coexist within the oocyte nucleus.

6. COUPLED TRANSCRIPTION-TRANSLATION

J.E. Mertz and E. De Robertis demonstrated that after injection of *Drosophila* histone DNA into *Xenopus* oocytes proteins with properties characteristic of *Drosophila* H2A histones appear within the oocyte (40). Similarly, sea urchin histone DNA gives rise to H2A, H2B proteins. The expression of SV40 is of particular interest since there is a clear cut regulation between early and late genes in permissive cells (reviewed in 41). Furthermore, RNA splicing events (42) are required for the production of functional messengers (42). The oocyte system appears to override many of the delicate viral regulatory patterns in that structural proteins for VP1, VP3, probably also VP2 as well as small t and large T-antigens are synthesized after injection of the SV40 DNA (43). Although these results do not necessarily mean that the oocyte is capable of recognizing specific transcriptional signals of the SV40 genome, it is clear that it must be capable of splicing the heterologous precursor RNA molecules to yield functional mRNAs.

7. SURROGATE GENETICS IN THE *XENOPUS* OOCYTE

By a combination of cloning, DNA sequencing, restriction and oocyte injection, the structural organization of the tRNA genes of *X.laevis* (15, 30-32) and *C.elegans* (33) has been investigated. These experiments have served to define the sequences promoting transcription of eukaryotic tRNA genes. In the case of *C.elegans* a small DNA fragment containing some 300 bases near the 5' end of the structural gene for a distinct tRNA was shown to still yield faithful tRNA.

A cloned tRNA fragment of *Xenopus laevis*, 3.18 kb long and containing eight genes coding for seven tRNA species was dissected (30-32). By injecting sub-fragments of the DNA molecule the monocistronic mode of transcription for these tRNA genes became apparent. In another series, the 5' sequences of one of these genes, the $tRNA^{met}_{1}$ gene A were removed in stages and the effects of this truncation on gene expression studied. Finally, a short DNA segment was isolated which contained besides the structural gene 22 bp at the 5' terminus and 88 bp at the 3' terminus of the structural gene. This DNA unit, when cloned in pCRI or ligated to another foreign DNA produced mature $tRNA^{met}_{1}$ at a high rate, when injected into the oocyte nucleus (31). Hence, much of the 5' DNA lying outside the structural gene is dispensable for the expression of this gene. Of the remaining 22 nucleotides near the 5' terminus of the structural gene some will code for the prelude sequences of the precursor tRNA. This leaves an even shorter sequence for possible promoter function. This extraordinary situation led us to consider that either the promoter for tRNA transcription is very short and primitive or that the information directing transcription extends into or is actually part of the structural gene.

In order to delimit the promoter of this gene even further, this 185bp DNA unit was cleaved into an anterior and a posterior portion by restriction with Hae III endonuclease. Both restriction segments were recloned in pCR1 using EcoRI linkers. Starting from these tDNA subclones a series of new recombinants were constructed, one of which consisted of a novel tRNA gene containing an artificial intron sequence.

None of these clones containing the anterior (5') or the posterior (3') section of the $tDNA^{met}_{1}$ gene by itself was capable of directing RNA synthesis (32). This observation, combined with those obtained from *in vitro* experiments, have suggested that promotion of the tDNA transcription requires the presence of both the anterior and posterior portion of the tRNA gene, hence that there are at least two DNA sites in this tRNA gene controlling its expression. Interestingly, the *in vitro* modified $tRNA^{met}_{1}$ gene containing an EcoRI linker as an intron was transcribed at high rate, although in this case the intron sequence was not cleaved out of the RNA molecule (32). Instead a modified tRNA accumulated which, presumably because of its altered secondary and tertiary structure, proved to be unstable within the oocyte.

An elegant method for preparing deletion mutants in the spacer preceding the 5S gene of *Xenopus laevis* has been reported by N.V. Federoff (29). A transposable element carrying a chloramphenicol resistance marker was introduced into an AT rich spacer 5S DNA which was then cloned in a plasmid containing a tetracycline resistance gene. This tetracycline resistance was destroyed by the construction of the recombinant. Revertance to chloramphenicol sensitivity and tetracycline resistance frequently involved not only loss of the transposable element but also of part of the 5S gene spacer unit. Several of these mutants carrying deletions of different lengths mapped as close as 50 nucleotides to the structural gene. All of them generated 5S RNA with similar efficiency when injected into the oocyte; hence as shown in the case of tDNA, the spacer immediately preceeding the structural gene appears not to be of major importance for the transcriptional activity of the injected DNA unit.

Most recently we have been able to obtain short deletion mutants of the prelude regions of the H2A gene of *Psammechinus*. Such mutant histone DNA clones, when injected into the oocyte, elicit specific effects for the expression of the H2A. Thus, deletion of a conserved GC rich DNA block upstream of the histone messenger gene leads to accellerated expression of the H2A gene, hence representing an up mutation. On the other hand, deletion of the TATAAA motif thought to be the equivalent of the bacterial Pribnow box, represents a down mutation and leads to the appearance of a plurality of H2A mRNA sequences with differing 5' termini (R. Grosschedl, unpublished results). We consider the "Hogness box" to represent a sequence instrumental in the "phasing" of initiation or capping of the mRNAs rather than in the promotion of transcription *per se*. The strongest down mutation obtained todate is elicited by a deletion of the spacer DNA immediately preceding the conserved GC rich sequence block. A possible model for the functional organization of the H2A gene resulting from these experiments has been discussed in detail elsewhere (44).

8. OUTLOOK

The few examples of Surrogate Genetics quoted above are probably just the beginning of a long series of experiments to come. One can envisage that this technique will ultimately be complemented by *in vitro* systems in which the various steps for gene expression will be reconstituted biochemically. Many of the systems used for the expression of the transferred genes are clearly very permissive and quite possibly, it will be necessary to introduce the same modified genes back to the whole animal to study the impact of manipulation on the regulation, and not just transcription, of these modified genes.

While the early Surrogate Genetics experiments have centered around the description of effects on RNA synthesis, these studies can be extended to include aspects of processing of precursor RNA, of RNA splicing, of RNA transport, of packaging of the RNA into informosomes of their partition in the various cytoplasmic compartments of protein synthesis and processing (45) and, finally, to the excretion of gene products from the oocyte into the surrounding medium. To give an example: Sequence manipulated genes will probably be able to explain why after the injection of sea urchin histone DNA in the oocyte genuine histone mRNAs move into the cytoplasm, while unfaithful transcripts of the same DNA are sequestered within the oocyte nucleus (see above).

Hardly anything has as yet been done to characterize the chromatin structure of injected genes and the proteins associated with it. We have also pointed out the importance of circularity of the DNA molecules for the expression of faithful H2B mRNA. This might ultimately turn out to be a consequence of chromatin assemblage and the DNA constraints introduced by circularity of the DNA molecule. There are obvious applications of the microinjection techniques to the study of viral genoms. As viral DNA can be brought to expression in the *Xenopus* oocyte, mutation which otherwise would be lethal to the virus can be studied in depth. The studies of the longevity of mRNA after removal of poly-A and polyadenylation of mRNA (reviewed in Ref.46) is another elegant example of how biochemical intervention can be used to further dissect the pathway of gene expression in the oocyte system. Because of its size, oocyte systems may provide not only a natural environment for the expression of genes in isolated, injected nuclei, it may also be useful for biochemical complementation in which regulatory proteins are identified when injected in conjunction with defined genes.

These few examples underline the importance of the *Xenopus* oocyte system for further research in Molecular Biology. While ultimately genes will have to be studied within the natural genetic background, implanted in the chromosomes, the technique of Surrogate Genetics will provide a useful alternative to the classical genetical analysis, at least in the near future.

9. ACKNOWLEDGEMENTS

We are grateful to Prof . G. Malacinski (Bloomington) and E. Triplett (Santa Barbara) for having introduced us generously and patiently to the basics of microinjection of frog oocytes and eggs. We wish to thank Mr. Paul Wettstein who has established and maintained a healthy *Xenopus* colony and has provided us with a long series of *Xenopus* females. Dr. Margaret Chipchase has critically read the manuscript and has made many useful comments. We wish to thank her and Frau Silvia Oberholzer who has typed the manuscript and Mr. Fritz

Ochsenbein who provided Figure 1.

10. REFERENCES

1) GANNON, F., O'HARE, K., PERRIN, F., LE PENNEC, J.P., BENOIST, C., COCHET, M., BREATHNACH, R., ROYAL, A., GARAPIN, A., CAMI,B. and CHAMBON, P. (1979). Organization and sequences at the 5' end of a cloned complete ovalbumin gene. Nature, 278, 428.
2) BUSSLINGER, M., PORTMANN, R. and BIRNSTIEL, M.L. (1979). A regulatory sequence near the 3' end of sea urchin histone genes. Nucleic Acids Res., 9, 2997.
3) BIRNSTIEL, M.L., and CHIPCHASE, M. (1977). Current work on the histone operon. Trends in Biochemical Sciences, 2, 149.
4) WIGLER, M., PELLICER, A., SILVERSTEIN, S. and AXEL, R. (1978). Biochemical transfer of single-copy eucaryotic genes using total cellular DNA as Donor. Cell, 14, 725.
5) SCHAFFNER, W., TOPP, W. and BOTCHAN, M. (1979). Movement of foreign DNA into and out of somatic cell chromosomes by linkage to SV40. In: Specific eukaryotic genes, Alfred Benzon Symposium 13, Munksgaard.
6) DUMONT, J.N. (1972). Oogenesis in Xenopus laevis. J. Morphol., 136, 153.
7) CABADA, M.O., DARNBROUGH, C., FORD, P.J. and TURNER, P.C. (1977). Differential accumulation of two size classes of poly(A) associated with messenger RNA during oogenesis in Xenopus laevis. Dev. Biol., 57, 427.
8) ANDERSON, D.M. and SMITH, L.D. (1978). Patterns of synthesis and accumulation of heterogeneous RNA in lampbrush stage oocytes of Xenopus laevis. Dev.Biol., 67, 274.
9) ROEDER, R.G. (1974). Multiple forms of deoxyribonucleic acid-dependent ribonucleic acid polymerase in Xenopus laevis. J.Biol. Chem., 249, 249.
10) ADAMSON, E.D. and WOODLAND, H.R. (1977). Changes in the rate of

11) LANE, C.D. and KNOWLAND, J. (1975). The injection of RNA into living cells: The use of frog oocytes for the assay of mRNA and the study of the control of gene expression. In: The biochemistry of animal development. Vol. III, 145.

12) COLMAN, A. (1975). Transcription of DNAs of known sequence after injection into the eggs and oocytes of Xenopus laevis. Eur. J. Biochem., 57, 85.

13) MERTZ, J.E. and GURDON, J.B. (1977). Purified DNAs are transcribed after microinjection into Xenopus oocytes. Proc.Natl.Acad.Sci.USA, 74, 1502.

14) GURDON, J.B. (1976). Injected nuclei in frog oocytes: Fate, enlargement, and chromatin dispersal. J. Embryol. Exp. Morph.,36, 523.

15) KRESSMANN, A., CLARKSON, S.G., TELFORD, J.L. and BIRNSTIEL, M.L. (1977). Transcription of Xenopus $tDNA^{met}_{1}$ and sea urchin histone DNA injected into the Xenopus oocyte nucleus. Cold Spring Harbor Symp. Quant. Biol.,42, 1077.

16) GURDON, J.B. (1974). The control of gene expression in animal development. Clarendon Press.

17) BILLET, F.S. and WILD, A.E. (1975). Practical studies of animal development. Chapman.

18) WYLLIE, A.H., GURDON, J.B. and PRICE, J. (1977). Nuclear localization of an oocyte component required for the stability of injected DNA. Nature, 268, 150.

19) WYLLIE, A.H., LASKEY, R.A., FINCH, J. and GURDON, J.B. (1978). Selective DNA conservation and chromatin assembly after injection of SV40 DNA into Xenopus oocytes. Dev. Biol., 64, 178.

20) GURDON, J.B. and BROWN, D.D. (1978). The transcription of 5S DNA injected into Xenopus oocytes. Dev. Biol., 67, 346.

21) TRENDELENBURG, M.F. and GURDON, J.B. (1978). Transcription of cloned Xenopus ribosomal genes visualised after injection into oocyte nuclei. Nature, 276, 292.

22) GURDON, J.B. (1967). On the origin and persistance of a cytoplasmic

state inducing nuclear DNA synthesis in frog eggs. Proc. Natl. Acad. Sci.USA, 58, 545.

23) GURDON, J.B., BIRNSTIEL, M.L. and SPEIGHT, V.A. (1969). The replication of purified DNA introduced into living egg cytoplasm. Biochim. Biophys. Acta, 174, 614.

24) LASKEY, R.A. and GURDON, J.B. (1973). Induction of Polyoma DNA synthesis by injection into frog-egg cytoplasm. Eur. J. Biochem., 57, 467.

25) BENBOW, R.M., KRAUSS, M.R. and REEDER, R.H. (1978). DNA synthesis in a multi-enzyme system from Xenopus laevis eggs. Cell, 13, 307.

26) BROWN, D.D. and GURDON, J.B. (1977). High-fidelity transcription of 5S DNA injected into Xenopus oocytes. Proc. Natl. Acad. Sci. USA, 74, 2064.

27) BROWN, D.D. and GURDON, J.B. (1978). Cloned single repeating units of 5S DNA direct accurate transcription of 5S RNA when injected into Xenopus oocytes. Proc. Natl. Acad. Sci.USA, 75, 2849.

28) KORN, L.J. and BROWN, D.D. (1978). Nucleotide sequence of Xenopus borealis oocyte 5S DNA: Comparison of sequences that flank several related eukaryotic genes. Cell, 15, 1145.

29) FEDOROFF, N.V. (1979). Deletion mutants of Xenopus leavis 5S ribosomal DNA. Cell, 16, 551.

30) KRESSMANN, A., CLARKSON, S.G., PIROTTA, V. and BIRNSTIEL, M.L. (1978). Transcription of cloned tRNA gene fragments and subfragments injected into the oocyte nucleus of Xenopus laevis. Proc. Natl. Acad. Sci. USA, 75, 1176.

31) TELFORD, J.L., KRESSMANN, A., KOSKI, R.A.,GROSSCHEDL, R., MUELLER, F., CLARKSON, S.G. and BIRNSTIEL, M.L. (1979). Delimitation of a promoter for RNA polymerase III by means of a functional test. Proc. Natl. Acad. Sci. USA, 76, 2590.

32) KRESSMANN, A., HOFSTETTER, H., DI CAPUA, E., GROSSCHEDL, R. and BIRNSTIEL, M. (1979). A tRNA gene of Xenopus laevis contains at least two sites promoting transcription. Nucl. Acids Res., 7,

December issue, in press.

33) CORTESE, R., MELTON, D., TRANQUILLA, T. and SMITH, J.D. (1978). Cloning of nematode tRNA genes and their expression in the frog oocyte. Nucl. Acids Res., 5, 4593.

34) DE ROBERTIS, E.M. and OLSON, M.V. (1979). Transcription and processing of cloned yeast tyrosine tRNA genes microinjected into frog oocytes. Nature, 278, 137.

35) PROBST, E., KRESSMANN, A. and BIRNSTIEL, M.L. (1979). Expression of sea urchin genes in the oocyte of Xenopus laevis. J. Mol. Biol., 135, 709.

36) LASKEY, R.A., HONDA, B.M., MILLS, A.D., MORRIS, N.R., WYLLIE, A.H., MERTZ, J.E., DE ROBERTIS, E.M. and GURDON, J.B. (1977). Cold Spring Harbor Symp. Quant. Biol., 42, 171.

37) BIRNSTIEL, M.L., KRESSMANN, A., SCHAFFNER, W., PORTMANN, R. and BUSSLINGER, M. (1978). Aspects of the regulation of histone genes. Phil. Trans. R. Soc. Lond. B., 283, 319.

38) BIRNSTIEL, M.L., PORTMANN, R., BUSSLINGER, M., SCHAFFNER, W., PROBST, E. and KRESSMANN, A. (1979). Functional organization of the histone genes in the sea urchin Psammechinus: A progress report. In: Specific eukaryotic genes, Alfred Benzon Symposium, Munksgaard.

39) TRENDELENBURG, M.F., JENTGRAF, H., FRANKE, W.W. and GURDON, J.B. (1978). Transcription patterns of amplified Dytiscus genes coding for ribosomal RNA after injection into Xenopus oocyte nuclei. Proc. Natl. Acad. Sci. USA, 75, 3791.

40) DE ROBERTIS, E.D. and MERTZ, J.E. (1977). Coupled transcription-translation of DNA injected into Xenopus oocytes. Cell, 12, 175.

41) FAREED, G.C. and DAVOLI, D. (1977). Molecular biology of papovaviruses. Ann. Rev. Biochem., 46, 471.

42) ALONI, Y., DHAR, R., LAUB, O., HOROWITZ, M. and KHOURY, G. (1977). Novel mechanism for RNA maturation. The leader sequences of simian virus 40 mRNA are not transcribed adjacent to the coding sequences. Proc. Natl. Acad. Sci.USA, 74, 3686.

43) RUNGGER, D. and TUERLER, H. (1978). DNAs of simian virus 40 and polyoma direct the synthesis of viral tumor antigens and capsid proteins in Xenopus oocytes. Proc. Natl. Acad. Sci. USA, 75, 6073.

44) GROSSCHEDL, R. and BIRNSTIEL, M.L. (1980). Deletions in the prelude of the sea urchin H2A histone gene elicit quantitative and qualitative changes in gene expression. Proc. Natl. Acad. Sci. USA, in press.

45) HUEZ, G., GHYSDAEL, J., TRAVNICEK, M., BURNY, A., CLEUTER, Y., KETTMANN, R., MARBAIX, G. and PORTETELLE, D. (1978). Post-translational processing of oncornavirus proteins. In: Processing and turnover of proteins and organelles in the cell. 12th FEBS Meeting, 1978, 53, 3.

46) MARBAIX, G., HUEZ, G., SOREQ, H., GALLWITZ, D., WEINBERG, E., DEVOS, R., HUBERT, E. and CLEUTER, Y. (1978). Role of the polyadenylate segment in the stability of eukaryotic messenger RNAs. In: Gene functions. 12th FEBS Meeting, 1978, 51, 427.

GRAFTS AND TRANSFER OF CELL CONSTITUENTS INTO THE GIANT UNICELLULAR ALGA *ACETABULARIA**

S. Bonotto and A. Lüttke

Department of Radiobiology
C.E.N.-S.C.K., 2400 Mol
Belgium

1. INTRODUCTION

The transfer of cell constituents into eukaryotic cells has been realized by nature long before the scientists had developed appropriate experimental procedures. For instance, chloroplasts occur within the cells of the digestive diverticula of the marine gastropod molluscs *Elysia atroviridis* (1,2), *Tridachia crispata, Tridachiella diomedea* and *Placobranchus ianthobapsus* (3, 4). Moreover, chloroplasts with stalked pyrenoids and mitochondria most probably belonging to a cryptomonad endosymbiont were found in the marine planktonic ciliate *Mesodinium rubrum* (5).

Successful transfers have been performed in the laboratory with animal or plant cells having a large size: *Amoeba* (6-8), *Stentor* (9-11) , *Micrasterias* (12), *Chara* and *Nitella* (13) and *Acetabularia* (14).

---

*Work dedicated to Professor Joachim Hämmerling, pioneer of transfer of cell constituents into *Acetabularia*.

Sea-urchin and amphibian eggs were also utilized for obtaining anucleate fragments (15). These latter, however, undergo a limited development compared with the extensive regeneration capability of anucleate *Acetabularia*. This paper is thought to demonstrate the unique suitability of *Acetabularia* for grafts and for transfer of cell constituents : experiments already performed and possibilities.

2. *ACETABULARIA* AND THE OTHER DASYCLADALES

Acetabularia is a unicellular uninucleate marine alga with a very peculiar morphology during its biological cycle (16). It belongs to the Dasycladales, which is a conspicuous group of 40 living species within the Chlorophyceae. Experiments are mainly done with *A. mediterranea* (Fig. 1a) . Other species less often used but equally well suited are *A. crenulata* (Fig. 1b), *A. major, A. peniculus* (Fig. 1c, d) and *Batophora oerstedii*.

A considerable amount of literature has been accumulated on *Acetabularia* and on the other Dasycladales (17-21). According to current ideas (16), the morphological differentiation of the cell is controlled by the nucleus. The products of nuclear genes - "morphogenetic substances" (22) - migrate into the cytoplasm, where they can be stored for several weeks. The nuclear mRNAs specify the synthesis of the enzymes necessary for the morphogenetic events. Morphogenesis is thought to be regulated at the level of translation (23). Post-translational processes, as emphasized by Werz (24), may also be important for the co-ordinated realization of morphogenesis in *Acetabularia*.

Fig. 1. *Morphological traits of 3 Acetabularia species*. A: 2 *A. mediterranea* cells with a cap; B: *A. crenulata*; C: Apical region of an *A. peniculus* cell showing cap's primordia and the numerous hairs of a whorl; D: Reproductive cap of *A. peniculus*. The nucleus is located in the rhizoid (r).
Bar: A and B = 5 mm; C = 5 mm; C = 1 mm; D = 2.5 mm.

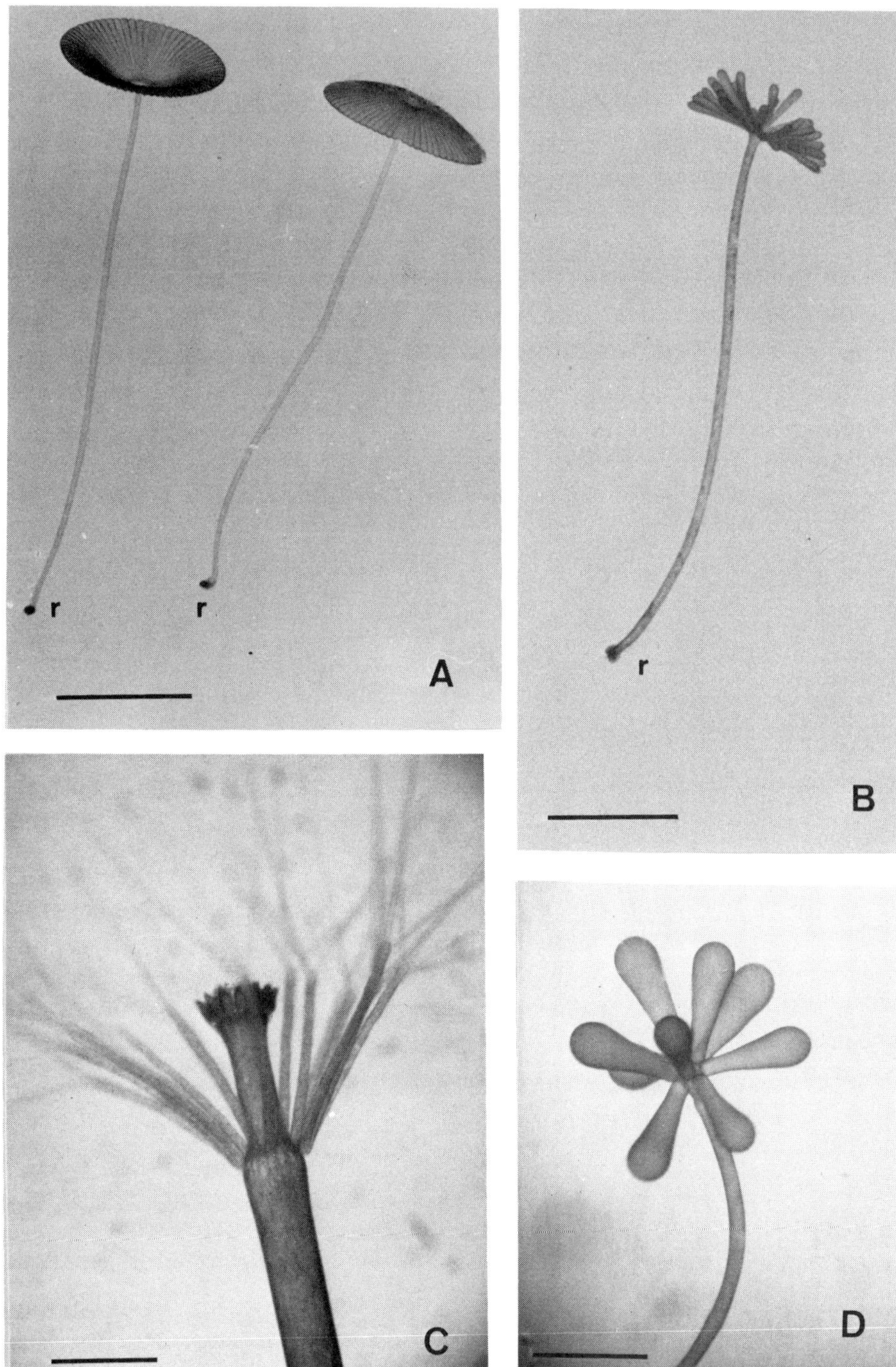
r
r
A
r
B
C
D

3. MANIPULATIONS WITH *ACETABULARIA* AND RELATED SPECIES

For the large size of *A. mediterranea* (3-4 cm) and several related species different types of manipulations are possible, which are essentially based on microsurgery and microinjection (25).

(i) Preparation of nucleate and anucleate fragments

Since in *Acetabularia* the nucleus is located in the rhizoid, enucleation may be made by simply cutting off the basal end (1-2 mm) of the stalk (26). This operation provides a long anucleate fragment (often called anucleate cell) and a very short nucleate basal part, which regenerates again to a whole cell (Fig. 2a). Anucleate fragments are capable of forming such complex structures as stalk, sterile whorls and a species specific cap (26). For investigations on the morphological and physiological apicobasal gradient, *Acetabularia* cells may be dissected into defined segments (Fig. 2b).

(ii) Preparation of whorls

During the vegetative growth, *Acetabularia* cells develop several whorls (27), which contain elongated chloroplasts. Whorl preparation is obtained by cutting the stalk above and beneath the first order articles (Fig. 2c). The stalk cytoplasm flows into the medium, whereas that of the hairs is maintained in position thanks to their constrictions. Isolated whorls are useful for studies on their physiology and metabolic activity.

Fig. 2. *Classification of manipulations with Acetabularia.* A: Preparation on nucleate and anucleate fragments; B: Dissection into 4 segments having a different morphogenetic capability; C: Preparation of whorls; D: Uninucleate grafts; E: Binucleate graft obtained by joining telescopically two basal parts; F: Anucleate cytoplasmic graft; G: Double graft of anucleate stalks to a rhizoid; H: Double graft of rhizoids to an anucleate stalk; I: Graft with branched cells.

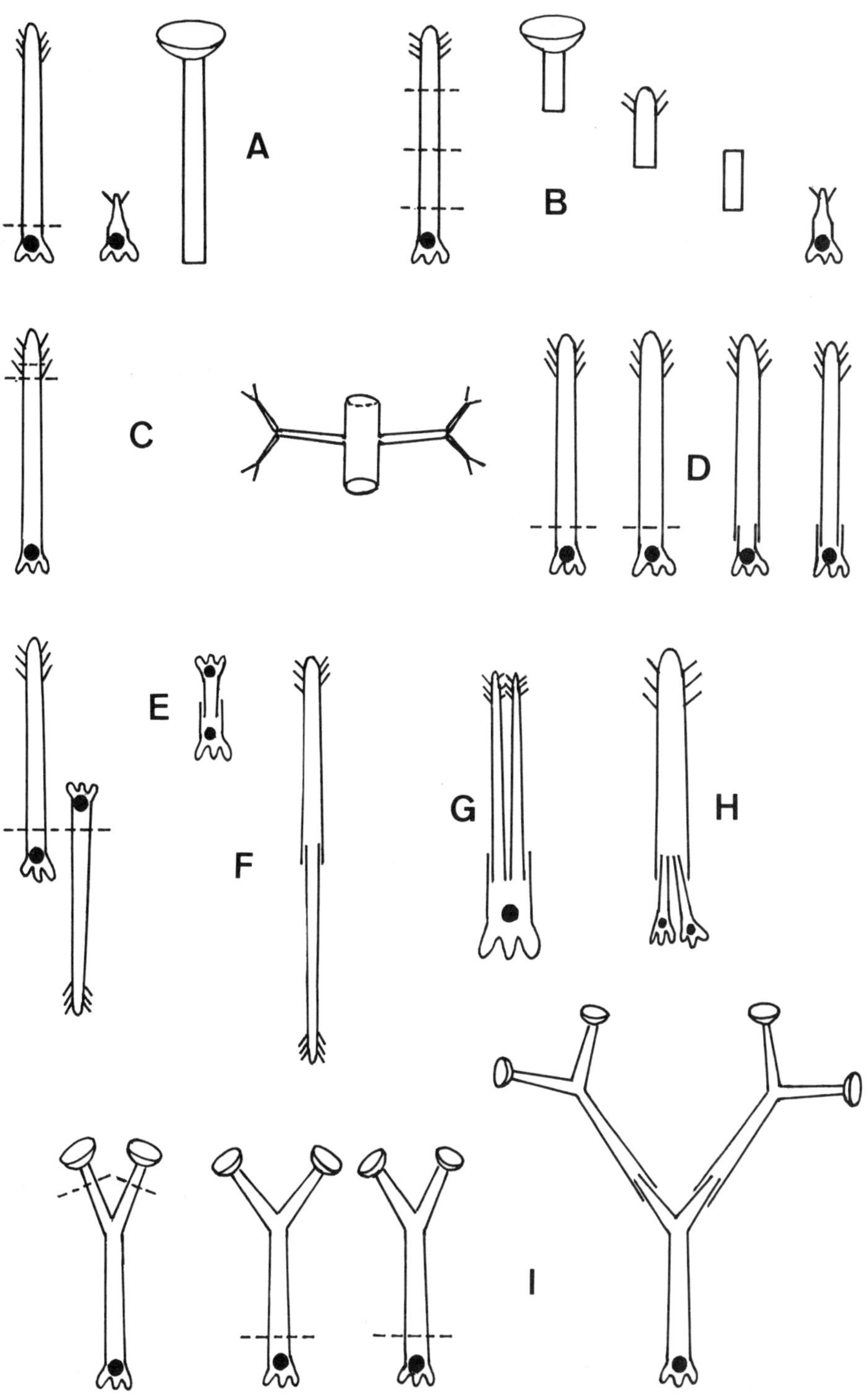
A
B
C
D
E
F
G
H
I

(iii) Isolation of cytoplasts and of protoplasts

Cut *Acetabularia* fragments release small droplets of cytoplasm, which contain all the constituents of a living cell except for the nucleus and the cell wall. These droplets, called cytoplasts by Gibor (28), are able to survive for at least two weeks but can not synthesize a new cell wall. They may be useful for *in vitro* physiological studies, such as investigations on the duration of functional chloroplasts in a normal cellular environment but free of nuclear control, or nucleus implantation studies.

Treatment of "haploid" *Acetabularia* (29) with papain and proteinase K induces protoplast extrusion (30). Fusion of two protoplasts or of a protoplast and an anucleate cytoplast (28) was artificially induced. However, fusion of the two "haploid" nuclei has never been observed (30). Fusion of protoplasts from *Acetabularia* may offer the possibility of obtaining homozygous diploid algae or diploid genomes. However, it is not yet ascertained that fused protoplast are able to regenerate a whole cell. It is to be noted that intra- and interspecific fusions of protoplasts have already been obtained with higher plants (31, 32).

(iv) Intraspecific and interspecific grafts

Two or more parts of *Acetabularia* may be grafted together by joining telescopically the cut ends (Fig. 2, d-h). The first intraspecific graft has been made with *Acetabularia mediterranea* by Hämmerling already in 1932 (26). Later on, several types of intraspecific and of interspecific grafts were undertaken by Hämmerling (14-22) and his collaborators as well as by other authors (33). Four species were mainly used for preparing interspecific grafts:

A. mediterranea, A. crenulata, A. peniculus and *A. wettsteini*.

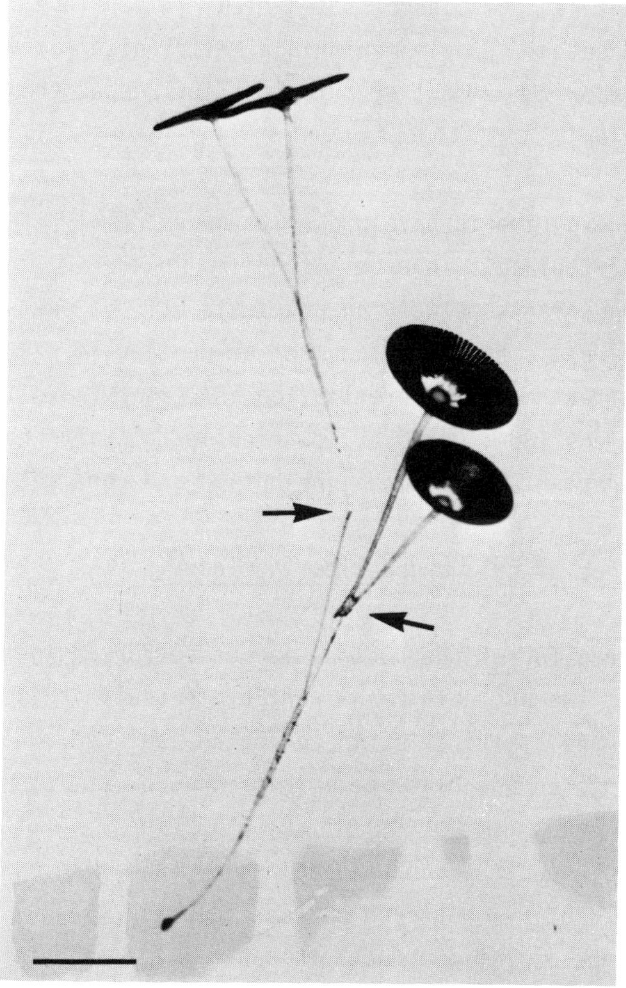

Fig. 3. *A. mediterranea*. Grafted cell showing 4 reproductive caps with cysts. The arrows indicate the site where the stalks are joined. Bar = 5 mm.

Extraordinarily large cells of *A. mediterranea* were obtained by grafting apical cell fragments into a branched stalk containing the rhizoid with one nucleus (Fig. 2i). These cells, which had been investigated in our laboratory (34), have shown normal development until cyst formation in their caps (Fig. 3). Cells of this type should be interesting for questions like: "Is there a positive correlation between the size of the nucleus (higer level of polyploidy) and the amount of cytoplasm within a cell"? Alternatively, it can be asked, whether the amount of cytoplasm influences the physiology of the nucleus.

Graft experiments have proven to be extremely useful for studying nucleocytoplasmic interrelationships in *Acetabularia*. More than 40 years ago grafts between an anucleate half of one species (*A. mediterranea*) and a nucleate fragment of another (*A. wettsteini*) demonstrated that cell differentiation in *Acetabularia* is controlled by the nucleus (35). Moreover, plurinucleate grafts have permitted to gain important insight on gene dosage and gene interactions (36).

(v) Transfer of cell organelles: Nucleus

The transfer of the nucleus may be performed in two ways: 1) by grafting the nucleate basal part of the cell (rhizoid) to the cut end of the stalk; 2) by injecting an isolated nucleus into a whole or into an anucelate cell (Fig. 4 a, b).

A viable nucleus can be obtained by squeezing out the content of the rhizoid in a buffered sucrose solution (37-39). Recent improvement of the isolation procedure has allowed to keep a nucleus alive *in vitro* for one day (40). The isolated nucleus is picked up by suction and injected by means of a glass capillary (40). Theoretically any anucleate portion of the stalk receiving a nucleus acquires the capability of regenerating a whole cell and of forming a reproductive cap (Fig. 4c).

It is to be noticed that an isolated nucleus remains more or less contaminated by chloroplasts (41, 42) and probably also by mitochondria. Nevertheless, the number of contaminating organelles surrounding an isolated nucleus is very low with respect to the seve-

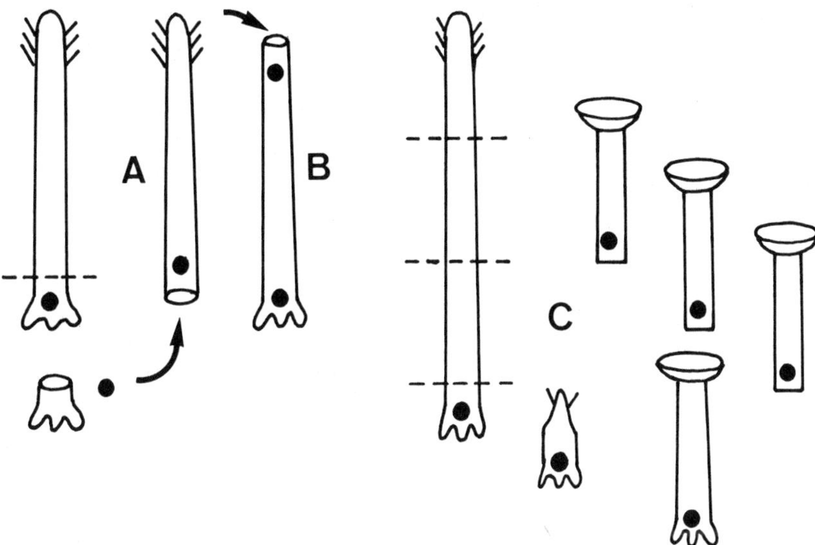

Fig. 4. *Transfer of the nucleus in Acetabularia.* A: Into an anucleate stalk; B: Into a nucleate stalk, giving a binucleate cell; C: Into 3 anucleate fragments of the stalk, which acquire the capability of regenerating a whole cell and of forming a reproductive cap.

ral million chloroplasts of a recipient anucleate cell.

(vi) Transfer of cell organelles: Chloroplasts and mitochondria

It is known that chloroplasts and mitochondria possess their own genome (43). Recent investigations have shown that these organelles are not fully autonomous in that several of their proteins being coded for by the nucleus (44). Transfer of chloroplasts and mitochondria into an heterologous cytoplasm may reveal interesting aspects concerning the specificity of their nuclear dependency.

An *Acetabularia* cell has several million chloroplasts, which are distributed along the stalk according to an apicobasal morphological and physiological gradient (16). Their genome can be visualized in the intact organelle by staining with the DNA specific fluorochrome DAPI (4'6-diamidino-2-phenylindole) (45) (Fig. 5). The flourescent image of the DAPI-DNA complex suggests that inside the chloroplasts the nucleoids are linked. Intact chloroplasts may be obtained by cutting whole *Acetabularia* cells into small pieces: the cytoplasm with the plastids flows into the medium from the cut ends of the stalk. The chloroplasts may then be isolated from the other cell constituents by differential centrifugation. However, chloroplast preparations are always more or less contaminated by mitochondria, which fairly often stick to the plastidal envelope (46). Consequently, when clots of chloroplasts are injected into whole or anucleate *Acetabularia*, some mitochondria are invariably implanted together. In recent work (42), nuclei and chloroplasts of *A. crenulata* have been transferred into anucleate fragments of *A. mediterranea*, for studying the effect of the nucleus on the synthesis of plastidal malate dehydrogenase (MDH).

Although the nuclear dependency of chloroplast MDH has been confirmed (see Ref. 47), the mechanism involved has not been entirely elucidated. Theoretically, the nuclear dependency of chloroplasts for MDH may be explained in various ways: 1) the mRNA synthesized in the nucleus is translated on cytoplasmic 80S ribosomes and the protein is transported into the chloroplasts; 2) the nuclear mRNA is transported into the chloroplasts (48), where it is translated on chloroplastic 70S ribosomes, giving the protein; 3) the nucleus produces specific substances which stimulate the division of species specific chloroplasts, where the synthesis of MDH occurs; 4) the nucleus produces aspecific substances which stimulate the division of homologous as well as of heterologous chloroplasts capable of synthesizing their own MDH; 5) the nucleus modifies the electrophoretic mobility of the MDH without changing its amino acid sequence. The first possibility -- transport of the nuclear gene originated 80S ribosome translation product into the plastids -- seems at present the most plausible. Nevertheless, new transfer experiments

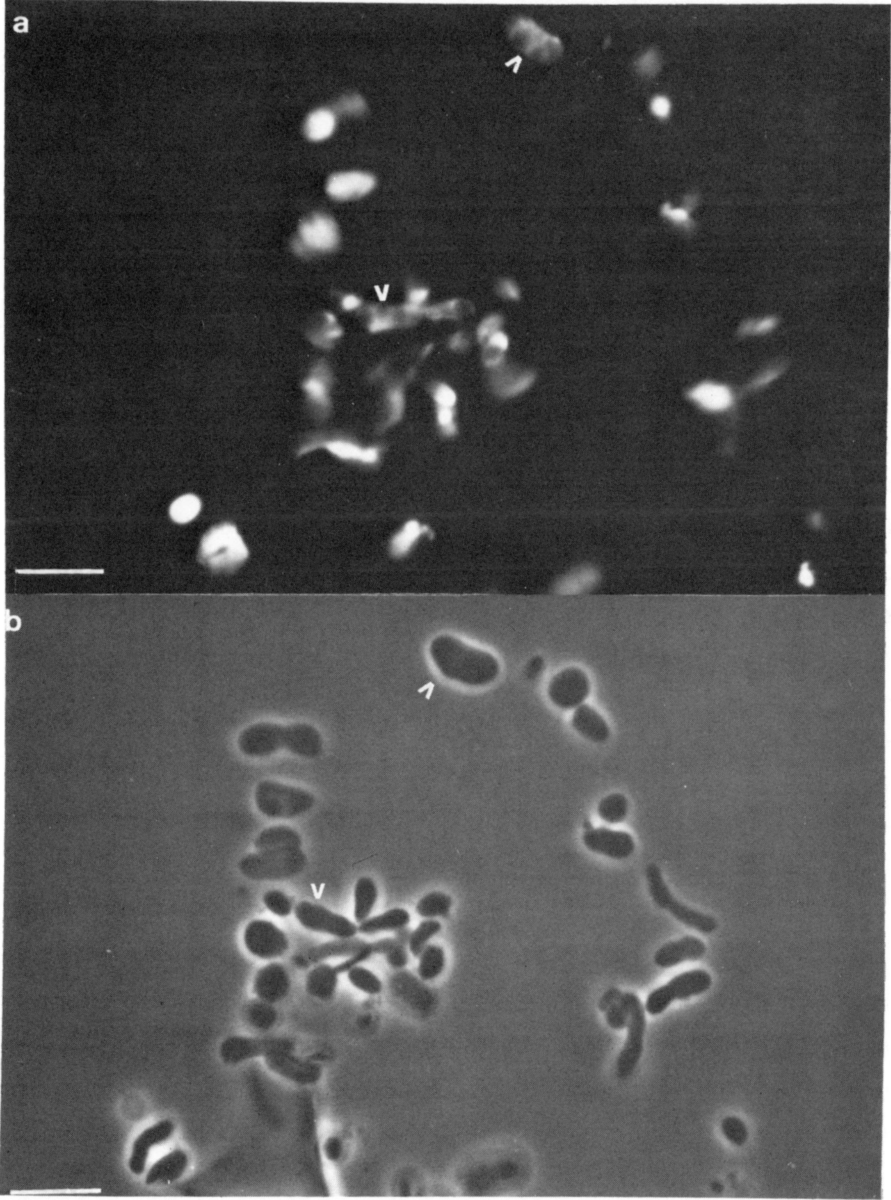

Fig. 5. *A. mediterranea*. Fluorescence (a) and phase contrast (b) photomicrograph of isolated chloroplasts stained with the DNA specific fluorochrome DAPI. Inside the plastids, the nucleoids seem to be linked (arrowheads). The same preparation under phase contrast (b) clearly demonstrates the different size (heterogeneity) of the organelles. Dry mounts. Bar = 10 μm.

seem necessary to throw light on this subject, particularly on account of the "contamination" of the transplanted nucleus by homologous chloroplasts (41, 42).

(vii) Microinjection of virus, viral RNA and polyribosomes

Recent studies have shown that *Acetabularia* cells may be used as an experimental test system for investigating the expression of a heterologous genetic material. Injection of TMV virus or of TMV RNA into anucleate fragments of *A. mediterranea* leads to a *de novo* synthesis of virus nucleic acids and proteins (49). Moreover, an animal virus RNA (Mengovirus) is also translated in *Acetabularia*: isolated nuclei of *A. crenulata* are injected with virus RNA and then transferred into anucleate fragments of *A. mediterranea* or fused with *A. ryukyuensis* cytoplasts (50, 51). After injection of rat polyribosomes an accumulation of albumine and of tyrosine aminotransferase is observed in the recipient anucleate fragments of *A. mediterranea* (49). It is not known if the rat mRNA is translated on the injected animal ribosomes or on the *Acetabularia* ribosomes or on both. Theoretically, an exogenous mRNA transferred into *Acetabularia* may be translated on cytoplasmic 80S or on organelle 70S ribosomes.

It is likely that *Acetabularia* species will be used in future research also for the study of the expression of exogenous DNAs (nuclear, chloroplast, mitochondrial and perhaps plasmid DNA).

(viii) Transfer of proteins

For the progress of research on cellular and molecular biology, it is of interest to know which kind of biological processes are induced by exogenous proteins transferred into living cells. Werz has found that the injection of a gelatine sheet in *A. mediterranea* induces the synthesis of a cell wall around the protein

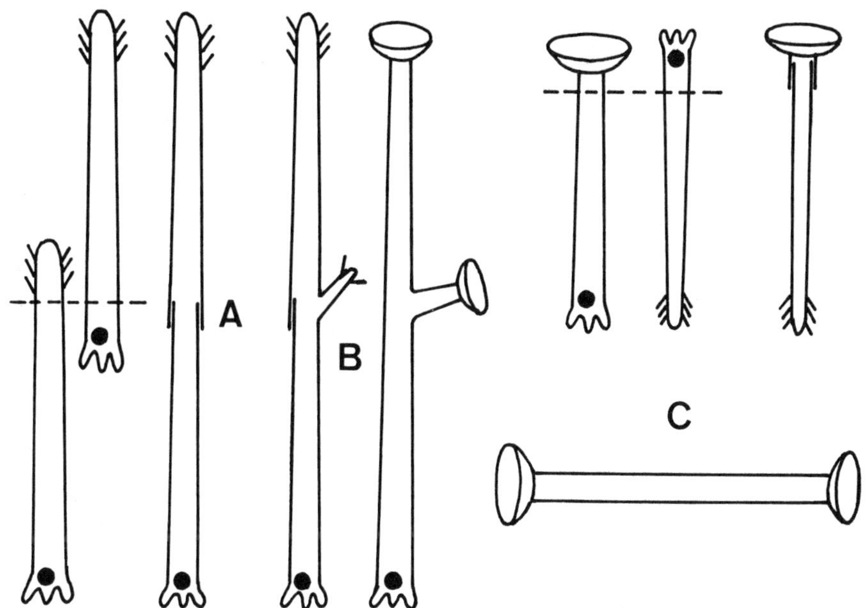

Fig. 6. *A. mediterranea*. New types of intraspecific grafts. A: Uninucleate cell, 8 cm long; B: Regeneration of a new apex at the joining site; in this case the cell develop 2 reproductive caps; C: Grafting of a vegetative anucleate fragment to an old cap already having secondary nuclei in its rays; the anucleate fragment forms a reproductive cap.

(52). New investigations on this subject would be particularly useful.

4. NEW INTRASPECIFIC GRAFTS WITH *A. MEDITERRANEA*

The large size of a normal *Acetabularia* and the availability of branched cells permit to perform new intraspecific grafts. A very long nucleate cell may be obtained by joining a whole cell to an anucleate fragment (Fig. 6a). These cells may be indicated with the formula med_1 med_0 med_0, since they have a twofold amount of cytoplasm. Often a new stalk regenerates at the joining of the two stalk ends, forming later a reproductive cap (Fig. 6b). We have found that se-

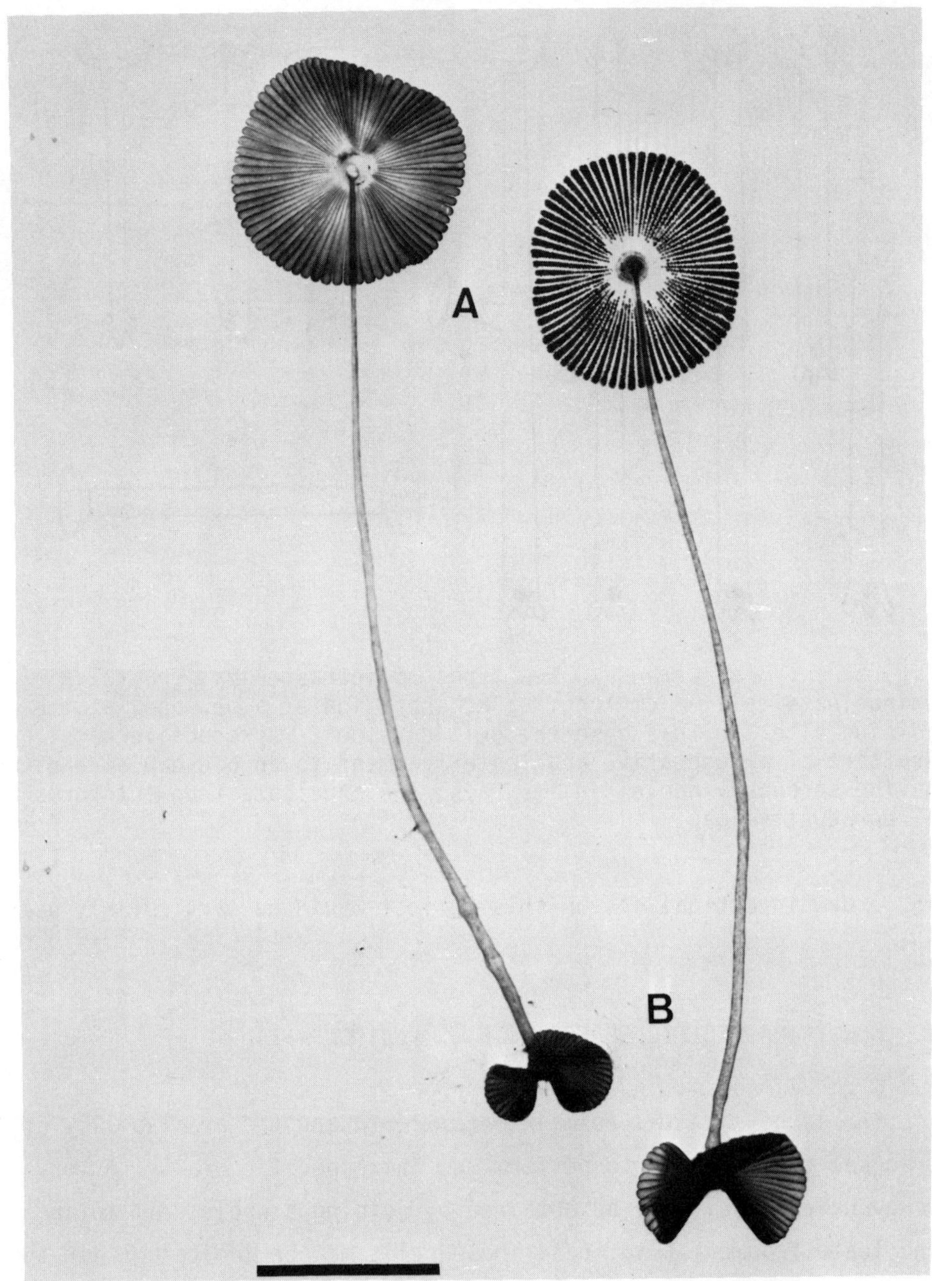

Fig. 7. *A. mediterranea*. Grafting of a vegetative anucleate fragment to an old cap with secondary nuclei in its rays. A: Old caps; B: New caps formed by the grafted anucleated fragments. Bar = 5 mm.

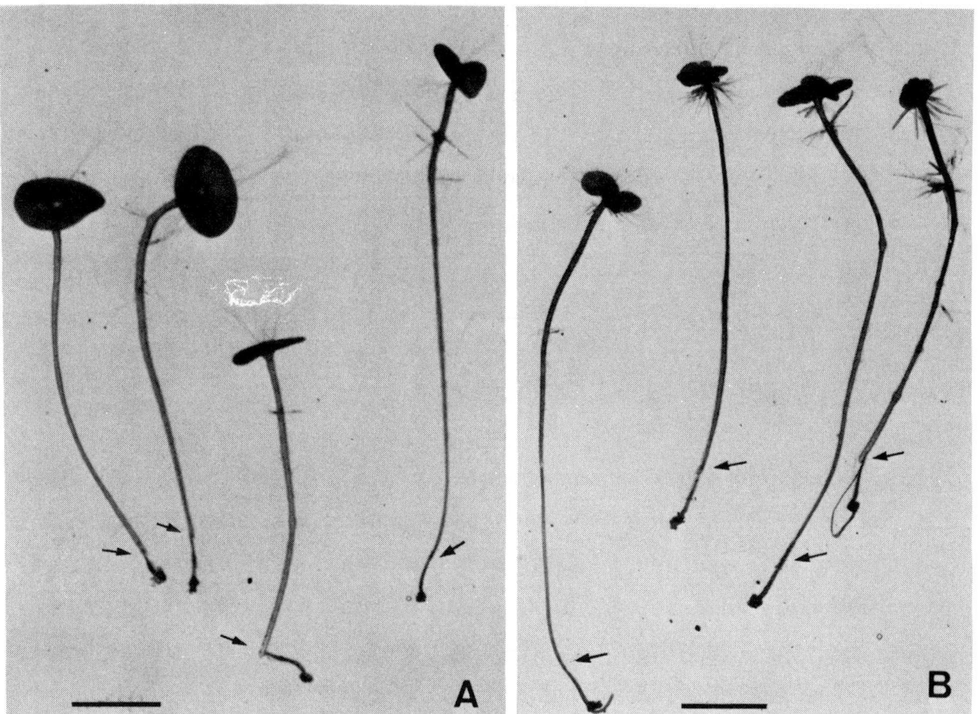

Fig. 8. *A. mediterranea.* Grafts between irradiated (X-rays) and non-irradiated plants (med_1 med_0) according to the scheme shown in Fig. 2D. Rhizoids of about 5 mm length from control plants were transplanted into anucleate cells (50 Kr) 34 days after the irradiation. A: Grafted cells having developed a normal cap; B: Grafted cells having formed an irregularly shaped cap. 20 days after transplantation. The arrows show the joining site. Bar = 5 mm.

condary nuclei are able to cover a distance of 7-8 cm, from the rhizoid to the reproductive cap. However, the regulation of their transport may be disturbed since in some cells numerous secondary nuclei remain in the stalk, where later cysts develop.

Another interesting type of graft may be made between a whole cell possessing a full grown cap and an anucleate vegetative fragment (Fig. 6c). This type of graft may indicate if one or more of the haploid secondary nuclei originally migrated into the cap, acquire the capability of moving again into a new transplanted stalk. Fig. 7 shows a grafted cell, in which the secondary nuclei remain in the old cap in spite of the fact that the anucleate fragment has formed a reproductive cap. Possibly, the secondary nuclei present in an old cap are incapable of moving because they are anchored by microtubules (53). However, as our investigations are still at a preliminary stage, it is too early to come to a definite interpretation.

5. RADIOBIOLOGY AND GRAFT EXPERIMENTS

Graft experiments are particularly valuable for studying several radiobiological problems (54, 55). Grafts with one irradiated and one control partner (nucleate and/or anucleate) may answer such important questions as: 1) Is the nucleus or the cytoplasm the main target for the radiation?; 2) How stable is the effect of the radiation in the nucleus and in the cytoplasm?; 3) Can irradiated nuclei and cytoplasm recover by grafting unirradiated cell constituents?; 4) Which is the contribution of cytoplasmic organelles to cell differentiation?

In previous work (16, 18) it has been found that the morphological differentiation of *Acetabularia* cells is strongly inhibited by increasing doses of radiations. A dose of 50 Kr inhibits the differentiation in 40-50% of the cells, probably by destroying the morphogenetic substances (55). We have observed that cells irradiated with a dose of 50 Kr acquire the capability of differentiation after transplanting a normal rhizoid, even if a long lapse of time (34 days) is passed after the irradiation (Fig. 8 a, b). However, some cells show several anomalies (Fig. 9 a, b) indicating that part of the radiation damage can not completely be restored in all the cells. The rhizoids cut from irradiated cells (50 Kr) show a different degree of regeneration: Some regenerate as normal cells, others per-

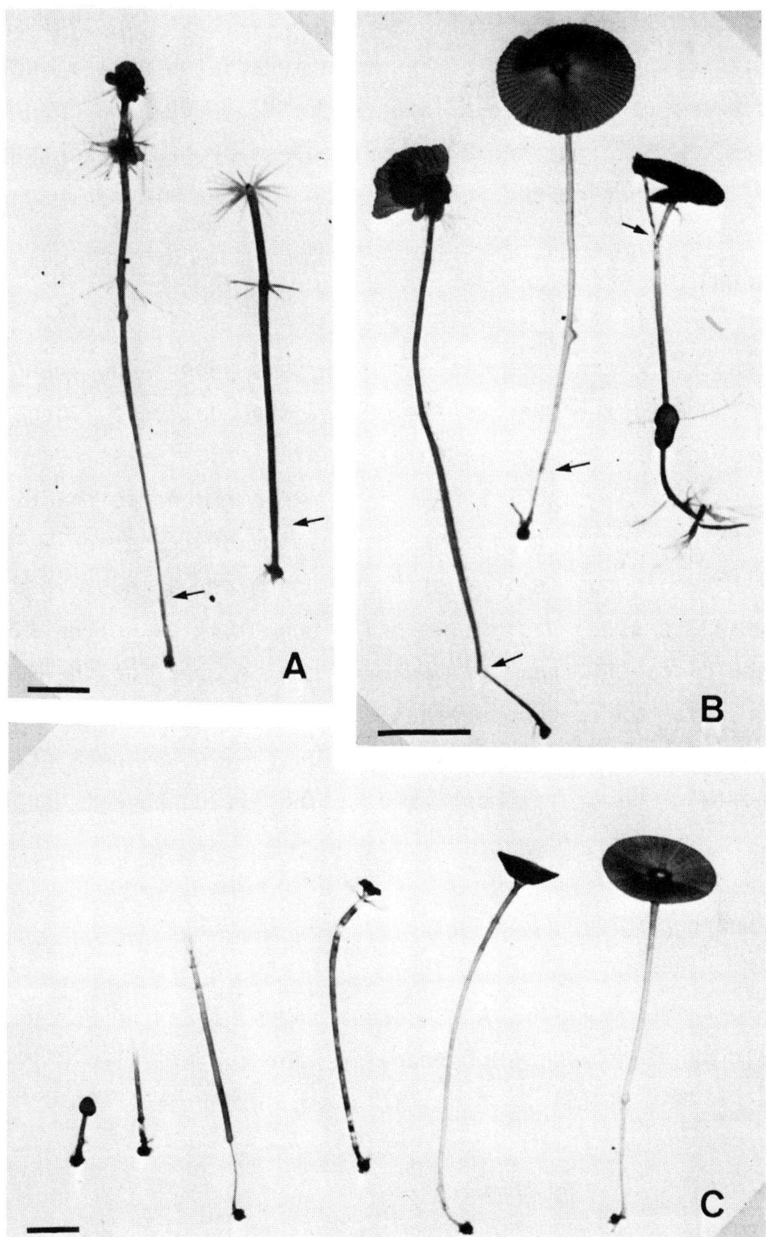

Fig. 9. *A. mediterranea*. A and B: Grafted cells ($med_1\ med_{OR}$) having regenerated more or less irregular caps; one of them (A) has regenerated only sterile whorls. C: Regenerated rhizoids of the irradiated plants (X-rays; 50 Kr). The arrows show the joining site. Bar = 5 mm.

form only a limited regeneration (Fig. 9c). These findings suggest that cutting the stalk may revive some irradiated nuclei and at the same time show that: 1) Irradiated nuclei (50 Kr) have not lost their potentialities; 2) The irradiated cytoplasm probably exerts an inhibitory influence on the nucleus.

6. CONCLUSIONS

Results and concepts discussed in this paper show that *Acetabularia* (and related species) is one of the most useful organisms for investigating the subtle relationships which exist between nucleus and cytoplasm and for examining the intergenomic co-operation inside the eukaryotic cell. The possibility of transferring homologous or heterologous cell constituents permits various types of *in vivo* and *in vitro* biological and biochemical experiments. Moreover, the discovery that *Acetabularia* can be used for the study of the expression of exogenous genetical material increases even more the value of this giant unicellular alga, which was once called by Brachet (18) "one of the most fascinating living objects in the world".

7. ACKNOWLEDGEMENTS

We wish to thank Mr. A. Bossus and Mrs. Jeannine Romeyer for kind help and The European Communities for support. The DAPI was a generous gift of Prof. O. Dann, Erlangen University.

8. REFERENCES

1) KAWAGUTI, S. and YAMASU, T. (1965). Electron microscopy of the symbiosis between an elysioid gastropod and chloroplasts of a green alga. Biol. J. Okayama Univ., 11, 57.
2) TAYLOR, D.L. (1968). Chloroplasts as symbiotic organelles in the

digestive gland of *Elysia viridis* (Gastropoda: Opisthobranchia). J. Mar. Biol. Ass. U.K., 48, 1.

3) TRENCH, R.K. (1969). Chloroplasts as functional endosymbionts in the mollusc *Tridachia crispata* (Bërgh), (Opisthobranchia, Sacoglossa). Nature, 222, 1071.

4) TRENCH, R.K., GREENE, R.W. and BYSTROM, B.G. (1969). Chloroplasts as functional organelles in animal tissues. J. Cell Biol., 42, 404.

5) TAYLOR, F.J.R., BLACKBOURN, D.J. and BLACKBOURN, J. (1969). Ultrastructure of the chloroplasts and associated structures within the marine ciliate *Mesodinium rubrum* (Lohmann), Nature, 224, 819.

6) ORD, H.J. (1968). The viability of the anucleate cytoplasm of *Amoeba proteus*. J. Cell Sci., 3, 81

7) JEON, K.W. and LORCH, I.J. (1969). Lethal effect of heterologous nuclei in *Amoeba* heterokaryons. Exptl. Cell Res., 56, 233.

8) LORCH, I.J. and JEON, K.W. (1969). Character changes induced by heterologous nuclei in *Amoeba* heterokaryons. Exptl. Cell Res., 57, 22.

9) TARTAR, V. (1961). "The Biology of *Stentor*". Pergamon Press, Oxford, p. 413.

10) TARTAR, V. (1968). Micrurgical experiments of cytokinesis in *Stentor coeruleus* . Amer. J. Exptl. Zool, 167, 21.

11) TARTAR, V. (1972). Anucleate Stentors: Morphogenetic and behavioral capabilities. In: "Biology and Radiobiology of Anucleate Systems. I. Bacteria and Animal Cells". (eds., S. Bonotto, R. Goutier, R. Kirchmann and J.R. Maisin), Academic Press, New York and London, p. 125.

12) WARIS, H. and KALLIO, P. (1972). Effects of enucleation of *Micrasterias*. In: "Biology and Radiobiology of Anucleate Systems. II. Plant Cells". (eds., S. Bonotto, R. Goutier, R. Kirchmann and J.R. Maisin), Academic Press, New York and London, p. 137.

13) KURODA, K. and KAMIYA, N. (1968). Cell operation in *Nitella*. V. Implantation of foreign bodies into an internodal cell. Proc. Japan Acad., 44, 823.

14) HÄMMERLING, J. (1963). Nucleocytoplasmic interactions in *Acetabularia* and other cells. Ann. Rev. Plant Physiol., 14, 65.

15) BRACHET, J. (1972). Morphogenesis and synthesis of macromolecules in the absence of the nucleus. In: "Biology and Radiobiology of Anucleate Systems. I. Bacteria and Animal Cells". (eds., S. Bonotto, R. Goutier, R. Kirchmann and J.R. Maisin), Academic Press, New York and London, p. 1.

16) BONOTTO, S., LURQUIN, P. and MAZZA, A. (1976). Recent advances in research on the marine alga *Acetabularia*. Adv. Mar. Biol., 14, 123.

17) PUISEUX-DAO, S. (1970). "*Acetabularia* and Cell Biology". Logos Press, London, p. 162.

18) BRACHET, J. and BONOTTO, S. (eds.) (1970). "Biology of *Acetabularia*", Academic Press, New York and London, p. 300.

19) PUISEUX-DAO, S. (ed.) (1977). "Molecular Biology of Nucleocytoplasmic Relationships", Elsevier, Amsterdam and New York, p. 328.

20) WOODCOCK, C.L.F. (ed.). (1970). "Progress in *Acetabularia* Research", Academic Press, New York, San Francisco and London, p. 341.

21) BONOTTO, S., KEFELI, V. and PUISEUX-DAO, S. (eds.). "Developmental Biology of *Acetabularia*", Elsevier/North-Holland Biomedical Press, Amsterdam, New York and Oxford, p. 312.

22) HÄMMERLING, J. (1934). Über formbildende Substanzen bei *Acebularia mediterranea*, ihre räumliche und zeitliche Verteilung und ihre Herkunft. Archiv Entwicklungsmech. Organis., 131, 1.

23) ZETSCHE, K. (1966). Regulation der zeitlichen Aufeinanderfolge von Differenzierungsvorgängen bei *Acetabularia*. Z. Naturforsch., 21b, 375.

24) WERZ, G. (1974). Fine structural aspects of morphogenesis in

Acetabularia. Int. Rev. Cytol, 38, 319.

25) KECK, (1964). Culturing and experimental manupulation of *Acetabularia*. In: "Methods in Cell Physiology", Vol. I, (ed., D.M. Prescott), Academic Press, New York, p. 189.

26) HÄMMERLING, J. (1932). Entwicklung und Formbildungsvermögen von *Acetabularia mediterranea*. II. Das Formbildungsvermögen kernhaltiger und kernloser Teilstücke. Biol. Zentralbl., 52, 42.

27) BONOTTO, S. (1969). Quelques observations sur les verticilles d'*Acetabularia mediterranea*. Bull. Soc. roy. Bot. Belgique, 102, 165.

28) GIBOR, A. (1965). Surviving cytoplasts *in vitro*. Proc. Natl. Acad. Sci., 54, 1527.

29) GREEN, B.R. (1976). Abnormal cells resulting from asexual reproduction in *Acetabularia* . Phycologia, 15, 161.

30) PRIMKE, M., BERGER, S. and SCHWEIGER, H.G. (1978). Protoplasts from *Acetabularia*:Isolation and fusion. Cytobiologie, 16, 375.

31) POTRYKUS, I. (1971). Intra and interspecific fusion of protoplasts from petals of *Torenia baillonii* and *Torenia fournieri*. Nature New Biology, 231, 57.

32) GILES, K.L. (1977). Chloroplast uptake and genetic complementation. In: "Applied and Fundamental Aspects of Plant Cell, Tissue Organ Culture" (eds., J. Reinert and Y.P.S. Bajaj), Springer Verlag, Berlin, Heidelberg and New York, p. 536.

33) PUISEUX-DAO, S., VALET, G. and BONOTTO, S. (1970). Greffes interspécifiques uninucléés, *Acetabularia mediterranea* et *A. peniculus* et mobilité des substances morphogénétiques dans le cytoplasme, C.R. Acad. Sci. Paris, 271, 1354.

34) BONOTTO, S., KIRCHMANN, R. and MANIL, P. (1971). Cell engineering in *Acetabularia*: A graft method for obtaining large cells with two or more reproductive caps. Giorn. Bot. Ital., 105, 1.

35) HÄMMERLING, J. (1935). Über Genomwirkungen und Formbildingsfähigkeit bei *Acetabularia*. Archiv. Entwicklungsmech. Organis., 132, 424.

36) WERZ, G. (1955). Kernphysiologische Untersuchungen an *Acetabularia*. Planta, 46, 113.

37) RICHTER, G. (1959). Die Auslösung kerninduzierter Regeneration bei gealterten kernlosen Zellteilen von *Acetabularia* und ihre Auswirkungen auf die Synthese von Ribonucleinsäure und Cytoplasmaproteinen. Planta, 52, 554.

38) WERZ, G. (1962). Zur Frage der Elimination von Ribonucleinsäure und Protein aus dem Zellkern von *Acetabularia mediterranea*. Planta, 57, 636.

39) BRÄNDLE, E. and ZETSCHE, K.(1973). Zur Lokalisation der α-Amanitin sensitiven RNA-Polymerase in Zellkernen von *Acetabularia*. Planta, 111, 209.

40) BERGER, S., NIEMANN, R. and SCHWEIGER, H.G. (1975). Viability of *Acetabularia* nucleus after 24 hours in an artificial medium. Protoplasma, 85, 115.

41) SCHWEIGER, H.G., BANNWARTH, H., BERGER, S. and KLOPPSTECH, K. (1975). *Acetabularia*, a cellular model for the study of nucleocytoplasmic relationships" (ed., S. Puiseux-Dao), Elsevier, Amsterdam and New York, p. 203.

42) ASTAUROVA, O.B., AFANASOVA, L.A., SALAMAKHA, O.V. and YAZYKOV, A.A. (1979). Isozyme composition of malate dehydrogenase in two species of *Acetabularia*, in normal conditions and after nuclear implantation. In: "Developmental Biology of *Acetabularia*". (eds., S. Bonotto, V. Kefeli and S. Puiseux-Dao), Elsevier/North-Holland Biomedical Press, Amsterdam, New York and Oxford, p. 259.

43) GIBOR, A. and GRANICK, S. (1964). Plastids and mitochondria: Inheritable systems. Science, 145, 890.

44) CIFERRI, O. (1978). The chloroplast DNA mystery. Trends in Biochem. Sci., 3, 256.

45) JAMES, T.W. and JOPE, C. (1978). Visualization by fluorescence of chloroplast DNA in higher plants by means of the DNA-specific probe 4'6-diamidino-2-phenylindole. J. Cell Biol., 79, 623.

46) D'EMILIO, M.A., HOURSIANGOU-NEUBRUN, D., BAUGNET-MAHIEU, L., GILLES, J., NUYTS, G., BOSSUS, A., MAZZA, A. and BONOTTO, S. (1979). Apicobasal gradient of protein synthesis in *Acetabularia*, In: "Developmental Biology of *Acetabularia*". (eds., S. Bonotto, V. Kefeli and S. Puiseux-Dao), Elsevier/North-Holland Biomedical Press, Amsterdam, New York and Oxford, p..269.

47) SCHWEIGER, H.G., MASTER, R.W.P. and WERZ, G. (1967). Nuclear control of a cytoplasmic enzyme in *Acetabularia*, Nature, 216, 554.

48) KHOLMATOVA, M.D., MAHMADBEKOVA, L.M. and ALIJEV, K.A. (1979). Preliminary indications on a possible transport of nuclear RNA into chloroplasts of regenerating *Acetabularia* cells. In: "Developmental Biology of *Acetabularia*". (eds., S. Bonotto, V. Kefeli and S. Puiseux-Dao), Elsevier/North-Holland Biomedical Press, Amsterdam, New York and Oxford, p. 233.

49) BELYAYEV, N.D., GAVRILOVSKAYA, I.N., GORBUNOVA, E.E., MAMAYEVA, O.A. and SANDAKHCHIEV, L.S. (1979). Biosynthesis of nucleic acids and proteins after injection of heterologous templates into *Acetabularia* . In: "Developmental Biology of *Acetabularia*". (eds., S. Bonotto, V. Kefeli and S. Puiseux-Dao), Elsevier/North-Holland Biomedical Press, Amsterdam, New York and Oxford, p. 295.

50) CAIRNS, E. (1978). Translation of animal virus RNA in *Acetabularia*. Cytobiologie, 18, 207.

51) CAIRNS, E, GSCHWENDER, H.H., PRIMKE, M., YAMAKAWA, M., TRAUB, P. and SCHWEIGER, H.G. (1978). Translation of animal virus RNA in the cytoplasm of a plant cell. Proc. Natl. Acad. Sci., 75. 5557.

52) WERZ, G. (1967). Induktion von Zellwandbildung durch Fremdprotein bei *Acetabularia* . Naturwissenschaften, 14, 374.

53) WOODCOCK, C.L.F. (1971). The anchoring of nuclei by cytoplasmic microtubules in *Acetabularia*. J. Cell Sci., 8, 61.

54) WERZ, G. and HÄMMERLING, J. (1961). Über die Beeinflussung

artspezifischer Formbildungsprozesse von *Acetabularia* durch UV-Bestrahlung. Z. Naturforsch., 16b, 829.

55) SIX, E. and PUISEUX-DAO, S. (1961). Die Wirkung von Strahlen auf Acetabularien. IV. Röntgenstrahlenwirkungen in zweikernigen Transplantaten. Z. Naturforsch., 16b, 832.

CONTRIBUTORS

BEIGEL, M., Department of Biological Sciences, Institute of Life Sciences, The Hebrew University of Jerusalem, Israel. p. *143*.

BIRNSTIEL, M.L., Institut für Molekularbiologie II, der Universität Zürich, Switzerland. p. *383*.

BONOTTO, S., Department of Radiobiology, C.E.N./S.C.K., Mol, Belgium. p. *409*.

BRAVO, R., Division of Biostructural Chemistry, Chemistry Department, Aarhus University, Denmark. p. *1*, p. *275*.

BRUCK, C., Laboratoire de Chimie Biologique, Département de Biologie Moléculaire, Université Libre de Bruxelles, Rhode St-Genèse, Belgium. p. *55*.

CABANTCHIK, Z.I., Department of Biological Sciences, Institute of Life Sciences, The Hebrew University of Jerusalem, Israel, p. *143*.

CELIS, A., Division of Biostructural Chemistry, Chemistry Department, Aarhus University, Denmark. p. *275*.

CELIS, J.E., Division of Biostructural Chemistry, Chemistry Department, Aarhus University, Denmark. p. *1*, p. *75*, p. *275*.

CLEUTER, Y., Laboratoire de Chimie Biologique, Département de Biologie Moléculaire, Université Libre de Bruxelles, Rhode St-Genèse, Belgium. p. *55*.

EGE, T., Institut of Medical Cell Research and Genetics, Medical Nobel Institut, Karolinska Institut, Stockholm, Sweden. p. *201*.

GINSBURG, H., Department of Biological Sciences, Institute of Life Sciences, The Hebrew University of Jerusalem, Israel. p. *143*.

GRAESSMANN, A., Institut für Molekularbiologie und Biochemie, Freien Universität Berlin, West Germany. p. *61*.

GRAESSMANN, M., Institut für Molekularbiologie und Biochemie, Freien Universität Berlin, West Germany. p. *61*.

GREGORIADIS, G., Division of Clinical Sciences, Clinical Research Centre, Harrow, Middlesex, England. p. *173*.

HUEZ, G., Laboratoire de Chimie Biologique, Département de Biologie Moléculaire, Université Libre de Bruxelles, Rhode St-Genèse, Belgium. p. *55*, p. *347*.

ISENBERG, G., Max-Planck-Institute for Psychiatrie, Munich, West Germany. p. *75*.

KALTOFT, K., Division of Biostructural Chemistry, Chemistry Department, Aarhus University, Denmark. p. *1*, p. *275*.
KLEIN, G., Department of Tumor Biology, Karolinska Institutet, Stockholm, Sweden. p. *235*.
KRESSMANN, A., Institut für Molecularbiologie II, der Universität Zürich, Switzerland. p. *383*.
LOYTER, A., Department of Biological Chemistry, The Hebrew University of Jerusalem, Israel. p. *143*.
LÜTTKE, A., Department of Radiobiology, C.E.N./S.C.K., Mol, Belgium. p. *409*.
MARBAIX, G., Laboratoire de Chimie Biologique, Département de Biologique Moléculaire, Université Libre de Bruxelles, Rhode St-Genèse, Belgium. p. *347*.
MUELLER, C., Institut für Molekularbiologie und Biochemie, Freien Universität Berlin, West Germany. p. *61*.
PAPAHADJOPOULOS, D., Department of Biology, University of Utah, Salt Lake City, Utah, U.S.A.. p. *155*.
PORTETELLE, D., Chaire de Zootechnie, Faculté Agronomique de l'Etat, Gembloux, Belgium. p. *55*.
RECHSTEINER, M., Department of Biology, University of Utah, Salt Lake City, Utah, U.S.A.. p. *113*.
RUDDLE, F.H., Department of Biology, Kline Biology Tower, Yale University, New Haven, Connecticut, U.S.A.. p. *295*.
STACEY, D.W., Rockefeller University, New York, U.S.A.. p. *29*.
SMALL, J.V., Institute of Molecular Biology, Austrian Academy of Sciences, Salzburg, Austria. p. *75*, p. *275*.
SCHELL, J., Rijksuniversiteit-Gent, Lab. voor Genetica, Gent, Belgium. p. *325*.
TABER, R., Department of Viral Oncology and Experimental Pathology, Roswell Park Memorial Institute, Buffalo, New York, U.S.A. p. *155*.
VOLSKY, D.J., Department of Biological Sciences, Institute of Life Sciences, The Hebrew University of Jerusalem, Israel. p. *143*.
VAN MONTAGU, M., Laboratory for Genetics, State University-Gent, Belgium. p. *325*.
WILLECKE, K., Institut für Zellbiologie, Universität Essen, West Germany. p. *311*.
WILSON, T., Department of Physiology and Biophysics, CMDNJ-Rutgers Medical School, Piscataway, New Jersey, U.S.A. p. *155*.
ZEUTHEN, J., Institute of Human Genetics, Bartholin Bygningen, Aarhus University, Denmark. p. *235*.

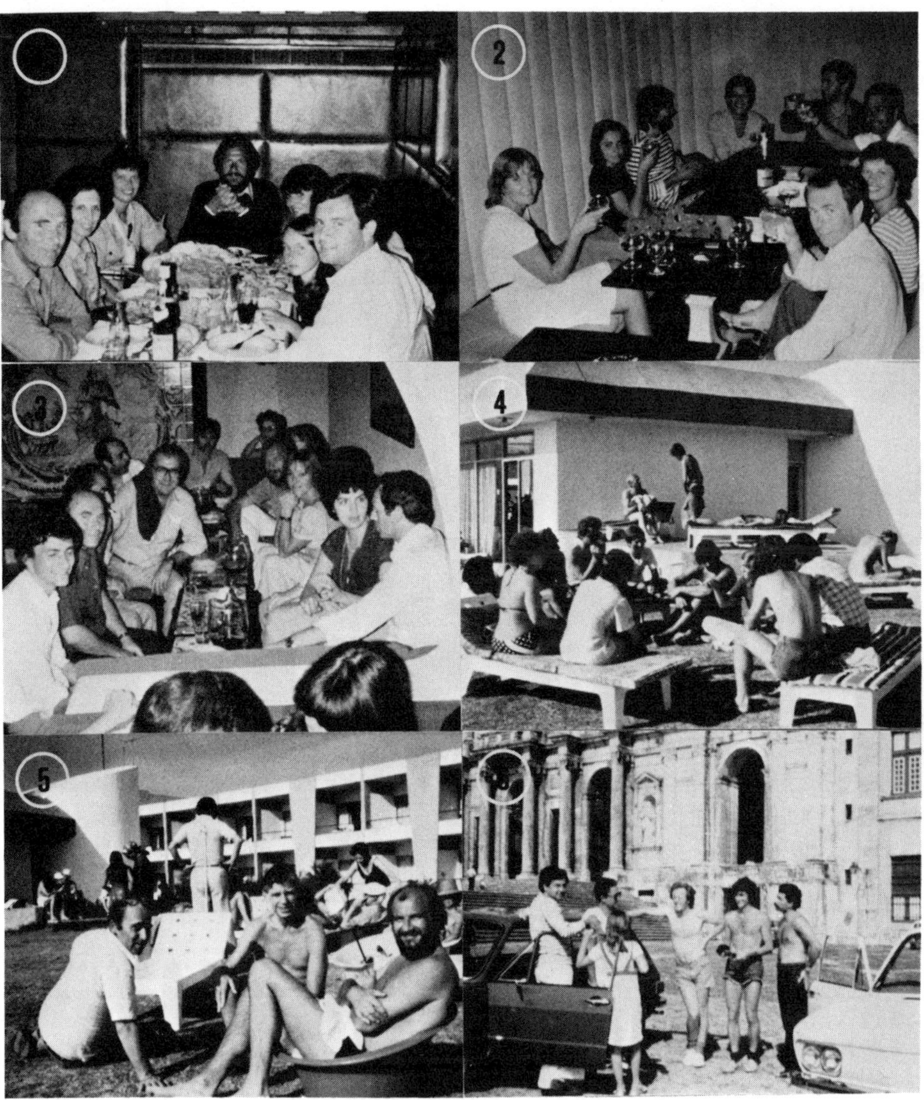

(From left to right)

1) The organising committee: A. Loyter, M.C. Lechner, L. Heilesen, A. Graessmann, H. Gata, C. Celis & J. Celis.

2) R. Schmid, E. Giulotto, R. Jaggi, M. Stefanini, E. Magnien, P.F. Pignatti, L. Heilesen & T. Ege.

3) D. Schmid, A. Loyter, G. Gregoriadis, D. Papahadjopoulos, A. Graessmann, R. Schmid, P. Caskey & T. Ege.

4) M. Barros, L. Sperling, R. Bravo, G. Gregoriadis, E. Wawra, M. Stefanini, P. Uster, M. Rechsteiner, D. Spandidos & S. Fey.

5) A. Loyter, F. Ruddle & A. Graessmann.

6) C. Celis, J. Celis, P. Andersen, V. Small, S. Fey & R. Bravo.

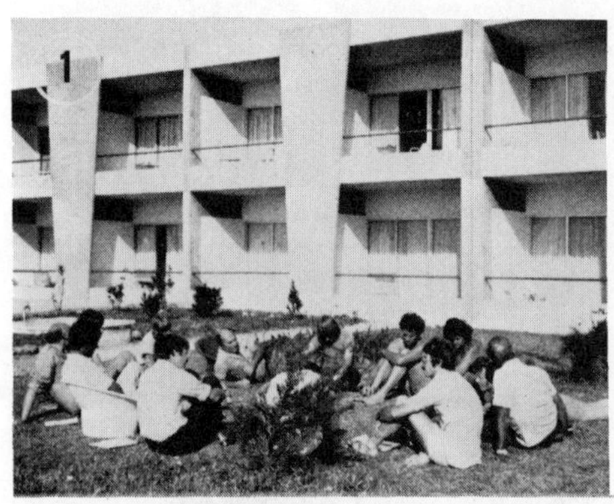

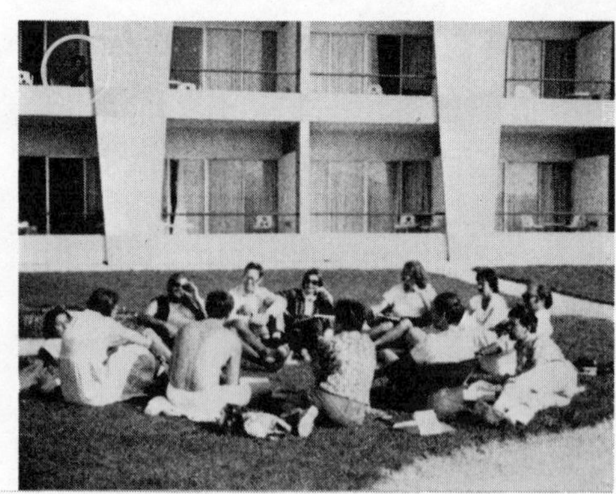

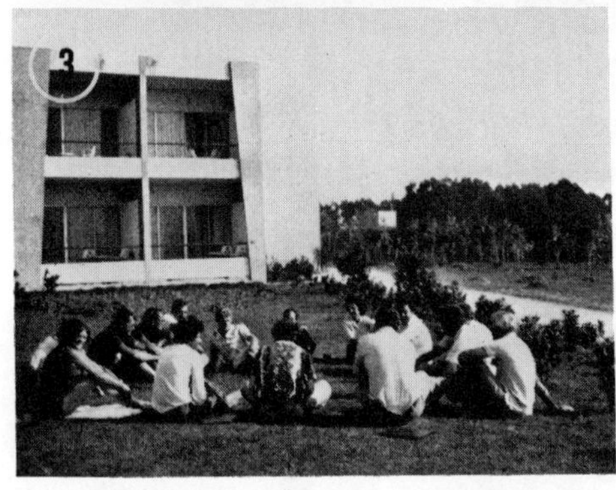

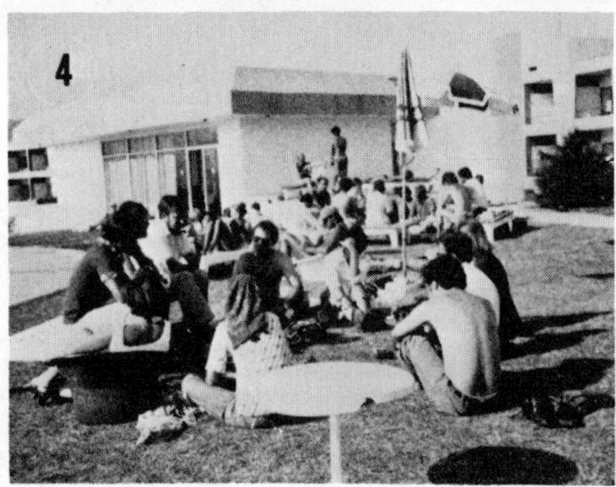

1) R. Contreras, D.E. Griffiths, A. Mottura, A. Loyter, D. Melton, R. Shields, M. Menezes-Ferreira, V. Small, L. Archer, A. Mitchell & D. Stacey.

2) S. Oldfield, E. Guilotto, A. Graessmann, K. Hendil, A. Lüttke, C. Boogaard, D. Neerunjun, D. Papahadjopoulos, E. Magnien, B. Wasylyk, J. Atidia & T. Caskey.

3) S. Metcalfe, P.F. Pignatti, L. Medrano, G. Huez, A. Miller, P. Moradas-Ferreira, M.C. Lechner, J.E. Celis, T. Ege, K. Willecke, T. Truelsen, G. Jonak, M. Horisberger & D. Schmid.

4) R. Wyndaele, M. Capecchi, R. Jaggi, G. Marbaix, J. Zeuthen, M. Perrot, M. Cyrne, M. Freire, C. Sinogas & J. Bellatin.

SUBJECT INDEX